Medical Emergencies

Essentials for the Dental Professional

Ellen B. Grimes
RDH, MA, MPA, Ed.D.
Vermont Technical College

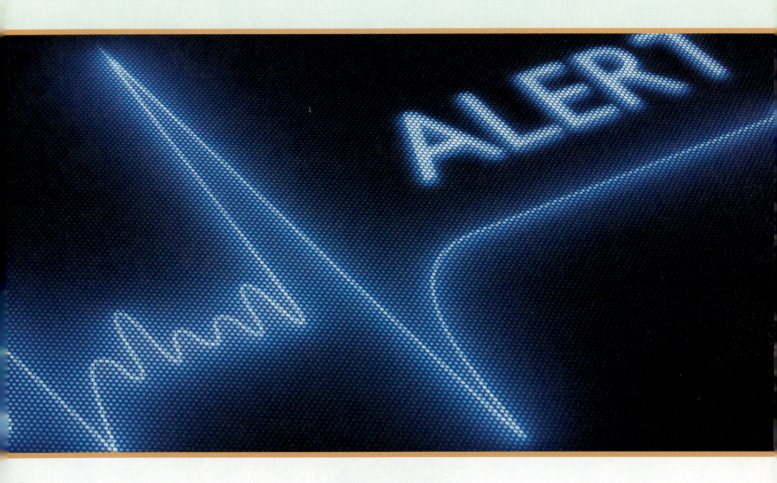

PEARSON

Boston   Columbus   Indianapolis   New York   San Francisco   Upper Saddle River   Amsterdam
Cape Town   Dubai   London   Madrid   Milan   Munich   Paris   Montréal   Toronto   Delhi
Mexico City   São Paulo   Sydney   Hong Kong   Seoul   Singapore   Taipei   Tokyo

Publisher: Julie Levin Alexander
Editor In Chief: Marlene McHugh Pratt
Executive Editor: John Goucher
Associate Editor: Nicole Ragonese
Editorial Assistant: Erica Viviani
Director of Marketing: David Gesell
Marketing Manager: Katrin Beacom
Production Manager: Tom Benfatti
Creative Director: Jayne Conte
Cover Designer: Suzanne Duda

Art Director - Interior: Christopher Weigand
Media Editor: Amy Peltier
Media Project Manager: Lorena Cerisano
Media Coordinator: Ashley De Jong
Full-Service Project Management:
    Murugesh Rajkumar Namasivayam/PreMediaGlobal
Composition: PreMediaGlobal
Printer/Binder: Courier/Kendalville
Cover Printer: Courier/Kendalville
Text Font: 10/12 Times Ten Roman

Credits and acknowledgments borrowed from other sources and reproduced, with permission, in this textbook appear on the appropriate page within text.

Microsoft® and Windows® are registered trademarks of the Microsoft Corporation in the U.S.A. and other countries. Screen shots and icons reprinted with permission from the Microsoft Corporation. This book is not sponsored or endorsed by or affiliated with the Microsoft Corporation.

Many of the designations by manufacturers and sellers to distinguish their products are claimed as trademarks. Where those designations appear in this book, and the publisher was aware of a trademark claim, the designations have been printed in initial caps or all caps.

Library of Congress Cataloging-in-Publication Data
Grimes, Ellen B.
    Medical emergencies : essentials for the dental professional / Ellen B.
Grimes.—2nd ed.
        p. ; cm.
    Includes bibliographical references and index.
    ISBN-13: 978-0-13-306562-6 (alk. paper)
    ISBN-10: 0-13-306562-6 (alk. paper)
    I. Title.
    [DNLM: 1. Dental Care—methods.   2. Emergencies.   3. Emergency Treatment—methods. WU 105]
    LC Classification not assigned
    616.02'5—dc23
                                                                                    2012039056

10 9 8 7 6 5 4 3 2 1

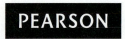

ISBN 10: 0-13-306562-6
ISBN 13: 978-0-13-306562-6

Dedication

This book is dedicated to my husband, Jeff, my family, friends, colleagues, and students for their support and encouragement during the writing of the first and second editions. I am so very fortunate to have you all in my life.

Contents

Preface

I considered writing this book for some time as I saw a need for a concise yet complete textbook on medical emergencies for the dental professional and particularly for dental hygiene and dental assisting students. I knew that the writing must be easily understandable, practical, and readily applicable to the dental clinical setting. I hope readers will find the second edition of this text meets all of these criteria.

The purpose of this book is to present fundamental information regarding medical emergencies that may be encountered in the dental practice setting. Presently, there are few textbooks on medical emergencies. The ones that are available either tend to be extremely detailed or are so simplistic that they do not provide the essential knowledge that will enable dental professionals to adequately diagnose and treat patients in emergency situations.

Following an introductory chapter and chapters discussing vital signs and the emergency kit, the chapters are sequenced according to the body system affected by the emergency. Although almost all emergencies are potentially fatal, this text begins with the neurological emergencies and leads off with syncope, which is the most common and an often benign medical emergency. It then progresses to cardiac, respiratory, endocrine, and bleeding emergencies. Two of the three final chapters discuss emergencies that are particular to individuals in the dental profession (intraocular foreign object and broken instrument tip). The final chapter discusses drug toxicity, which is becoming more prevalent in dental offices because of increased drug use in U.S. society.

In this text, many chapters begin with a "Case Scenario" whose purpose is to allow readers to apply their critical thinking strategies to the signs and symptoms presented by the hypothetical patient and determine from which medical emergency the patient might be suffering. This section is followed by an "Introduction" to the emergency. For example, in the discussion of diabetes-related emergencies in Chapter 16, a thorough review of diabetes is presented so that the reader has the key information related to the disease. The next section reports the "Signs and Symptoms" that are usually exhibited by a patient experiencing this emergency. In addition, some differential diagnosis information is described in this section to help readers better determine other emergencies that exhibit similar symptoms. The appropriate "Treatment" for the emergency is presented in the next section. All chapters end with a "Conclusion" (and Case Resolution section, for chapters with case studies), which pulls together all the pertinent information presented in the chapter and related to the case studies scenario. In each chapter, there is a flowchart that uses the acronym R.E.P.A.I.R. to help the practitioner understand each step involved in a medical emergency. *R* represents *r*ecognizing the signs and symptoms; *E* represents *e*valuating the patient's level of consciousness and vital signs; *P* represents *p*lacing the patient in the appropriate position; *A* represents the CABs (*c*irculation, *a*irway, and *b*reathing) of cardiopulmonary resuscitation; *I* represents *i*mplementing the appropriate emergency treatment; and the second *R* represents *r*eferring the patient to the appropriate healthcare professional, if necessary. A "Review Question" section provides multiple-choice questions to ensure a thorough grasp of the material presented. Lastly, references used to develop the text are included in the "Bibliography" section.

The information presented in this text provides the reader with a working knowledge of medical emergencies and may help the dental practitioner prevent serious debilitation or save a patient's life.

New to This Edition

Medical Emergencies: Essentials for the Dental Professional has been revised so that it provides for an even more valuable teaching and learning experience. Here are the enhancements we have made:

- New full color design with color photos and illustrations to capture the attention of students and enhance their overall learning experience.
- Videos depicting several of the most common medical emergencies students may encounter when going into practice.
- New images have been included to help learners better visualize the concepts presented in the text.
- Additional information and clarification in the vital signs chapter (chapter 3) which will allow students to have better grasp of this important topic.

Acknowledgments

I would like to acknowledge several people for their support in the preparation of this textbook:

My contributing authors, Leslie Hills, Tina Marshall, Sheila Bannister, Laura Mueller-Joseph, and Barbara Bennett, without whose help this text would never have been completed on time.

My librarians, Jane Kearns, Carolyn Barnes, and Nancy Bianchi, who performed endless searches on the topics for this text.

My editors, Mark Cohen and John Goucher, who believed that this book would be successful and continually encouraged me to complete the project.

My assisting editor, Nicole Ragonese, who assisted me through the second edition process.

My sister, Diana Hoppe, who has always made me feel like I could do just about anything.

My parents, Norman and Shirley Briggs, who provided me with the education I needed to write this textbook.

My husband, Jeffrey Grimes, who has continuously supported all of my professional endeavors.

I would also like to thank the reviewers for this second edition. Their keen insights aided in strengthening the text.

Grimes Reviewers

Charles A. Crosby, DDS
York Technical College
Rock Hill, South Carolina

Jan Greenlee, RDH, MS
Harcum College
Bryn Mawr, Pennsylvania

Pam Kawasaki, RDH, MBA
Pacific University
Hillsboro, Oregon

Jennifer McKeon, CDA, CPFDA, RDH, MEd
Quinsigamond Community College
Worcester, Massachusetts

Terry Sigal Greene, RDH, BSc Dentistry, MEd
Northampton Community College
Bethlehem, Pennsylvania

Dawn P. Southerly, RDH, BSHS
Northern Virginia Community College-MEC
Springfield, Virginia

Cynthia Wampler, RDH, MS
Florida State College at Jacksonville
Jacksonville, Florida

Contributing Authors

Sheila C Bannister, RDH, MEd

Assistant Professor, Dental Hygiene

Vermont Technical College

Williston, Vermont

Chapter 20

Barbara L. Bennett, CDA, RDH, MS

Co-Division Director, Allied Health Programs Dental Hygiene

Chair, Dental Assisting Program

Texas State Technical College

Harlingen, Texas

Chapter 8

Leslie K. Hills, RDH, MEd

Assistant Professor, Dental Hygiene

Vermont Technical College

Williston, Vermont

Chapters 10 and 11

Tina Marshall, RDH, MEd

Assistant Professor, Dental Hygiene

Vermont Technical College

Williston, Vermont

Chapter 23

Laura Mueller-Joseph, RDH, MS, EdD

Program Director, Dental Hygiene

Farmingdale State College of New York

Farmingdale, New York

Chapter 13

1

Introduction

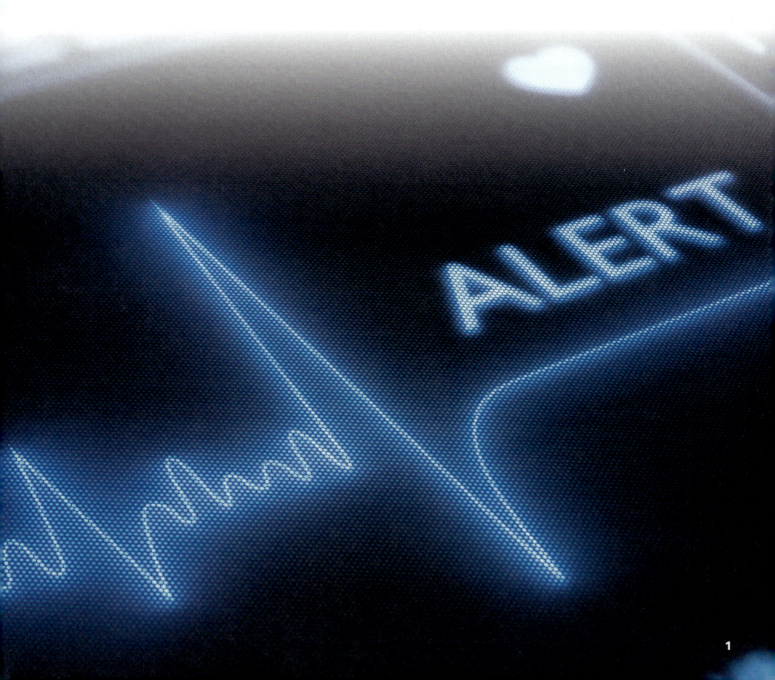

Medical emergencies can and do occur in the dental setting. The most common emergency reported was **syncope** (50%), followed by mild allergic reaction (8%), **angina pectoris** (8%), and **orthostatic hypotension** (8%). Medical emergencies were most likely to occur after the administration of **local anesthetics** and during tooth extraction or endodontic treatment. Approximately one-third of all medical emergencies in the dental office are potentially life threatening. It is predicted that due to the increasing age of the patient population, as well as advances in healthcare (such as pharmaceuticals, surgery, and life-prolonging treatments), there will be an increase in the number of medical emergencies seen in the dental setting; therefore, it is essential that all dental office personnel be familiar with the prevention and management of medical emergency situations and can effectively manage such situations until the patient can be transported to a medical facility.

There are some procedures that may help in preventing emergencies, such as taking a thorough and accurate medical history and taking and recording vital signs. Preparation for a medical emergency in the dental office is essential. This chapter discusses procedures for medical emergency prevention and preparation.

Medical History

Taking a complete and accurate medical history is essential to the possible prevention of a medical emergency. Often a patient will report a medical condition that should signal the dental practitioner of the increased risk of a possible emergency. Examples of medical conditions for which the medical history provides important evidence include, but are not limited to, the following:

- **A heart condition**—Be alert to a myocardial infarction (MI), congestive heart failure, or cerebrovascular accident (CVA).
- **Asthma**—Be alert to a possible asthma attack.
- **A stroke, frequent headaches, or dizziness**—Be alert to a possible CVA.
- **Epilepsy**—Be alert to a seizure.
- **Thyroid problems**—Be alert to myxedema coma or thyroid storm.
- **Diabetes**—Be alert to hypoglycemia or diabetic coma.
- **Corticosteroid use**—Be alert to signs of adrenal insufficiency.
- **Allergy**—Be alert to an allergic reaction.
- **Bleeding disorders**—Be alert to signs of bruising, hemorrhage, or hemophilia.

If patients report any of these conditions on their medical history, the dental practitioner should dialogue with the patient further to gain information for the prevention of a medical emergency. The frequency, severity, and triggers of the condition should be assessed to determine the likelihood of an emergency and/or to postpone treatment until the patient has been examined by his or her medical physician or the treatment provided has been modified in light of the patient's condition.

Vital Signs

Another important aspect in the prevention and management of medical emergencies is the taking and recording of the patients' vital signs. Vital signs include pulse, respiration, blood pressure, and temperature. These topics will be discussed extensively in Chapter 3. Hypertensive or hypotensive patients are more likely to experience various medical emergencies. This is also true for patients who exhibit **tachycardia**, **bradycardia**, **tachypnea**, **bradypnea**, or **dyspnea**.

ASA Physical Status Classification

A classification system to determine a patient's physical status was developed by the American Society of Anesthesiologists (ASA) and was amended in 1962 at the ASA's House of Delegates. (See Table 1.1 ■) This system is still used today and is as follows:

Table 1.1   ASA PS Classifications

ASA PS Classification	Patient Characteristics	Examples of Conditions
ASA PS I	Normal healthy patient	
ASA PS II	Mild systemic disease	Controlled type 2 diabetes Controlled epilepsy Controlled hypertension (Stage 1) Allergies Fearful dental patient Pregnancy
ASA PS III	Severe systemic disease that limits activity but is not incapacitating	Stable angina Myocardial infarction (MI) longer than six months ago Controlled type 1 diabetes Renal failure Controlled heart failure Poorly controlled hypertension with BP > 160/100 (Stage 2) Morbid obesity
ASA PS IV	Incapacitating systemic disease that is a constant threat to life	MI or CVA within past six months Unstable angina Heart failure Uncontrolled diabetes Uncontrolled epilepsy Hypertension with blood pressure > 180/110 Uncontrolled thyroid conditions
ASA PS V	Moribund patient not expected to survive 24 hours with or without operation	Multiorgan failure Poorly controlled coagulopathy Sepsis with hemodynamic instability
ASA PS VI	A declared brain-dead patient whose organs are being harvested for donation	

ASA PS I: Normal, healthy patient. No organic, physiologic, or psychiatric disturbance; excludes the very young and very old; healthy with good exercise tolerance.

ASA PS II: Patients with a mild systemic disease or a risk factor for a systemic disease, for example, tobacco use, alcohol abuse, mild obesity. No functional limitations; has a well-controlled disease. Patients who may be categorized as ASA PS II are those with controlled hypertension or type 2 diabetes without systemic effect, cigarette smoking without **chronic obstructive pulmonary disease** (COPD), mild obesity, pregnancy.

ASA PS III: Patients with a severe systemic disease with some functional limitations; a controlled disease of more than one body system; no immediate danger of death. Patients who may be categorized as ASA PS III are those with controlled heart failure, stable angina, controlled type 1 diabetes, poorly controlled hypertension, morbid obesity, chronic renal failure, poorly controlled asthma, and those who have had an MI longer than six months ago, but who have no signs or symptoms.

ASA PS IV: A patient with an incapacitating systemic disease that is a constant threat to life. These patients have at least one severe disease that is poorly controlled or at end stage and have a possible risk of death. Patients who may be categorized as ASA PS IV are those who have had an MI within the past six months and those who have unstable angina, symptomatic heart failure, COPD, or **hepatorenal** failure.

ASA PS V: A moribund patient not expected to survive without operation. Patients who may be categorized as ASA PS V are patients with multiorgan failure, poorly controlled coagulopathy, or sepsis with hemodynamic instability.

In the event of an emergency operation, precede the number with an E (e.g., E III) (American Society of Anesthesiologists, 1963).

ASA PS VI: A declared brain-dead patient whose organs are being harvested for donation.

The dental professional will commonly see patients classified as ASA PS I, II, and III. ASA IV and V classified patients will most likely be hospitalized or bedridden. ASA PS III patients are more likely to experience a medical emergency, and therefore the dental healthcare provider needs to be more alert to possible emergency situations and be prepared with a team approach for emergency management. In all cases a thorough and accurate medical history is a necessity and is required legally.

Regardless of the patient's ASA PS classification, the dental practitioner should be cognizant of the patient's external presentation. Behavior changes are common in many emergencies. For example, patients suffering from severe hypoglycemia often present with aggressive behavior. In addition, skin color should be noted. Hypoxia often manifests as a bluish tone to the skin tissues, whereas hypertensive individuals may appear flushed or red.

Preparation for Medical Emergencies in the Dental Office

Dental professionals should be prepared for any emergency that might occur in their office. A well-equipped medical emergency kit, automated external defibrillator (AED) unit, and a portable oxygen tank are a necessity and will be discussed in subsequent chapters.

Current cardiopulmonary resuscitation (CPR) training for all dental professionals is imperative to appropriately treat any medical emergency in or out of the dental office and is required by many state dental and dental hygiene practice acts. As CPR guidelines change (new guidelines were released in 2010 by the American Heart Association), it is important that the dental practitioner continuously maintain a current healthcare provider CPR card and be familiar with CPR techniques for all age levels. In addition, clinicians should be trained on the proper use of the AED. Malamed (2010) states that CPR recertification every two years is not adequate to properly perform CPR. He recommends annual CPR training for dental office personnel.

Medical Emergency Simulations

Emergencies do not occur on a regular basis and can happen without warning, so practicing simulated medical emergencies within the office is an important preparatory step. These simulations ensure that each individual understands his or her role should an emergency arise and will reduce the anxiety associated with emergency situations when they do occur.

A recommended format for the emergency team structure is as follows: (See Table 1.2 ■)

Table 1.2   Emergency Team Structure

Person	P1, P2 , P3, OR	Responsibility
Person 1	P1	Stays with patient; performs appropriate emergency treatment
Person 2	P2	Assists P1; takes vital signs and administers oxygen, records events and time of medication delivery
Person 3	P3	Retrieves emergency kit; prepares emergency drugs
Office receptionist	OR	Makes necessary phone calls

The person in whose operatory the emergency is occurring is Person 1 (P1) and stays with the patient and performs the appropriate treatment. The next most available person is Person 2 (P2), who assists P1 directly and is responsible for taking vital signs and administering oxygen. In addition, P2 is responsible for recording events, such as time at which vital signs were taken and the results, amount of oxygen provided, medications administered, and dosages. P2 also informs P1 of time elapsed since any medications were administered. Other items that should be recorded are time Emergency Medical Services (EMS) is contacted if necessary and by whom. The date and time of the event should also be documented. A sample emergency treatment record is included as Figure 1.1 ■. The next available person (P3) retrieves the emergency kit, prepares emergency drugs, and does whatever else P1 decides. The office receptionist is responsible for making all necessary phone calls.

Accurate communication between personnel during a medical emergency situation is essential. The American Heart Association (2006) recommends using a closed-loop approach whereby P1 sends instruction to P2, P3, or the office receptionist and the recipient acknowledges that he or she has understood the message, thereby reducing ambiguity. For example, P1 would say to P3, "Please get the emergency kit." P3 would respond "I am getting the emergency kit." Remaining calm and working as a team is extremely important in managing medical emergencies.

Management of Medical Emergencies

This text will utilize the R.E.P.A.I.R. system for the management of medical emergencies: **R**, recognize the signs and symptoms of the emergency and stop all treatment; **E**, evaluate the patient's level of consciousness; **P**, place the patient in the appropriate position; **A**, activate the CABs of CPR by checking the circulation, airway, and breathing; **I**, implement the appropriate emergency protocol for the specific emergency; and **R**, refer the patient to the appropriate healthcare professional, if necessary. If dental healthcare providers are unsure if they are able to handle an emergency that is occurring, they should not hesitate to seek medical assistance by contacting EMS by calling 9-1-1. Essentially dental healthcare providers are responsible for keeping the patient alive until someone with more training arrives.

Continuing Education Courses

Attending continuing education courses that review proper treatment of medical emergencies will help the dental professional be better prepared to handle emergency situations. In addition, education will ensure that the practitioner has the most current information available regarding the prevention and management of medical emergencies.

Emergency Treatment Record

White - File copy
Yellow - EMS copy

NOTE: Fill out and keep White copy for your records. Give Yellow copy to EMS.

Person's Name:______________________ Date:__________________ Time:____________

Allergies:____

List all medications taken prior to emergency:_____________________________________

____

Time	Blood Pressure	Pulse	Resp	Oxygen Saturation Percentage	Oxygen Flow L/min	Medications Administered	Medication Dosage	Medication Route (IV, IM, PO, SL)

Called 911 EMS at (time):____

EMS arrived at (time):____

EMS called by (who):____

Person taken to what hospital:____

Condition of person when transported from site:_______________________________

EMS personnel:____

People present:____

Signature of person recording events:_______________________Phone:______________

FIGURE 1.1 Emergency treatment record. © Institute of Medical Emergency Preparedness.

Conclusion

Taking and recording an accurate medical history and checking and recording vital signs are critical steps in preventing medical emergencies in the dental office. All dental office staff need to be prepared in the event of an emergency; such preparation includes current CPR certification, practice in office emergency drills, and participation in didactic and clinical continuing education courses in medical emergencies. Skill in using the emergency kit and administering oxygen is essential for managing medical emergencies.

Review Questions

1. Your patient is a controlled type 2 diabetic. What ASA PS classification would you assign to this patient?

   A. I
   B. II
   C. III
   D. IV

2. The person who records all medications provided to the patient is

   A. P1
   B. P2
   C. P3
   D. office receptionist

3. The most common medical emergency that occurs in the dental office is

   A. angina pectoris
   B. myocardial infarction
   C. syncope
   D. obstructed airway

Bibliography

American Heart Association. "Part 3: effective resuscitation team dynamics." In *Advanced Cardiovascular Life Support Provider Manual: Professional*, 11–17. Dallas: American Heart Association, 2006.

American Society of Anesthesiologists. "New Classification of Physical Status." *Anesthesiology* 24 (1963): 111.

ASA Physical Status (PS) Classification System. Retrieved from http://my.clevelandclinic.org/services/anesthesia/hic_asa_physical_classification_system.aspx.

Emery, R. W., and S. A. Guttenberg. "Management Priorities and Treatment Strategies for Medical Emergencies in the Dental Office." *Dental Clinics of North America* 43 (1999): 401–19.

Fast, T. B., M. D. Martin, and T. M. Ellis. "Emergency Preparedness: A Survey of Dental Practitioners." *Journal of the American Dental Association* 112 (1986): 499–501.

Haas, D. A. "Management of Medical Emergencies in the Dental Office: Conditions in Each Country, the Extent of Treatment by the Dentist." *Journal of Japanese Dental Society of Anesthesiology* 33 (2005): 153–57.

Hall, J. L. "Medical Emergency in Your Office One Year Later: You've Been Served! What Do You Do Now?" *Dental Assistant* 77(2008): 44–47.

Institute of Medical Emergency Preparedness. Emergency treatment record [Form]. Retrieved October 21, 2011, from http://www.emergencyactionguide.com/.

Malamed, S. G. "Emergency Medicine." *Dental Economics* (2010): 38–43.

Malamed, S. F. "Managing Medical Emergencies." *Journal of the American Dental Association* 124 (1993): 40–53.

Morrison, A. D., and R. H. B. Godday. "Preparing for Medical Emergencies in the Dental Office." *Journal of the Canadian Dental Association* 65 (1999): 284–86.

Pickett, F., and J. Gurenlian. *The Medical History: Clinical Implications and Emergency Prevention in Dental Settings* (1st ed.). Philadelphia, PA: Williams & Wilkins, 2005.

Pickett, F., and J. Gurenlian. *Preventing Medical Emergencies: Use of the Medical History.* (2nd ed.). Philadelphia, PA: Williams & Wilkins, 2010.

Rutland, C. "Management of Medical Emergencies in Dental Practice." *Dental Nursing* 7(2011): 274–77.

Shampaine, G. "Patient Assessment and Preventive Measures for Medical Emergencies in the Dental Office." *Dental Clinics of North America* 43 (1999): 383–400.

PEARSON
myhealthprofessionskit™

Use this address to access the Companion Website created for this textbook. Simply select "Dental Hygiene" from the choice of disciplines. Find this book and log in using your username and password to access interactive activities, videos, and much more.

2

The Emergency Kit

LEARNING OBJECTIVES

Upon reading the material in this chapter, the reader will be able to:

☑ Explain the essential components of an emergency kit in the dental office.

☑ List the nonessential components of an emergency kit in the dental office.

☑ Discuss adult and pediatric doses of essential emergency drugs.

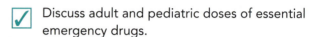

Introduction

The emergency kit in a dental office should be custom designed and readily available for use. There are numerous commercial emergency kits available, and they do offer automatic shipping of drugs as they near their expiration date. In many instances they do not meet the individual needs and capabilities of every dental team; therefore, development of a self-designed emergency kit is the most desirable approach to meet these requirements. In addition, it is usually more cost-effective to purchase emergency equipment and drugs separately.

The emergency kit should be mobile or transportable with an easily accessible oxygen apparatus. It should include a manual with emergency telephone numbers, names of persons responsible for the emergency kit update and emergency drills, emergency protocol, and an emergency treatment record. (See Figure 2.1 ■)

The key to designing an emergency kit is simplification. The simpler the kit, the more likely the dental professional will remember how to use the material included in the kit in an emergency situation. This chapter explains the equipment and drugs that are recommended for inclusion in the kit; however, the dental team should choose only those materials with which they are most familiar and willing to use. Moreover, the location of the dental office should be considered. An office proximal to a hospital emergency room or close to the Emergency Rescue Service need not contain numerous injectable drugs. Conversely, an office located in a rural setting should contain a full complement of injectable drugs because it will take considerable time for an emergency rescue squad to arrive at the office.

Fortunately, the majority of dental office emergencies can be handled without the use of injectable drugs. First and foremost in the management of these situations is basic life support. It is only after life-support steps have been taken that the use of drugs should be considered. One exception to this is in the management of an acute allergic reaction. In this situation, immediate injection of epinephrine followed by a histamine blocker is required.

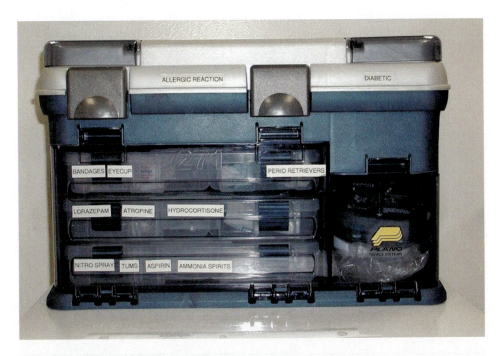

FIGURE 2.1 Emergency drug kit.

Essential Drugs

There are a few components that are considered essential for the emergency kit in the dental office. These include oxygen, epinephrine, nitroglycerin, histamine blocker, albuterol, aspirin, and oral glucose. Each of these components is discussed individually, and a chart with the common emergency drugs and their dosages is included in Table 2.1 ■.

Oxygen

The use of oxygen is indicated for most emergencies with the exception of hyperventilation. Because of the importance of oxygenation of patients during medical emergencies, oxygen administration is discussed in depth in Chapter 4. (See Figure 2.2 ■)

Epinephrine

Epinephrine is the drug of choice for the emergency treatment of anaphylaxis (severe allergic reaction) as it counteracts the major physiological events that occur with this life-threatening emergency. Epinephrine has some potentially serious side effects, so it should be used cautiously and only when there is certainty that anaphylaxis is

Table 2.1   Common Emergency Drugs and Their Dosages

Medication	Dosage	Emergency
Epinephrine	0.3 mg 1:1,000 adult 0.25 mg 1:1,000 age 6–12 0.12 mg 1:1,000 age six months to six years	Anaphylaxis
Nitroglycerine	0.2–0.6 mg every five minutes maximum of three doses	Angina, heart failure or myocardial infarction
Diphenhydramine	Mild: adult: 25–50 mg every six to eight hours Children >10 kg: 12.5–25 mg three to four times/day Moderate: 25–50 mg IM	Mild to moderate allergic reaction with urticaria and pruritus
Chlorpheniramine	Children: two to six years: 1 mg every four to six hours 6–12 years: 2 mg every four to six hours Children > 12 years and Adults: 4 mg every 4–6 hours	Mild allergy
Albuterol	Children: one spray 90 mcg/spray Adult: two sprays 90 mcg/spray	Asthma attack
Aspirin	162–325 mg chewed and absorbed in mouth	Myocardial infarction
Oral carbohydrate (glucose)	15–20 gm	Hypoglycemia
Lorazepam	0.5–1 mg IM	Seizures or hyperventilation
Glucagon	Children < 20 kg: 0.5 mg or 20–30 mcg/kg/dose Children ≥ 20 kg and adults: 1 mg	Hypoglycemia with unconscious patient
Hydrocortisone	100–500 mg IM	Anaphylaxis

occurring. Epinephrine is extremely beneficial for this emergency as it will reduce the risk of **hypotension**, **bronchospasm**, and **laryngeal edema** and prevents the further release of **histamine** and other **chemical mediators**. It has a very rapid onset, but a short duration of action. The usual dosage is 0.3 mg of a 1:1,000 concentration for intramuscular (IM) injections. Because of the short duration of action, it is recommended that more than one ampule or autoinjector system be available. In addition, a pediatric formulation of 0.15 mg of a 1:1,000 concentration is recommended. These doses should be repeated until the anaphylaxis symptoms subside. Another emergency for which an IM injection of epinephrine is indicated is a severe asthma attack that has not responded to the first drug of choice, albuterol. The dosage is the same as that for anaphylaxis.

Epinephrine should not be given to a patient with ischemic heart disease or severe hypertension as it can exacerbate these conditions. It should, however, be given to a patient with cardiac problems if the anaphylactic episode or asthmatic bronchospasm is imminently life threatening. (See Figure 2.3 ■)

Nitroglycerin

Nitroglycerin is indicated for acute angina, myocardial infarction (MI), or heart failure. The drug works by dilating the coronary blood vessels to provide additional oxygenation to the heart muscle. Because of its rapid onset, it is extremely effective for these emergencies. Nitroglycerin is available in both tablet and spray form; however, it is important to note that if the tablets are exposed to air or light, their shelf life is reduced to 12 weeks. Therefore, if a patient uses his or her own nitroglycerin tablet, it may be ineffective, and the use of the drug from the emergency kit may be necessary (the kit must contain a fresh supply of nitroglycerin). One tablet (0.2–0.6 mg) sublingually or one spray translingually or sublingually should be administered, and if the condition is angina, relief should occur in minutes. Two additional doses can be administered at five-minute intervals. If the systolic blood pressure falls below 90 mmHg, nitroglycerin is contraindicated. (See Figure 2.4 ■) Nitroglycerin is also contraindicated in patients who have taken an erectile dysfunction medication within the past 24 hours as it can cause an unsafe drop in blood pressure.

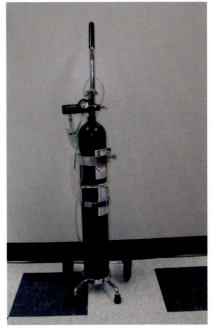

FIGURE 2.2 Portable size E oxygen cylinder.

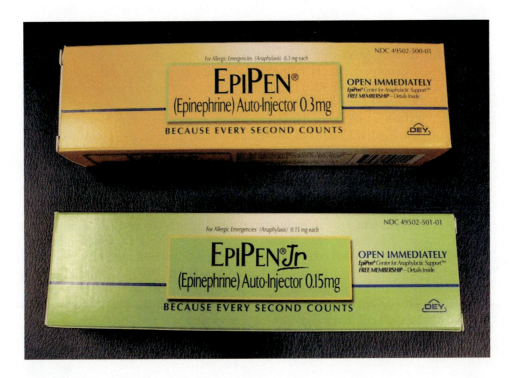

FIGURE 2.3 Adult and child EpiPens.

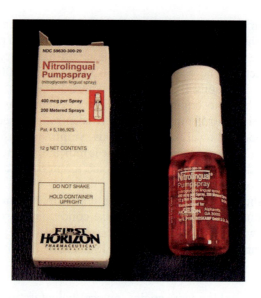

FIGURE 2.4 Nitroglycerin spray.

Diphenhydramine or Chlorpheniramine

A histamine blocker is recommended for management of allergic reactions. For a mild, non-life-threatening allergic reaction, an oral histamine blocker is recommended. Chlorpheniramine (10 mg) or diphenhydramine (25–50 mg) is the recommended dosage. An injectable histamine blocker is recommended for moderate allergic reactions with primarily dermatologic signs (e.g., **urticaria** and **pruritus**) and with some respiratory symptoms (e.g., **wheezing**). Diphenhydramine (25–50 mg) or Chlorpheniramine (10–20 mg) IM is the recommended dosage for adults. Chlorpheniramine seems to cause less drowsiness than does diphenhydramine. The pediatric dose of diphenhydramine is 1 mg/kg of body weight and should not exceed the adult dose. (See Figures 2.5 and 2.6 ■)

Albuterol

A bronchodilator is used to treat an asthma attack or bronchospasm. It is administered via an inhaler and provides dilation of the bronchioles while causing minimal cardiovascular effects. Albuterol is the drug of choice as it has a quick onset, with a peak effect of 30–60 minutes and a long duration of action (four to six hours). The adult dose is two sprays, which can be repeated as necessary, and the pediatric dose is one spray, which can also be repeated if necessary to reduce symptoms. (See Figure 2.7 ■) If the initial dose is ineffective, the use of a spacing device is recommended as it allows for more effective distribution of the drug in the lungs. (See Figure 2.8 ■)

Aspirin

Aspirin is an important drug to include in the emergency kit as it has been shown to be effective in reducing overall mortality from MI. If aspirin is administered early enough during the MI, the drug will help prevent the progression from cardiac ischemia to cardiac injury to cardiac tissue death. The minimum effective dose of aspirin is not known; however, at least 162 mg or two baby aspirins should be given to any patient with pain suggestive of MI. As many patients are allergic to aspirin, the medical history should be reviewed prior to administration. (See Figure 2.9 ■)

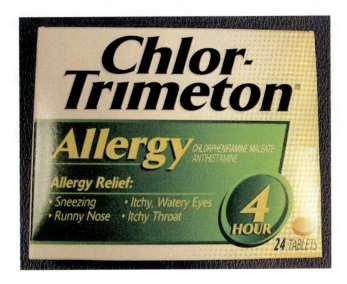

FIGURE 2.5 Chlorpheniramine tablets.

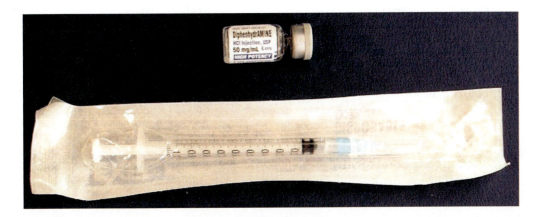

FIGURE 2.6 Diphenhydramine with disposable syringe.

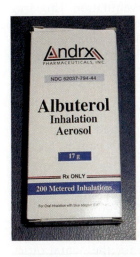

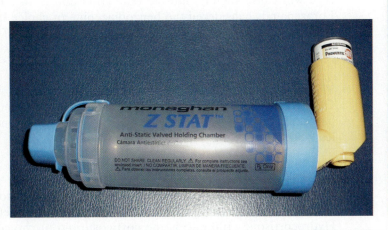

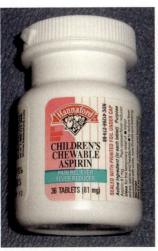

FIGURE 2.7 Albuterol inhaler. **FIGURE 2.8** spacing device. **FIGURE 2.9** Children's aspirin.

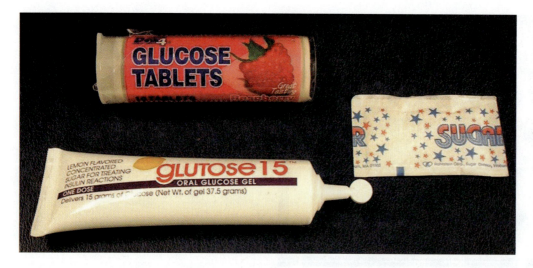

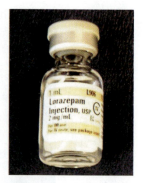

FIGURE 2.11 Injectable lorazepam.

FIGURE 2.10 Oral glucose: tablets, gel, and sugar packet.

Oral Carbohydrate

The emergency kit should include some oral carbohydrate source for conscious patients suffering from hypoglycemia. Glucose paste and tablets are recommended as they do not require refrigeration and they have long shelf lives; however, juice or soda (not diet) can be used if tablets and paste are unavailable. (See Figure 2.10 ■)

Supplemental Drugs

There are a few drugs that are beneficial, but not essential, to have in a dental office emergency kit. These supplemental drugs are injectable benzodiazepine, glucagon, and corticosteroids.

Injectable Benzodiazepine

The administration of an injectable benzodiazepine may be necessary for the management of prolonged or recurrent seizures or hyperventilation. This drug type will cause skeletal muscle relaxation and is an effective anticonvulsant. Lorazepam is considered the benzodiazepine of choice for use with seizures as it can be administered intramuscularly. The adult dose of lorazepam is 4 mg IM. (See Figure 2.11 ■)

Glucagon

Glucagon administered IM is the drug of choice for the unconscious hypoglycemic patient. The recommended dosage for an adult is l mg IM, and for a patient weighing less than 20 kg, 0.5 mg should be used. (See Figure 2.12 ■)

Corticosteroid

Administration of a corticosteroid may be indicated for the prevention of a recurrence of an anaphylactic reaction and the management of adrenal crisis. Hydrocortisone (100 mg) is the corticosteroid of choice for the dental office emergency kit. Also, steroids will reduce histamine release, which is important in the management of allergic reactions. The major drawback of the use of corticosteroids in emergency situations is their slow onset of action (greater than one hour); therefore, they are not considered essential drugs in the emergency kit. (See Figure 2.13 ■)

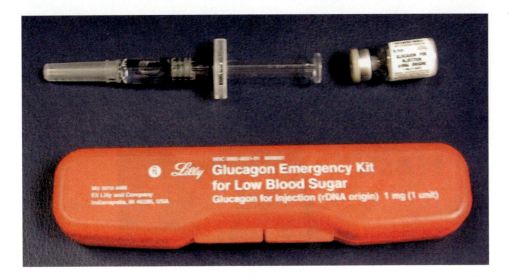

FIGURE 2.12 Injectable glucagon.

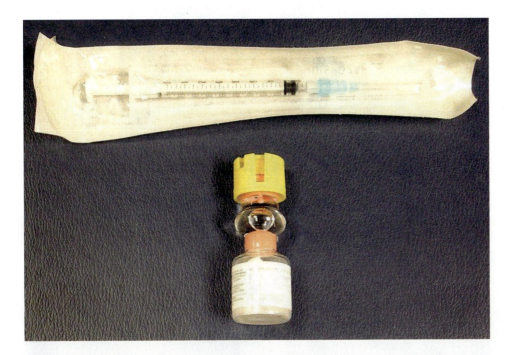

FIGURE 2.13 Injectable Solu-Cortef (hydrocortisone).

Additional Items for the Emergency Kit

There are a few additional items that should be included in a dental office emergency kit. A blood pressure cuff and stethoscope should be readily available, as well as a pocket mask with a one-way valve. (See Figure 2.14 ■) Syringes should be available for the delivery of IM drugs that are not in preloaded syringes. A perioretriever, a magnetized device for the removal of broken instrument tips, should be included. (See Figure 2.15 ■) Band-Aids and sterile gauze should be available for minor cuts or burns. An ice pack is necessary for burns or hematomas (bruises). (See Figure 2.16 ■) A thermometer is useful to determine if the patient is suffering from pyrexia (fever), particularly in the event of thyroid storm. Many dental offices are now including an AED (automated external defibrillator) in case of an MI. (See Figure 2.17 ■) A glucometer to measure blood glucose levels in patients suspected of suffering from hypoglycemia or hyperglycemia is recommended. (See Figure 2.18 ■)

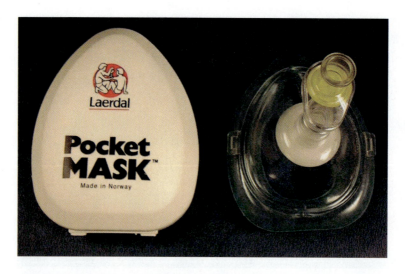

FIGURE 2.14 Pocket mask with one-way valve.

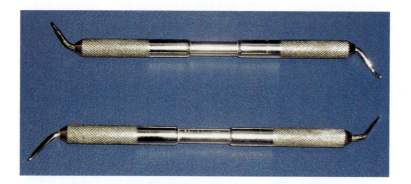

FIGURE 2.15 Perioretrievers.

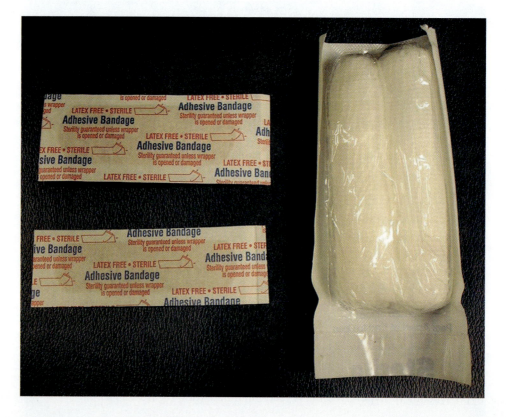

FIGURE 2.16 Assorted bandages.

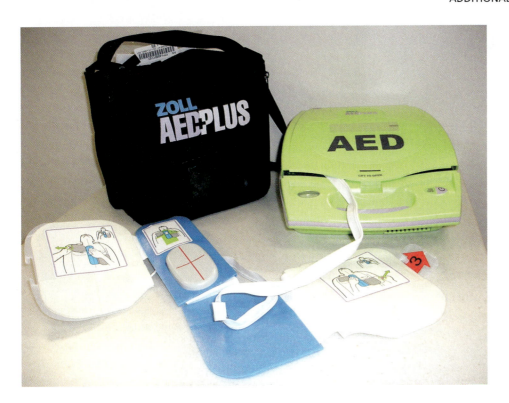

FIGURE 2.17 AED—automated external defibrillator.

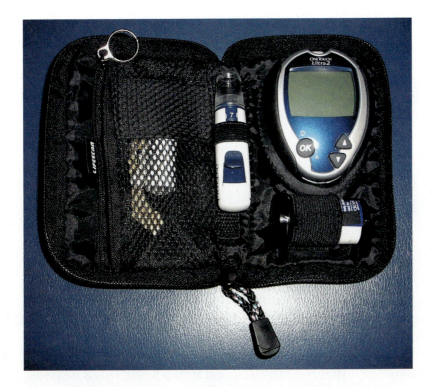

FIGURE 2.18 Glucometer.

Conclusion ···→

A well-prepared emergency kit is an essential component of the twenty-first-century dental office. Each office should design its kit based on its knowledge and skill level, location, and patient base. The drugs and additional items discussed is this chapter may be needed in an emergency situation in order to save a patient's life.

Review Questions

1. What is the drug of choice for a severe allergic reaction?

   A. Chlorpheniramine 10 mg orally
   B. diphenhydramine 50 mg IM
   C. epinephrine 1:1,000 0.3 mg IM
   D. nitroglycerin one tablet sublingually

2. For which medical emergency would you administer albuterol?

   A. adrenal insufficiency
   B. asthma attack
   C. angina attack
   D. epileptic seizure

3. A patient who is hypoglycemic would benefit from which emergency item?

   A. aspirin
   B. atropine IM
   C. corticosteroid injection
   D. oral carbohydrate

4. Nitroglycerin aids in the treatment of angina pectoris by

   A. increasing blood pressure
   B. increasing pulse rate
   C. dilating coronary arteries
   D. constricting cerebral arteries

5. All of the following are essential items for the dental office emergency kit *except* one. Which one is the *exception*?

   A. atropine
   B. epinephrine
   C. glucose
   D. albuterol

Bibliography

ADA Council on Scientific Affairs. "Office Emergencies and Emergency Kits." *Journal of the American Dental Association* 133 (1999): 364–65.

Alberto, P. L. "Office Preparation and Your Medical Emergency Kit: What You Should Know." *Access* 22 (2008): 26–29.

American Society of Anesthesiologists. "New Classification of Physical Status." *Anesthesiology* 24 (1963): 111.

Balmer, C., and L. Longman. *The Management of Medical Emergencies: A Guide for Dental Professionals* (1st ed.), 2008. London: Quay Books.

Chapman, P. J. "An Overview of Drugs and Ancillary Equipment for the Dentist's Emergency Kit." *Australian Dental Journal* 48 (2003): 130–33.

Emery, R. W., and S. A. Guttenberg. "Management Priorities and Treatment Strategies for Medical Emergencies in the Dental Office." *Dental Clinics of North America* 43 (1999): 401–19.

Haas, D. A. "Emergency Drugs." *Dental Clinics of North America* 46 (2006): 815–30.

Haas, D. A. "Management of Medical Emergencies in the Dental Office: Conditions in Each Country, the Extent of Treatment by the Dentist." *Anesthesia Progress* 53 (2006): 20–24.

Malamed, S. F. "Emergency Medicine." *Dental Economics* (2010): 38–43.

Morrison, A. D., and R. H. B. Godday. "Preparing for Medical Emergencies in the Dental Office." *Journal of the Canadian Dental Association* 65 (1999): 284–86.

Pickett, F., and J. Gurenlian. *The Medical History: Clinical Implications and Emergency Prevention in Dental Settings* (1st ed.), 2005. Philadelphia, PA: Williams & Wilkins.

Santini, M., F. Ammirati, F. Colivicchi, G. Gentilucci, and V. Guido. "The Effect of Atropine in Vasovagal Syncope Induced by Head-Up Tilt Testing." *European Heart Journal* 20 (1999): 1745–51.

Shampaine, G. "Patient Assessment and Preventive Measures for Medical Emergencies in the Dental Office." *Dental Clinics of North America* 43 (1999): 383–400.

Wheeler, D. S., M. L. Kiefer, and W. B. Poss. "Pediatric Emergency Preparedness in the Office." *American Family Physician* 61 (2000): 3333–42.

Wynn, R. L., T. M. Meiller, and H. L. Crossley. (Eds.). *Drug Information Handbook for Dentistry*, 2010. Hudson, OH: Lexicomp.

3

Vital Signs and Hypertensive Urgency and Emergency

LEARNING OBJECTIVES

Upon reading the material in this chapter, the reader will be able to:

☑ Discuss the importance of taking and recording the body's vital signs.

☑ Describe the process for taking pulse, respiration, and blood pressure.

☑ Differentiate normal from abnormal vital sign readings.

☑ Discuss hypertension, including its predisposing factors and prevention strategies.

☑ Differentiate between hypertensive urgency and emergency.

Case Studies ·······························➤

Scenario 1

Your 1:00 P.M. oral prophylaxis patient, John Brown, is a 79-year-old male retired service salesman for an automobile dealership. He is in fair health and suffered from a previous myocardial infarction four years ago. You take his vital signs (pulse, respiration, and blood pressure) and find the following readings:

> *Pulse: 102 beats/minute*
>
> *Respiration: 22 respirations/minute and exaggerated*
>
> *Blood pressure: 150/98 mmHg*
>
> *What can you conclude from the vital signs?*

Scenario 2

Your 2:00 P.M. patient, Harry Fredericks, is a 62-year-old male postal worker and is new to your practice. His history indicates daily intake of hypertension medications, but he states that he does not like to take them due to the side effects. Other than hypertension, his medical history is negative.

> *Blood pressure: 188/112 mmHg*
>
> *Pulse: 86 beats/minute*
>
> *Respiration: 16 respirations/minute*
>
> *What is the medical significance of the information stated by the patient and the recorded blood pressure?*

Introduction

The accurate taking and recording of vital signs for each patient is essential to comprehensive patient care. The vital signs typically recorded in a dental office include pulse, respiration, and blood pressure. These measurements determine the body's ability to pump blood and breathe, which are essential elements for sustaining human life. Determining baseline vital signs enables the healthcare provider to compare normal readings for a patient with readings that are occurring during a medical emergency, which will help determine the severity of the emergency. In addition, vital signs are taken to determine the health status of the patient. Temperature is also considered a vital sign, and an elevated temperature may indicate the presence of infection. With infection, pain may be causing an increased stress level for the patient and therefore could be an indicator of an emergency.

Pulse

A person's pulse indicates the speed and force of his or her heartbeat and the expansion and contraction of an artery as blood is forced out of the heart muscle. A pulse can be felt in various locations in the body where an artery lies close to the skin surface and can be compressed over a hard structure, such as bone or muscle tissue. The most common areas to take a pulse are the carotid pulse in the neck, the radial pulse in the wrist, and the brachial pulse in the arm. The femoral pulse felt in the groin area is another site used to take a pulse in an emergency situation.

The most common pulse taken in a dental practice is the radial pulse. To determine the rate of the radial pulse be sure to first have the patient rest for 10 seconds, place the tips of the index and middle fingers along the groove at the base of the thumb on the patient's wrist. Press against the radial artery with your index and middle fingers to block the pulse, and gradually release the pressure until pulsations are felt. Do not use your thumb as it has a pulse of its own. Move the fingers until you discover the pulsing sensation. Count the number of times a beat is felt for 30 seconds and then multiply by 2 in order to determine the number of heartbeats per minute. (See Figure 3.1 ■) If the pulse seems irregular, count the beats for one full minute. The initial pulse sensation is counted as zero. In a healthy adult and children over 10 years of age the normal resting heart rate is between 60 and 100 beats/minute. Individuals who exercise routinely may have lower pulse rates in the range of 40–60 beats/minute. (See Table 3.1 ■) A slow pulse or a rapid pulse can indicate a serious illness or condition; however, as stated previously, a fit individual may naturally have a slow pulse rate. Knowing an individual's baseline pulse rate is particularly important for comparison during a medical emergency.

A rapid pulse rate of more than 100 beats/minute is termed tachycardia. A person's heart rate normally increases in response to fever, exercise, nervous excitement, medications, or stimulant-type drugs. Tachycardia can also be a result of disease states, such as heart failure, hemorrhage, or shock. Tachycardia attempts to increase the amount of oxygen delivered to the cells of the body by increasing the amount of blood circulated through the blood vessels.

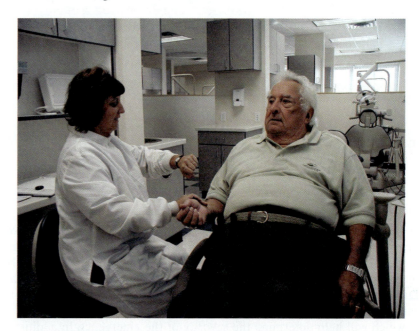

FIGURE 3.1 Taking a pulse rate.

Table 3.1   Normal Pulse Rates

Age or Fitness Level	Beats/Minute (bpm)
Babies to age 1	80–120
Children ages 1 to 10	70–130
Children age 10+ and adults	60–100
Well-conditioned athletes	40–60

Bradycardia occurs when the heart rate is less than 60 beats/minute. When this condition occurs as a result of disease or illness, it may cause lightheadedness, dizziness, chest pain, and possibly syncope (fainting) and circulatory collapse. (The latter two conditions will be discussed in subsequent chapters.) Bradycardia is often treated by the administration of the drug atropine, which increases a person's heart rate. If the patient continues to experience bradycardia, a medical referral is necessary to evaluate for possible implantation of a **pacemaker**.

In addition to pulse rate, the dental practitioner should assess the rhythm and strength or amplitude of the patient's pulse. The rhythm is the relationship of one impulse to another impulse as measured by regularity of action. Whether the pulse is regular or irregular should also be noted. An irregular pulse could be a sign of an **arrhythmia** (irregular heart beat). In addition, the strength of the pulse reflects the volume of blood pushing against the blood vessel walls with each heart contraction. This is known as the **stroke volume** (SV). An extremely strong pulse, often referred to as a bounding pulse, is an indication of an increased SV. A bounding pulse can be dangerous particularly if the patient has hypertension, which would increase her or his risk of cerebrovascular accident (CVA) or stroke. A weak pulse, often described as a thready pulse, indicates a decrease in the heart's stroke volume. In this case the pulse is present but may be difficult to detect.

If a patient has any of the problems discussed previously—tachycardia, bradycardia, irregular pulse, or increased or decreased stroke volume—the dental practitioner should refer him or her to a physician for further assessment. In addition, a determination should be made as to whether or not treatment should be performed in the dental office that day, because any of these conditions may increase the possibility of the occurrence of a medical emergency.

Respiration

Respiration is the process by which oxygen and carbon dioxide are exchanged within the body. The two processes involved in respiration are external and internal. **External respiration** occurs when oxygen is taken into the body and carbon dioxide is eliminated via the lungs. **Internal respiration** involves the use of oxygen, the production of carbon dioxide, and their exchange between cells and blood. (See Figure 3.2 ■)

Normal breathing is involuntary. The respiration rate (RR) is the number of times the patient breathes per minute. It is counted by the rise and fall of the chest. A normal RR for an adult at rest is 12–20 breaths/minute. Infants and children have much quicker RRs. Newborns can have an RR ranging from 40 to 50 breaths/minute. As the individual ages the RR declines, and by puberty the respirations are in the range of 15–20 breaths/minute. (See Table 3.2 ■ on page 25) Tachypnea is an abnormally fast respiratory rate above 20 breaths/minute in an adult. This condition is often seen in individuals experiencing **hyperventilation**. (Hyperventilation is discussed in Chapter 7.) Bradypnea is an abnormally slow respiratory rate, less than 12 breaths/minute in an adult. This condition is often seen in individuals experiencing syncope. **Apnea** is the absence of respirations and is often described by the length of time in which no respirations occur. If apnea continues, the condition is considered **respiratory arrest** and is not compatible with sustaining life, as brain tissue is the most sensitive tissue to oxygen deprivation. Brain tissue survives only a few minutes without oxygen. Brain damage and/or coma can occur if oxygen deprivation lasts 10 minutes or longer.

Determining a patient's respiratory rate can be a challenge. Patients can control their breathing, so they should not be aware that you are actually assessing their respiratory rate. The respiratory rate in the dental setting should be measured immediately following the procedure for pulse determination. Move the patient's arm over the patient's stomach and continue as if monitoring the patient's pulse rate. Instead of counting heartbeats, count the number of times the patient's chest rises and falls in a

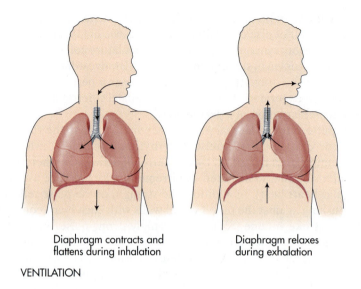

Diaphragm contracts and flattens during inhalation

Diaphragm relaxes during exhalation

VENTILATION

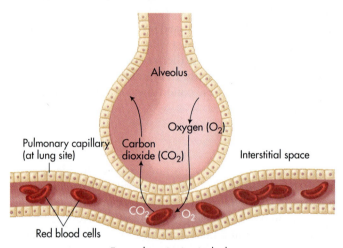

Alveolus

Oxygen (O_2)

Pulmonary capillary (at lung site)

Carbon dioxide (CO_2)

Interstitial space

CO_2 O_2

Red blood cells

External respiration in the lungs

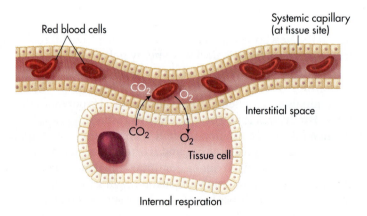

Red blood cells

Systemic capillary (at tissue site)

CO_2 O_2

Interstitial space

CO_2 O_2

Tissue cell

Internal respiration

RESPIRATION

FIGURE 3.2 Contrast of ventilation and external and internal respiration.

Table 3.2   Normal Respiratory Rate

Age Level	Respirations/Minute
Newborns	40–50
Infants	20–40
Preschool children	20–30
Older children	15–25
Adults	12–20

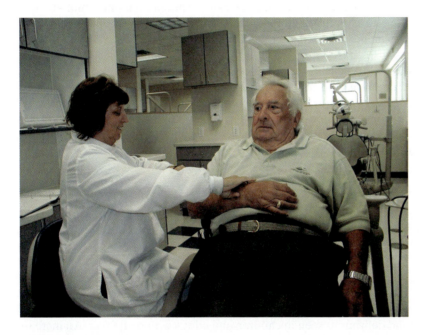

FIGURE 3.3 Taking a respiration rate.

30-second time frame and multiply this number by 2. (See Figure 3.3 ■) If the patient's respirations are irregular, count the number of respirations for one full minute.

In addition to rate, the rhythm, depth, and quality of respirations should be assessed. Respiratory rhythm should be regular in nature, with expiration being twice as long as inspiration. There are several abnormal respiratory patterns, such as **Biot's respirations**, **Cheyne–Stokes respirations**, and **Kussmaul respirations**. Biot's respirations are cyclic breathing patterns characterized by periods of shallow breathing alternating with periods of apnea. This type of respiration is often seen in individuals with neurological problems, head trauma, brain abscesses, and heat stroke. Cheyne–Stokes respirations are cyclic breathing patterns characterized by periods of respirations of increased rate and depth alternating with periods of apnea. This type of abnormal respiratory pattern is typically seen in individuals suffering from heart failure and drug overdose. Kussmaul respirations are an increased depth and rate of respirations of over 20 breaths/minute. This type of breathing pattern is seen in individuals with hyperventilation, metabolic acidosis, diabetic ketoacidosis, and renal failure.

Respirations should be quiet, automatic, and effortless. Abnormalities are usually characterized by problems with effort or noise. Dyspnea (labored breathing) is a general term describing respirations that require excessive effort. Any type of dyspnea needs to be recognized and the appropriate steps taken to alleviate the condition, such as providing oxygenation. There are several terms used to describe noises made during respiration. **Stridor**, wheezing, and **sighs** are common conditions with which a dental practitioner should be familiar. Stridor is a harsh sound made during inspiration that sounds like crowing. This is often associated with airway obstruction. Wheezing is a high-pitched sound that is usually heard on expiration but may be heard on inspiration, as well. This sound is often associated with individuals suffering from asthma. Sighs are breaths of deep inspiration and prolonged expiration. Frequent sighing may indicate an individual is under a great deal of stress or tension. Periodically, people unconsciously take single deep breaths or sighs to expand small airways prone to collapse.

There are several factors that can affect respirations, including age, medications, stress, exercise, altitude, gender, and body position. As lung capacity increases from childhood to adulthood, a lower respiratory rate is needed to exchange air, so respiratory rates decrease; however, as adults age their lungs become less elastic, and the respiratory rate increases to allow for adequate air exchange. Some medications, such as narcotics, will decrease respiratory rates, whereas sympathomimetic drugs that mimic the effects of organ stimulation, such as albuterol, will dilate the bronchioles, leading to an increase in the patient's ability to breathe.

Stress can cause an increase in the strength and depth of respirations, as will exercise. As altitude increases, the oxygen content of the air decreases. As a result, the rate and depth of respirations are increased at higher elevations. In most instances, men have a larger lung capacity than women, and thus will have a lower respiratory rate than women. Moreover, if patients are in a slumped or stooped body position, it is more difficult for them to exchange oxygen and carbon dioxide, so their rate and depth of respirations will increase.

Temperature

Temperature is the measure of heat associated with the metabolism of the body. It is normally maintained at a constant level of 98.6°F (37.5°C). Body temperature may actually be 1°F (0.6°C) or more above or below 98.6°F (37°C) and still be considered within the normal range.

Fever or **pyrexia** is an abnormal elevation in body temperature. Infection, neurological disease, **malignancy**, heart failure, severe trauma, and many drugs may cause the development of fever. **Convulsions** may occur in children with extremely high fevers, and delirium is seen in children and adults with high fever. An increased temperature is indicative of illness that may precede an emergency situation; therefore, it should be considered seriously in the patient evaluation process.

Hypothermia is a state in which an individual's body temperature is reduced below his or her normal range, but not below 96°F. Characteristics of hypothermia are mild shivering, cool skin, and pallor. Illness, trauma, malnutrition, and medications may all cause hypothermia; therefore, patients exhibiting this condition should be referred to their medical physician or the emergency department. (See Figure 3.4 ■)

Blood Pressure

Blood pressure is the force exerted by the blood against the blood vessel walls. A blood pressure reading is stated in millimeters of mercury (mmHg) and is recorded as a fraction of the **systolic blood pressure** reading over the **diastolic blood pressure** reading (systole/diastole; 120/80). The force of the blood against the blood vessel walls during ventricular contraction is termed systolic blood pressure. A normal adult reading for systolic pressure is 100–120 mmHg. The force of the blood against the blood vessel walls during ventricular relaxation is the diastolic reading. A normal adult reading for diastolic pressure is 60–80 mmHg. The difference between the systolic pressure and the diastolic pressure is termed the **pulse pressure**. The diastolic blood pressure is more significant in individuals aged 50 or younger. The higher the diastolic reading in this group the greater the risk for myocardial infarctions (MIs), CVAs, and kidney failure. As individuals age the diastolic pressure will begin to decrease and the systolic pressure will increase and become more important. For individuals aged 50 and older the systolic blood pressure gives a better diagnosis of hypertension. In addition, if left untreated, high systolic blood pressure can lead to a CVA (stroke), MI (heart attack),

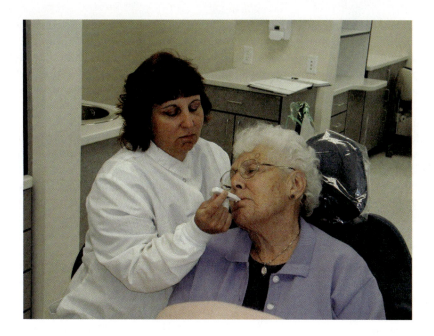

FIGURE 3.4 Taking a temperature.

heart failure, kidney damage, blindness, or other conditions. A normal adult pulse pressure reading is 30–40 mmHg. For example, if a patient's systolic blood pressure is 100 mmHg and the diastolic blood pressure is 70 mmHg, then the pulse pressure would be 30 mmHg (100 minus 70). This pulse pressure would be within the normal range. A higher or lower pulse pressure than normal may indicate some type of cardiac abnormality, and the patient should be referred to a physician for assessment.

Blood Pressure in Children

Unlike adults, blood pressure in children varies based on gender, age, and height. As a result, it is classified by percentile norms. Children are categorized into four groups according to percentile in which their average systolic or diastolic pressure falls based on their height. Normal blood pressure for children indicates that the child's average systolic or diastolic blood pressure is at the 89th percentile or lower, based on their gender, age, and height. In other words, 89% of children of that gender, age, and height would have blood pressure below this level.

Prehypertension in children indicates the child's average systolic or diastolic blood pressure is between the 90th and 94th percentile. In adolescents (ages 12 to 18) this means that the blood pressure exceeds 120/80 mmHg, up to the 95th percentile for their gender, age, and height. **Stage 1 hypertension** in children indicates high blood pressure in which the average systolic or diastolic pressure ranges from the 95th percentile, up to 5 mmHg above the blood pressure measurement at the 99th percentile. **Stage 2 hypertension** in children is more severe high blood pressure, which means the child's average systolic or diastolic blood pressure is 5 mmHg or more above the 99th percentile for his or her gender, age, and height. It is recommended that blood pressure monitoring begin at three years of age.

Factors Affecting Blood Pressure

Blood volume, cardiac output, blood viscosity, and blood vessel resistance are factors that influence blood pressure. An increase in blood volume, such as one would experience after a blood transfusion or pregnancy, will cause blood pressure to rise. Conversely, if there is a decrease in blood volume, such as during hemorrhaging, a reduction in blood pressure will occur.

As cardiac output (the amount of blood ejected by the heart) increases, so will blood pressure; conversely, as cardiac output decreases, so will blood pressure readings. When the thickness of the blood increases, the heart needs to contract more forcefully in order to move the blood through the circulatory system, so the blood pressure will increase. Blood vessel walls that are elastic can accommodate changes in blood pressure much more readily than blood vessel walls that are rigid. Therefore, patients who are suffering from atherosclerosis (thickening and calcification of the lumen of blood vessel) will tend to have higher blood pressure readings.

Other factors affecting blood pressure are patient age, gender, history of taking stimulants, and exercise. Elderly patients are more likely to experience hypertension because they are more prone to atherosclerosis. Men and postmenopausal women are more likely to exhibit hypertension. Individuals who use stimulants in any form, such as nicotine or caffeine, will also tend to have elevated blood pressure. Immediately following exercise blood pressure will rise; however, those individuals who exercise routinely will tend to have lower overall blood pressures.

Measuring Blood Pressure

To measure blood pressure, the clinician will need a **sphygmomanometer** and stethoscope. The sphygmomanometer consists of an inflatable cuff that is composed of a nonelastic material with a Velcro closing. There are different-sized cuffs for children, adults, and obese individuals. Using an incorrectly sized cuff can give inaccurate blood pressure readings. For example, using a cuff that is too large will lead to a lower than accurate reading; conversely, a cuff that is too small will lead to a higher than normal blood pressure reading. The cuff should cover two-thirds of the upper arm. The sphygmomanometer has a pressure gauge attached directly to the cuff or attached by a tube. (See Figure 3.5 ■)

There are essentially three different types of gauges: mercury, aneroid, and digital. The mercury gauge has proven to be the most accurate; however, aneroid gauges are acceptable in the dental office setting. Attached to the cuff is a hand control bulb to pump air into and out of the cuff. Digital blood pressure devices are easy to use, and their accuracy has improved over the years. Dental practitioners who are

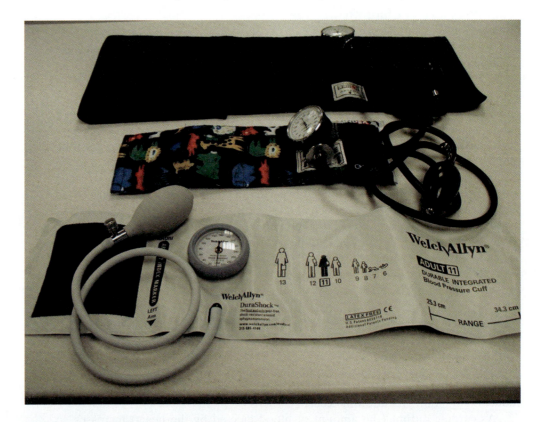

FIGURE 3.5 Pediatric, adult, and large adult blood pressure cuff.

considering an electronic device are encouraged to review the data regarding accuracy prior to purchase.

The stethoscope is a listening device that magnifies sound. It is composed of two earpieces and an endpiece that are connected by tubing.

The process for taking blood pressure is as follows:

- Explain the procedure to the patient.
- Seat the patient comfortably with the arm placed at heart level and the palm up.
- Ask the patient what is his or her normal blood pressure reading.
- Consistently take blood pressure on the same arm. There can be a 5–20 mmHg difference between the patient's right and left arm, with the right arm providing a slightly higher reading. Recent evidence suggests that the difference in blood pressure readings is unrelated to age, sex, ethnicity, arm circumference, handedness, being hypertensive, being diabetic, or a history of cardiovascular disease. As the differences are relatively small, either arm can be selected for blood pressure measurement, but the same arm should be used consistently for that patient.
- Have patient roll up sleeve for more accurate results as long as the sleeve is nonrestrictive.
- Apply the deflated cuff to the patient's arm—if the patient has a shunt in the arm (e.g., kidney dialysis), the other arm should be utilized.
- Place the lower edge of the cuff approximately 1 inch above the antecubital fossa (crease in the arm when bent).
- Adjust the position of the gauge so that it is easily visible to the clinician but not to the patient.
- Locate the brachial pulse approximately 1 inch below the antecubital fossa, toward the medial surface of the inner arm.
- Place the endpiece of the stethoscope over the brachial pulse directly on the skin (it may be necessary to have the patient hold the endpiece in place).
- Place the earpieces in ears facing toward the tip of the nose.
- Locate the radial pulse.
- Inflate the cuff by first closing the valve on the hand control bulb (make sure that it can be opened easily with one hand).
- Inflate the cuff until the radial pulse is no longer felt—remember this reading.
- Look at the sphygmomanometer and inflate the cuff 20 or 30 mmHg higher than the reading where you no longer felt the radial pulse.
- Deflate the cuff (2 mmHg at a time) so that the gauge drops gradually and an accurate reading can be obtained.
- Listen for the first sound—this is the systolic reading—and note the number on the gauge.
- Continue to release the pressure slowly until no more tapping sounds are heard; note the number on the gauge for the last sound heard—this will be the diastolic reading.
- Release all air out of the cuff rapidly.
- If unsure of the reading, be sure to deflate the cuff completely and wait at least 30 seconds before inflating the cuff again to retake the blood pressure. Failure to do so causes the veins to remain collapsed under the cuff and will increase the chance of having an **auscultatory gap**. An auscultatory gap refers to the disappearance and reappearance of the **Korotkoff sounds** that can occur during auscultatory blood pressure measurements, particularly in hypertensive individuals. If the clinician stops inflating the cuff in the middle of the auscultatory gap, the reappearance of the Korotkoff sounds as the cuff pressure is lowered will be misinterpreted as systolic blood pressure, causing significant underestimation of systolic blood pressure.
- Once an accurate reading is obtained, be sure to record the blood pressure in the patient's chart along with the date and which arm was used.
- If the blood pressure is being taken during a medical emergency, it is helpful to leave the blood pressure cuff in place until the emergency is resolved or EMS (emergency medical services) arrives. (See Figures 3.6 and 3.7 ■)

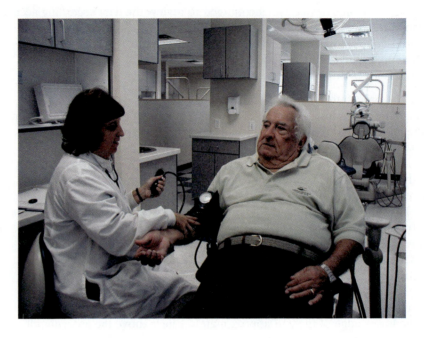

FIGURE 3.6 Taking a blood pressure.

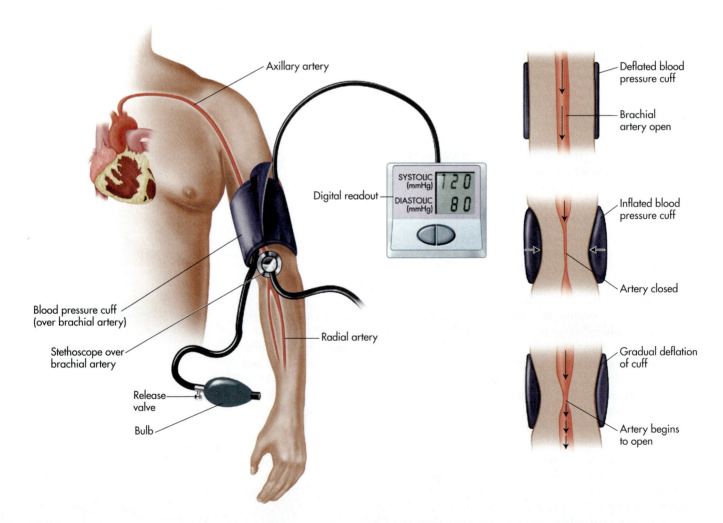

FIGURE 3.7 Blood pressure measurement.

Hypertension

Hypertension is a common disorder characterized by elevated blood pressure exceeding 140/90 mmHg. Hypertension is the most common primary diagnosis in the United States, affecting 60 million Americans. Seventy percent of Americans are unaware that they are suffering from hypertension, so it is incumbent on dental professionals to accurately assess the blood pressure for each patient they treat. The National Heart, Lung, and Blood Institute of the U.S. Department of Health has determined four classifications of blood pressure: normal, prehypertension, Stage 1 hypertension, and Stage 2 hypertension. Table 3.3 ■ illustrates the most current blood pressure classifications for adults, and Tables 3.4 and 3.5 ■ illustrate the most current blood pressure classifications for children.

Normal blood pressure in adults is any systolic blood pressure reading less than 120 mmHg and any diastolic blood pressure reading less than 80 mmHg; however, extremely low values are classified as hypotension. The prehypertension category includes individuals with a systolic blood pressure reading of 120–139 mmHg or a diastolic blood pressure reading of 80–89 mmHg. Individuals with prehypertension are at increased risk of progressing to hypertension and should be counseled to modify their lifestyle to incorporate more healthy choices. Lifestyle modifications include weight reduction for overweight individuals, sodium reduction, appropriate physical activity, and moderation of alcohol consumption. In addition, the consumption of a diet rich in fruits, vegetables, and low-fat dairy products is advised. Incorporating any or all of these concepts can lower blood pressure from 2 to 20 mmHg.

Stage 1 hypertension includes individuals with a systolic blood pressure of 140–159 mmHg or a diastolic blood pressure of 90–99 mmHg. These patients should be advised of healthy lifestyle choices and should also be referred to their physician for assessment. Often these patients are placed on antihypertensive medications, such as thiazides.

Stage 2 hypertension includes individuals with a systolic blood pressure of 160 mmHg or higher or a diastolic blood pressure above 100 mmHg. Patients exhibiting this blood pressure reading without any prior **target-organ damage**, such as a prior **myocardial infarction** or CVA, should have their blood pressure rechecked to ensure accuracy and then be referred to their physician for assessment. Patients exhibiting this level of blood pressure reading with prior target-organ damage should have their blood pressure rechecked to ensure accuracy and then be referred immediately for a medical evaluation. No additional dental treatment should be performed as these patients are at extreme risk for a CVA.

Individuals with untreated hypertension are at risk for many disorders. Hypertension underlies most cardiovascular diseases. In addition, it has been associated with kidney damage and CVA. For each 10-mmHg increase in systolic blood pressure

Table 3.3 **Blood Pressure Classification for Adults**

	Systolic Blood Pressure (mmHg)	Diastolic Blood Pressure (mmHg)
Normal	<120	< 80
Prehypertension	120–139	80–89
Stage 1 hypertension	140–159	90–99
Stage 2 hypertension	≥ 160	≥ 100

< means less than; ≥ means greater than or equal to; when systolic and diastolic blood pressures fall into different categories, the higher category should be used to classify blood pressure level.

Adapted from U.S. Department of Health and Human Services, National Institutes of Health, National Heart, Lung, and Blood Institute (2004). *The Seventh Report of the Joint National Committee on Prevention, Detection, Evaluation, and Treatment of High Blood Pressure.* Retrieved December 28, 2006, from http://www.nhlbi.nih.gov/guidelines/hypertension/jnc7full.pdf.

Table 3.4 Blood Pressure Levels for Girls and Boys by Age and Height Percentile

Girls SBP by Age and Height
(Normal SEP is less than the prehypertensive result.)

Age 1	BP Classification	Systotic BP(mm Hg)						
3	*Height(cm)*	*91*	*92*	*95*	*98*	*100*	*103*	*105*
	Prehypertension	100	100	102	103	104	106	106
	Stage–1 HTN	104	104	105	107	108	109	110
	Stage–2 HTN	106	116	118	119	120	121	122
4	*Height(cm)*	*97*	*99*	*101*	*104*	*108*	*110*	*112*
	Prehypertension	101	102	103	104	105	107	108
	Stage–1 HTN	105	106	107	108	110	111	112
	Stage–2 HTN	117	118	118	120	122	123	124
5	*Height(cm)*	*104*	*105*	*108*	*111*	*115*	*118*	*120*
	Prehypertension	103	103	105	106	107	109	109
	Stage–1 HTN	107	107	108	110	111	112	113
	Stage–2 HTN	119	119	121	122	123	125	126
6	*Height(cm)*	*110*	*112*	*115*	*118*	*122*	*126*	*128*
	Prehypertension	101	105	106	108	109	110	111
	Stage–1 HTN	100	109	110	111	113	114	115
	Stage–2 HTN	120	121	122	124	125	126	127
7	*Height(cm)*	*116*	*118*	*121*	*125*	*129*	*132*	*135*
	Prehypertension	106	107	108	109	111	112	113
	Stage–1 HTN	110	111	112	113	115	116	116
	Stage–2 HTN	122	123	124	125	127	128	129
8	*Height(cm)*	*121*	*123*	*127*	*131*	*135*	*139*	*141*
	Prehypertension	108	109	110	111	113	114	114
	Stage–1 HTN	112	112	114	115	116	118	118
	Stage–2 HTN	124	125	126	127	128	130	130
9	*Height(cm)*	*125*	*128*	*131*	*136*	*140*	*144*	*147*
	Prehypertension	110	110	112	113	114	116	116
	Stage–1 HTN	114	114	115	117	118	119	120
	Stage–2 HTN	126	126	128	129	130	132	132
10	*Height(cm)*	*130*	*132*	*136*	*141*	*146*	*150*	*153*
	Prehypertension	112	112	114	115	116	118	118
	Stage–1 HTN	136	116	117	119	120	121	122
	Stage–2 HTN	128	128	130	131	132	134	134
11	*Height(cm)*	*136*	*138*	*143*	*148*	*153*	*157*	*160*
	Prehypertension	114	114	116	117	118	119	120
	Stage–1 HTN	118	118	119	121	122	123	124
	Stage–2 HTN	130	130	131	133	134	135	136
12	*Height(cm)*	*143*	*146*	*150*	*155*	*160*	*164*	*165*
	Prehypertension	116	116	117	119	120	120	120
	Stage–1 HTN	119	120	121	123	124	125	126
	Stage–2 HTN	132	132	133	135	136	137	138
13	*Height(cm)*	*148*	*151*	*155*	*159*	*164*	*168*	*170*
	Prehypertension	117	118	119	120	120	120	120
	Stage–1 HTN	121	122	123	124	126	127	128
	Stage–2 HTN	133	134	135	137	138	139	140
14	*Height(cm)*	*151*	*153*	*157*	*161*	*166*	*170*	*172*
	Prehypertension	119	120	120	120	120	120	120
	Stage–1 HTN	123	123	125	126	127	139	1329
	Stage–2 HTN	135	136	137	138	140	141	141

Age 1	BP Classification	Systotic BP(mm Hg)						
15	*Height(cm)*	*152*	*154*	*158*	*162*	*167*	*171*	*173*
	Prehypertension	120	120	120	120	120	120	130
	Stage–1 HTN	124	125	126	127	129	130	131
	Stage–2 HTN	136	137	138	139	141	142	143
16	*Height(cm)*	*152*	*154*	*158*	*163*	*167*	*171*	*173*
	Prehypertension	120	120	120	120	120	120	120
	Stage–1 HTN	125	126	127	128	130	131	132
	Stage–2 HTN	137	138	139	140	142	143	144
17	*Height(cm)*	*152*	*155*	*159*	*163*	*167*	*171*	*174*
	Prehypertension	120	120	120	120	120	120	120
	Stage–1 HTN	125	126	127	129	130	131	132
	Stage–2 HTN	138	138	139	141	142	143	144

Boys SBP by Age and Height
(Normal SBP is less than the prehypertensive result.)

Age 1	BP Classification	Systotic BP(mm Hg)						
3	*Height(cm)*	*92*	*94*	*96*	*99*	*102*	*104*	*106*
	Prehypertension	100	101	103	105	107	108	109
	Stage–1 HTN	104	105	107	109	110	112	113
	Stage–2 HTN	116	117	119	121	123	124	125
4	*Height(cm)*	*99*	*100*	*103*	*106*	*109*	*112*	*113*
	Prehypertension	100	103	105	107	109	110	111
	Stage–1 HTN	106	107	109	111	112	114	115
	Stage–2 HTN	118	119	121	123	125	126	127
5	*Height(cm)*	*104*	*106*	*109*	*112*	*116*	*119*	*120*
	Prehypertension	104	105	106	108	110	111	112
	Stage–1 HTN	108	109	110	112	114	115	116
	Stage–2 HTN	120	121	123	125	126	128	128
6	*Height(cm)*	*110*	*112*	*115*	*119*	*122*	*126*	*127*
	Prehypertension	106	106	108	110	111	113	113
	Stage–1 HTN	109	110	117	114	115	117	117
	Stage–2 HTN	121	122	124	126	128	129	130
7	*Height(cm)*	*116*	*118*	*121*	*125*	*129*	*132*	*134*
	Prehypertension	106	107	109	111	113	114	115
	Stage–1 HTN	110	111	113	115	117	118	119
	Stage–2 HTN	122	123	125	127	129	130	131
8	*Height(cm)*	*121*	*123*	*127*	*131*	*135*	*139*	*141*
	Prehypertension	107	109	110	112	114	115	116
	Stage–1 HTN	111	112	114	116	118	119	120
	Stage–2 HTN	124	125	127	128	130	132	132
9	*Height(cm)*	*126*	*128*	*132*	*136*	*141*	*145*	*147*
	Prehypertension	119	110	112	114	115	117	118
	Stage–1 HTN	113	114	116	118	119	120	121
	Stage–2 HTN	125	126	128	130	132	133	134
10	*Height(cm)*	*130*	*133*	*137*	*141*	*146*	*150*	*153*
	Prehypertension	111	112	114	115	117	119	119
	Stage–1 HTN	115	116	117	119	121	122	123
	Stage–2 HTN	127	128	130	132	133	135	135
11	*Height(cm)*	*135*	*137*	*142*	*146*	*151*	*156*	*159*
	Prehypertension	113	114	115	117	119	120	120
	Stage–1 HTN	117	118	119	121	123	124	125
	Stage–2 HTN	129	130	132	134	135	137	137

(continued)

Age 1	BP Classification	Systotic BP(mm Hg)						
12	**Height(cm)**	**140**	**143**	**148**	**153**	**156**	**163**	**166**
	Prehypertension	115	116	118	120	120	120	120
	Stage–1 HTN	119	120	122	123	125	127	127
	Stage–2 HTN	131	132	134	136	138	139	140
13	**Height(cm)**	**147**	**150**	**155**	**160**	**166**	**171**	**173**
	Prehypertension	117	118	120	120	120	120	120
	Stage–1 HTN	121	122	124	126	128	129	130
	Stage–2 HTN	133	135	136	138	140	141	142
14	**Height(cm)**	**154**	**157**	**162**	**167**	**173**	**177**	**180**
	Prehypertension	120	120	120	120	120	120	120
	Stage–1 HTN	124	125	127	128	130	132	132
	Stage–2 HTN	136	137	139	141	143	144	145
15	**Height(cm)**	**159**	**162**	**167**	**172**	**177**	**182**	**184**
	Prehypertension	120	120	120	120	120	120	120
	Stage–1 HTN	126	127	129	131	133	134	135
	Stage–2 HTN	139	140	141	143	145	147	147
16	**Height(cm)**	**162**	**165**	**170**	**175**	**160**	**164**	**165**
	Prehypertension	120	120	120	120	120	120	120
	Stage–1 HTN	129	130	132	134	135	137	137
	Stage–2 HTN	141	142	144	146	148	149	150
17	**Height(cm)**	**164**	**166**	**171**	**176**	**181**	**185**	**187**
	Prehypertension	120	120	120	120	120	120	120
	Stage–1 HTN	131	132	134	136	138	139	140
	Stage–2 HTN	144	145	146	148	150	151	152

Adapted from the U.S. Department of Health and Human Services, National Institutes of Health, National Heart, Lung and Blood Institute. (2007). A Pocket Guide to Blood Pressure Measurement in Children. Retrieved October 5, 2011, from http://www.nhlbi.nih.gov/health/public/heart/hbp/bp_child_pocket/bp_child_pocket.pdf.

Table 3.5   Classification/Interpretation of Hypertension in Children

	SBP or DBP Percentile	Frequency of BP Measurement	Interpretation
Normal	<90th	Recheck at next scheduled physical examination.	No recommendations needed.
Prehypertension	90th to <95th or if BP exceeds 120/80 mmHg even if below 90th percentile up to <95th percentile	Recheck in six months.	Begin weight management (as appropriate).
Stage 1 hypertension	>95th percentile to <99th percentile +5 mmHg	Recheck in one to two weeks.	If BP remains at this level on recheck, begin evaluation and treatment including weight management if appropriate.
Stage 2 hypertension	>99th percentile +5 mmHg	Begin evaluation and treatment within one week, immediately if symptomatic.	

Adapted from the U.S. Department of Health and Human Services, National Institutes of Health, National Heart, Lung, and Blood Institute. (2007). A Pocket Guide to Blood Pressure Measurement in Children. Retrieved October 5, 2011, from http://www.nhlbi.nih.gov/health/public/heart/hbp/bp_child_pocket/bp_child_pocket.pdf.

above 160 mmHg, there is a 30% greater risk of a CVA as hypertension degenerates the cerebral blood vessels. Early detection of hypertension is imperative to a patient's total health as complications from prolonged hypertension include CVA, MI (heart attack), and kidney failure.

Hypertensive Urgencies and Emergencies

Severe hypertension can lead to some serious sequelae. There are two major categories of severe hypertension—**hypertensive urgency** and **hypertensive emergency**. In each case the patient presents with an extremely high blood pressure reading. The major difference is that in hypertensive emergency, formerly called hypertensive crisis, the patient would experience some form of target end organ damage. This condition is also referred to as malignant hypertension, because many of the patients did not recover. Types of target end organ damage include **aortic dissection**, **cerebral infarction** or hemorrhage, MI, and **renal insufficiency**. Patients suffering from hypertensive urgency will not have any form of target end organ damage. Patients presenting with hypertensive urgencies are usually newly diagnosed with hypertension, have poorly controlled blood pressure, or are noncompliant with previous therapy.

Signs and Symptoms of Hypertensive Urgency and Emergency

Signs and symptoms of hypertension urgency include headache (moderate to severe), anxiety, shortness of breath, **tinnitus**, **edema**, and **epistaxis**, with a sudden change in blood pressure greater than 180/110 mmHg. (See Table 3.6 ■). Many of these signs and symptoms are exhibited by Harry Fredericks in Case Scenario 2. Symptoms of hypertensive emergency include a sudden increase in blood pressure greater than 180/110 mmHg, but often as high as 220/140 mmHg, shortness of breath, chest pain, **nocturia**, **dysarthria** (difficulty speaking), weakness, and altered consciousness. In addition, there may be visual loss, seizures, heart failure, nausea, vomiting, and eventually **coma**. (See Table 3.7 ■)

Table 3.6 **Signs and Symptoms of Hypertensive Urgency**

- Headache (moderate to severe)
- Anxiety
- Shortness of breath
- Tinnitus
- Edema
- Epistaxis with a sudden change in blood pressure greater than 180/110 mmHg

Table 3.7 **Signs and Symptoms of Hypertensive Emergency**

- Sudden increase in blood pressure greater than 180/110 mmHg, but often as high as 220/140 mmHg
- Shortness of breath
- Chest pain
- Nocturia
- Dysarthria
- Weakness
- Altered consciousness
- Visual loss
- Seizures
- Heart failure
- Nausea
- Vomiting
- Eventually coma

Again, the dental healthcare professional needs to be vigilant of any symptom that could be attributed to some form of end organ damage. In addition, many of the symptoms of hypertensive emergency are similar to those in patients suffering from a CVA or MI, and therefore it is vital to determine exactly which emergency is occurring.

Treatment of Hypertensive Urgency and Emergency

Treatment for hypertensive urgency in the dental office would begin by retaking the blood pressure to ensure that the first reading was accurate. If the first reading is correct, the conscious patient should be seated upright and the unconscious patient supinely. EMS should be contacted, and the blood pressure should be routinely monitored every five minutes. Oxygen should be administered if the patient complains of shortness of breath. Once in the emergency department, the patient will be treated with some type of antihypertensive medication, particularly if his or her blood pressure level remains high. Presently, there are a variety of medication options, including furosemide (loop diuretic), captopril (ACE inhibitor), propranolol (beta-blocker), metoprolol (beta-blocker), and nicardipine (calcium channel blocker).

Patients experiencing a hypertensive emergency need to be treated quickly to reduce the blood pressure level to prevent further end organ damage. The primary objective is to treat whatever organ damage is occurring, such as acute MI, acute **glomerulonephritis**, aortic dissection, or CVA. Treating the severe hypertension is secondary. Although there is some controversy regarding the best medication to treat severe hypertension, the most common medications include sodium nitroprusside (arterial and venous vasodilator), nitroglycerin (coronary vasodilator), and nicardipine (calcium **antagonist**). Care must be taken when providing these drugs so the blood pressure is not reduced too severely or too rapidly. All of these drugs should be administered by appropriate medical personnel in a hospital setting.

Hypotension

Hypotension is an abnormal condition in which the blood pressure is not adequate for normal perfusion and oxygenation of the body tissues. Although hypotension can vary between patients, a reduction in systolic or diastolic pressure of 15–20 mmHg from baseline is indicative of this condition. Hypotension is often seen as a side effect of many medications that patients may take, particularly antihypertensive medications. Moreover, a sudden blood pressure reduction of this magnitude indicates a lack of perfusion of blood to the tissues, which can lead to emergent situations, such as shock. If a patient exhibits hypotension, the treatment would be to position the patient in a supine position with feet raised, assess the airway, and administer supplemental oxygen. Monitor vital signs, and if the patient does not improve, contact EMS for transport to the emergency department.

Orthostatic Hypotension

Orthostatic hypotension, or **postural hypotension**, is a sudden drop in systolic blood pressure caused by a change in body position, usually moving from a supine to a sitting position. This may cause a patient to lose consciousness after being repositioned from a reclined position to an upright position in the dental chair. Postural hypotension can follow prolonged bed rest or rehabilitation following acute illness. In addition, some medications, such as antihypertensives, can cause individuals to suffer from orthostatic hypotension.

Symptoms of orthostatic hypotension include dimming of vision, decreased hearing, and lightheadedness. Individuals who take antihypertensive medications and individuals with normally low blood pressure are prone to this condition. These patients should be repositioned from a reclined to a sitting position or from a sitting to a standing position very slowly and carefully. If a patient exhibits orthostatic hypotension, reposition the patient to a supine position with feet raised, assess the airway, and administer supplemental oxygen. In addition, monitor vital signs every five minutes, and if the patient does not improve, contact EMS for transport to the emergency department.

Other Patient Signs

In addition to the vital signs discussed thus far, the clinician should assess the patient's **gait**, eyes, speech, and skin color. Significant weight gain or loss is also an important piece of patient assessment. Changes in any of these areas could indicate a medical problem warranting emergency intervention, such as CVA or MI.

Case Resolutions and Conclusion

Vital signs are an extremely important aspect of the dental hygiene process of care. Determining a baseline blood pressure, respiration, and pulse rates for a patient will aid in determining the severity of an emergency and also may help to prevent an emergency. The patient's medical history should be thoroughly reviewed for cardiac or respiratory conditions. In addition, discussion with the patient regarding his or her vital signs is an important aspect of treatment. In some instances, consultation with a physician may be necessary to determine if treatment modifications are necessary, or treatment may need to be delayed until the patient has been examined and cleared to have dental care provided.

In Scenario 1, John Brown's vital signs are significantly elevated. His pulse is 102, and the normal range is 60–90 beats/minute. His respirations are 22 and exaggerated, whereas the normal RR is 12–20. His blood pressure places him in the Stage 1 hypertension range. Taken in combination, this individual should be referred to his physician for an examination prior to treatment.

The patient in Case Scenario 2, Harry Fredericks, indicated that he has a history of hypertension, but is noncompliant in the use of antihypertensives. His extremely high blood pressure and lack of any other form of target end organ damage should indicate to the clinician that he is most likely suffering from hypertensive urgency; however, the final determination on the diagnosis will be performed in the emergency department. The clinician retook Harry's blood pressure and determined it to be significantly elevated at 186/110 mmHg. Harry was seated upright, and EMS was contacted. Oxygen was administered via nasal cannula at 4 L/minute. Harry was treated in the emergency room for hypertensive urgency and was given Captopril, an angiotensin-converting enzyme inhibitor. He was administered the drug orally, and within 30 minutes his blood pressure had returned to a reasonable range. After this experience Harry was convinced that his hypertension was a serious concern and he took his antihypertensive medication as prescribed.

Review Questions

1. What is the normal pulse rate for an adult?

    A. 40–60 beats/minute
    B. 60–100 beats/minute
    C. 100–140 beats/minute
    D. greater than 140 beats/minute

2. An irregular pulse rate is often indicative of which of the following conditions?

    A. heart failure
    B. infective endocarditis
    C. hypertension
    D. cardiac arrhythmia

3. Tachypnea is an abnormally fast respiratory rate above 20 breaths/minute in an adult, whereas bradypnea is an abnormally slow respiratory rate less than 12 breaths/minute in an adult.

    A. The first statement is true, and the second statement is false.
    B. The first statement is false, and the second statement is true.
    C. Both statements are true.
    D. Both statements are false.

4. A high-pitched sound that is usually heard on expiration, but may be heard on inspiration, is referred to as

    A. stridor
    B. Kussmaul's respirations
    C. wheezing
    D. sigh

5. What is the term used for the force exerted by the blood against the blood vessel walls?

    A. blood pressure
    B. pulse rate
    C. stroke volume
    D. none of the above

6. All of the following factors affect blood pressure *except* one. Which one is the *exception*?

    A. cardiac input
    B. blood volume
    C. blood viscosity
    D. blood vessel resistance

7. Your adult patient has a blood pressure of 130/88 mmHg. You would classify this patient as

    A. normal blood pressure
    B. prehypertension
    C. Stage 1 hypertension
    D. Stage 2 hypertension

8. Hypertension can be a predisposing factor for all of the following conditions *except* one. Which one is the *exception*?

    A. diabetes mellitus
    B. myocardial infarction
    C. cerebrovascular accident
    D. kidney damage

Bibliography

Adelman, R. D., R. Coppo, and M. J. Dillon. "The Emergency Management of Severe Hypertension." *Practical Pediatric Nephrology* 14 (2000): 422–27.

American Heart Association. *BLS for Healthcare Providers*, 2001. American Heart Association. So. Deerfield, MA. Channing Bete Co, Inc.

Anderson, D. M., J. Keith, P. D. Novak, and M. A. Elliot (Eds.). *Mosby's Medical, Nursing & Allied Health Dictionary* (6th ed.), 2008. St. Louis, MO: Mosby-Year Book, Inc.

Bales, A. "Hypertensive Crisis." *Postgraduate Medicine* 105(1999): 119–26, 130.

Bennett, J. D., and M. B. Rosenberg. *Medical Emergencies in Dentistry* (1st ed.), 2002. Philadelphia, PA: W. B. Saunders.

Bergeron, J. D., C. Le Baudour, and K. Wesley. *First Responder* (8th ed.), 2008. Upper Saddle River, NJ: Prentice Hall.

Bledsoe, B. E., R. S. Porter, and R. A. Cherry. *Intermediate Emergency Care: Principles & Practice* (1st ed.), 2004. Upper Saddle River, NJ: Prentice Hall.

Cassidy, P., and K. Jones. "A Study of Inter-Arm Blood Pressure Differences in Primary Care." *Journal of Human Hypertension* 15 (2001): 519–22.

Cherney, D., and S. Straus. "Management of Patients with Hypertensive Urgencies and Emergencies." *Journal of General Internal Medicine* 17 (2002): 937–45.

Christensen, B. L., and E. O. Kockrow. *Foundations of Nursing* (6th ed.), 2011. St. Louis, MO: Mosby Publishing Company.

Craven, R. F. *Fundamentals of Nursing: Human Health and Function* (5th ed.), 2008. Philadelphia, PA: Lippincott Williams & Wilkins.

Dirckx, J. J. (Ed.). *Stedman's Concise Medical Dictionary for the Health Professions* (4th ed.), 2001. Philadelphia, PA: Lippincott Williams & Wilkins.

Elliott, W. J. "Clinical Features and Management of Selected Hypertensive Emergencies." *Journal of Clinical Hypertension* 6 (2004a): 587–92.

Elliott, W. J. "Hypertensive Emergencies." *Critical Care Clinics* 17 (2004b): 435–51.

Herbert, C. J., and D. G. Vidt. "Hypertensive Crises." *Primary Care: Clinics in Office Practice* 35 (2008): 475–87.

Herman, W. W., J. L. Konzelman, and L. M. Pisant. "New National Guidelines on Hypertension: A Summary for Dentistry." *The Journal of the American Dental Association* 135 (2004), 576–83.

Kazuo, E., M. Yacoub, J. Jhalani, W. Gerin, J. E. Schwartz, and T. G. Pickering. "Consistency of Blood Pressure Differences Between the Left and Right Arms." *Archives of Internal Medicine* 167 (2007): 388–93.

Lane, D., M. Beevers, N. Barnes, J. Bourne, A. John, S. Malins, and D. G. Beevers. "Inter-Arm Differences in Blood Pressure: When Are They Clinically Significant?" *Journal of Hypertension* 20 (2002): 1089–95.

Malamed, S. F. *Medical Emergencies in the Dental Office* (6th ed.), 2007. St. Louis, MO: Mosby Publishing Company.

Perry, A. G., and P. Potter. *Clinical Nursing Skills & Techniques* (6th ed.), 2010. St. Louis, MO: Mosby Publishing Company.

Pulse. *A.D.A.M. Medical Encyclopedia*. Retrieved from: http://www.nlm.nih.gov/medlineplus/ency/article/003399.htm.

Rosenow, D. J., and E. Russell. "Current Concepts in the Management of Hypertensive Crisis: Emergencies and Urgencies." *Holistic Nursing Practice* 15 (2001): 12–21.

Schottke, D. *First Responder: Your First Response in Emergency Care* (3rd ed.), 2001. Sudbury, MA: Jones & Bartlett Publishers.

Shafi, T. "Hypertensive Urgencies and Emergencies." *Ethnicity & Disease*, 14 (1999): 32–37.

Sproat, C., S. Beheshti, A. N. Harwood, and D. Crossbie. "Should We Screen for Hypertension in General Dental Practice?" *British Dental Journal* 207 (2009): 275–77.

Tanaby, P., R. Steinmann, M. Kippenhan, C. Stehman, and C. Beach. "Undiagnosed Hypertension in the ED Setting—An Unrecognized Opportunity by Emergency Nurses." *Journal of Emergency Nursing* 30 (2004): 225–29.

Timby, B. K. *Fundamental Skills and Concepts in Patient Care* (9th ed.), 2009. Philadelphia, PA: Lippincott Williams & Wilkins.

Tucker, S. M., M. M. Canobbio, E. V. Paquette, and M. F. Wells. *Patient Care Standards: Collaborative Planning and Nursing Interventions* (7th ed.), 2000. St. Louis, MO: Mosby Publishing Company.

U. S. Department of Health and Human Services, National Institutes of Health, National Heart, Lung and Blood Institute. (2004). *The Seventh Report of the Joint National Committee on Prevention, Detection, Evaluation, and Treatment of High Blood Pressure*. Retrieved December 28, 2006, from http://www.nhlbi.nih.gov/guidelines/hypertension/jnc7full.pdf.

U. S. Department of Health and Human Services, National Institutes of Health, National Heart, Lung and Blood Institute. (2007). *A Pocket Guide to Blood Pressure Measurement in Children*. Retrieved October 5, 2011, from http://www.nhlbi.nih.gov/health/public/heart/hbp/bp_child_pocket/bp_child_pocket.pdf.

Vaughn, C. J., and N. Delanty. "Hypertensive Emergencies." *The Lancet* 356 (2000): 411–17.

Vidt, D. G. "Hypertensive Crises: Emergencies and Urgencies." *Journal of Clinical Hypertension* 6(2004): 520–25.

White, G. C. *Equipment Theory for Respiratory Care* (4th ed.), 2005. Albany, NY: Thomson/Delmar Publishers.

Wilkins, E. M. *Clinical Practice of the Dental Hygienist* (10th ed.), 2009. Philadelphia, PA: Lippincott Williams & Wilkins.

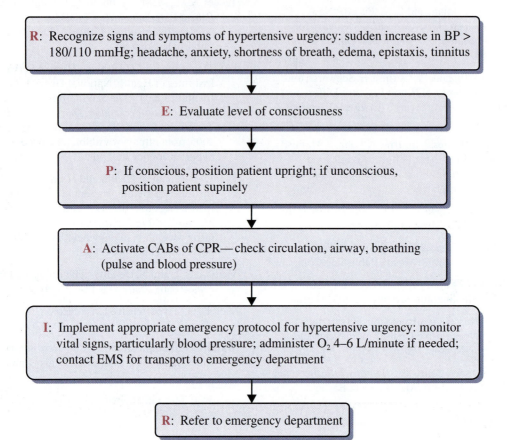

TREATMENT OF THE HYPERTENSIVE
URGENCY PATIENT
R.E.P.A.I.R.

R: Recognize signs and symptoms of hypertensive urgency: sudden increase in BP > 180/110 mmHg; headache, anxiety, shortness of breath, edema, epistaxis, tinnitus

E: Evaluate level of consciousness

P: If conscious, position patient upright; if unconscious, position patient supinely

A: Activate CABs of CPR—check circulation, airway, breathing (pulse and blood pressure)

I: Implement appropriate emergency protocol for hypertensive urgency: monitor vital signs, particularly blood pressure; administer O_2 4–6 L/minute if needed; contact EMS for transport to emergency department

R: Refer to emergency department

Oxygen Administration

LEARNING OBJECTIVES

Upon reading the material in this chapter, the reader will be able to:

- ☑ Explain the various methods of oxygen administration.

- ☑ Discuss the armamentarium associated with oxygen administration.

- ☑ Explain the proper operation of oxygen equipment and administration.

Oxygen Administration

When breathing is inadequate for keeping the blood saturated with oxygen, **hypoxaemia** results. Hypoxaemia is the condition when the oxygen level of arterial blood is below normal, and therefore the administration of oxygen or oxygen therapy is necessary. Administering oxygen to these patients will increase alveolar oxygen tension and decrease the effort of breathing. The oxygen content of room air is 21%, whereas patients requiring oxygen for emergency care will need a higher concentration of usually 40%–60%. Although the improper administration of oxygen can have serious side effects, if oxygen is administered properly in most instances it is life saving. As adequate oxygenation of body tissues and vital organs is essential, the major risk for most patients in an emergency situation is that they will be given too little oxygen. Insufficient oxygenation can lead to severe complications, such as cardiac arrhythmias, tissue injury, and damage to the vital organs.

In the dental office, oxygen is usually supplied by a portable oxygen tank, unless the office has oxygen piped into each individual operatory. In this situation, a wall outlet is used.

Portable oxygen tanks, which are green in color, have several parts with which the dental professional should be familiar: the cylinder, the regulator, and the flow meter. Oxygen cylinders come in various sizes and are based on the amount of oxygen they hold. A size E cylinder will supply 30 minutes of oxygen, with oxygen being delivered at its highest level, and is the recommended size for dental offices as Emergency Medical Services can arrive at most emergencies within that time frame. (See Figure 4.1 ■) The **regulator** is a common unit in which a **reducing valve** and **flow meter** are joined together. The reducing valve portion of the regulator allows for the safe release of the highly pressurized oxygen contained in the cylinder. The regulator must be turned to the "on" position for oxygen to be released. The flow meter portion of the regulator is the dial that allows the operator to determine how much oxygen is delivered to a patient. (See Figure 4.2 ■) Oxygen delivery rate is measured in liters per minute (L/minute), and the amount of oxygen provided to a patient is determined by the condition from which the patient is suffering and by the type of oxygen delivery device being used.

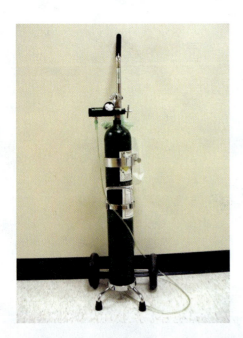

FIGURE 4.1 Portable size E oxygen cylinder.

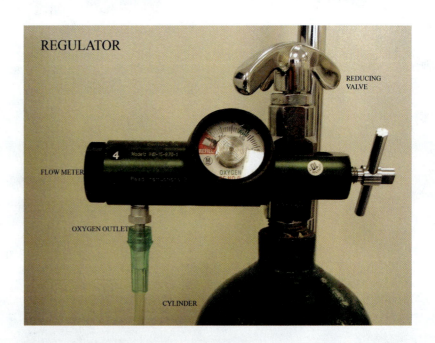

FIGURE 4.2 Regulator for oxygen tank.

Oxygen Tank Operation

The steps to operate the portable oxygen tank are as follows:

1. Open oxygen tank valve.
2. Adjust flow valve to appropriate level.
3. Place oxygen delivery device on patient.

Oxygen Delivery Devices

One method used to deliver oxygen in the dental office is a **nasal cannula**. The tube of the cannula rests on the patient's upper lip, with the prongs directed posteriorly into the nasal passages. The other portion of the cannula is looped around the patient's ears and tightened. (See Figure 4.3 ■) The flow of oxygen can be set between 1 and 6 L/minute and should be turned on prior to placement of the nasal cannula. This device would be used for a conscious patient suffering from MI or CVA, among other conditions.

The second method of oxygen delivery is the **non-rebreathing face mask**. This device is a plastic mask that has a reservoir bag attached to provide an additional reservoir of oxygen. The mask is placed over the patient's nose and mouth, and the straps are adjusted around the patient's head and over the ears. Often this type of device may cause patients to feel as if they are suffocating, so it is recommended to allow patients to place the mask over the nose and mouth in an effort to reduce their apprehension. This type of oxygen delivery device also has a one-way valve between the mask and the reservoir to prevent exhaled gas from mixing with the oxygen in the reservoir bag. In addition, there is a one-way valve on the exhalation port so that room air does not enter the mask. (See Figure 4.4 ■) The non-rebreather bag can deliver 6–12 L oxygen/minute. This device is recommended for conscious patients suffering from conditions, such as an asthma attack or angina pectoris.

The **bag-mask device** is used when the patient is in respiratory arrest and requires complete oxygen delivery. The bag mask consists of a bag and a non-rebreathing valve attached to a face mask. The most difficult aspect of using a bag mask is attaining a leak-proof seal around the patient's face. To attain a tight seal, the third, fourth, and fifth fingers should be placed on the bony portion of the mandible, and the thumb and index finger of the same hand should be placed on the mask. In addition, the

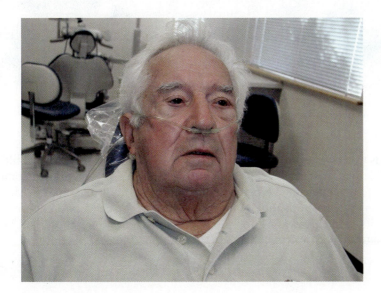

FIGURE 4.3 Placement of nasal cannula.

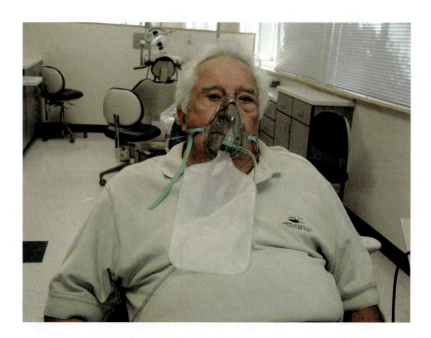

FIGURE 4.4 Placement of non-rebreather bag.

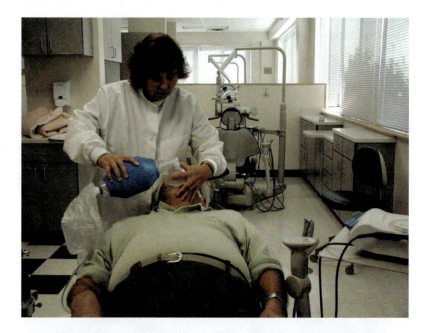

FIGURE 4.5 Bag mask.

bag needs to be squeezed while maintaining an open airway using a head tilt and jaw thrust. (See Figure 4.5 ■) Because of these difficulties, two rescuers are recommended when using a bag mask. The regulator should be set to 8–12 L/minute, and during ventilation the operator should see the chest rise. If the chest does not rise, the face mask position and airway position should be adjusted until the chest rises, indicating appropriate oxygen delivery.

Conclusion ···➤

Oxygen is consistently recommended in almost every medical emergency or situation of distress. Its use benefits most patients and is of low risk of causing harm to patients. Be advised that oxygen is classified as an accelerator, meaning that if there is a fire and oxygen is present, the fire will burn a larger area and it will spread more quickly.

Review Questions

1. Which portion of the oxygen tank has a dial that allows the operator to determine the amount of oxygen delivered to the patient?

   A. reducing valve
   B. cylinder
   C. flow meter
   D. nasal cannula

2. Which type of oxygen delivery device is used for a patient in respiratory arrest?

   A. bag-mask device
   B. nasal cannula
   C. non-rebreathing face mask
   D. regulator

3. The amount of oxygen recommended for use with a non-rebreathing bag is

   A. 3–6 L/minute
   B. 6–12 L/minute
   C. 12–15 L/minute
   D. > 15 L/minute

4. How many minutes of oxygen are supplied by a size E cylinder?

   A. 10 minutes
   B. 20 minutes
   C. 30 minutes
   D. 45 minutes

Bibliography

Bergeron, J. D., and G. Bizjak. *First Responder* (8th ed.), 2008. Upper Saddle River, NJ: Prentice Hall.

Bledsoe, B. E., R. S. Porter, and R. A. Cherry. *Intermediate Emergency Care: Principles & Practice* (1st ed.), 2004. Upper Saddle River, NJ: Prentice Hall.

Kelly, C., and A. Riches. "Emergency Oxygen for Respiratory Patients." *Nursing Times* 103 (2007): 40–42.

Malamed, S. F. *Medical Emergencies in the Dental Office* (6th ed.), 2007. St. Louis, MO: Mosby Publishing Company.

Murphy, R., K. Mackway-Jones, I. Sammy, P. Driscoll, A. Gray, R. O'Driscoll, et al. "Emergency Oxygen Therapy for the Breathless Patient. Guidelines Prepared by the North West Oxygen Group." *Emergency Medical Journal* 18 (2001): 6, 421–23.

Perry, A. G., and P. Potter. *Clinical Nursing Skills & Techniques* (7th ed.), 2010. St. Louis, MO: Mosby Publishing Company.

Smith, S. M., S. B. Roberts, M. Duggan-Brennan, K. D. Powrle, and R. Haffenden. "Emergency Oxygen Delivery in Adults 1: Updating Nursing Practice." *Nursing Times*, 105 (2009): 16–17.

White, G. C. *Equipment Theory for Respiratory Care* (4th ed.), 2005. Albany, NY: Delmar Publishers.

Wilkins, E. M. *Clinical Practice of the Dental Hygienist* (10th ed.), 2009. Philadelphia, PA: Lippincott Williams & Wilkins.

Syncope

LEARNING OBJECTIVES

Upon reading the material in this chapter, the reader will be able to:

- ☑ Compare and contrast the various types of syncope.

- ☑ Determine specific signs and symptoms associated with syncope.

- ☑ List suggested treatment modalities for syncope.

- ☑ Explain the steps needed to prepare an office for a patient experiencing a syncopal episode.

Case Study ·····································➤

Scenario

Your third patient this morning, David Michaels, is a 52-year-old male. He was seen last week for an initial examination. He has not received dental or dental hygiene care in approximately seven years. At his visit last week, it was determined that he has Class III periodontitis and moderate to heavy calculus deposits requiring four quadrants of periodontal debridement with anesthesia. The patient reluctantly agreed to this treatment plan and today is five minutes late for his 10:00 A.M. appointment to begin debridement of the mandibular right quadrant. You greet him in the reception area and accompany him to the operatory. You review his medical history and perform an intra/extra oral examination and find no significant findings or contraindications to treatment. His vital signs are within normal limits although slightly elevated, which you attribute to his anxiety (pulse 88, respirations 16, blood pressure 138/88 mmHg). Reviewing his personal oral hygiene seems to place him at ease.

You prepared the anesthetic syringe prior to his arrival and approach him with the topical anesthetic on a cotton-tipped applicator. You notice that he has become quite pale and the hairs on his arms are standing up. He is beginning to sweat profusely and frequently yawns. You ask him if he is feeling well, and he states that he is fine, just a little nervous and a bit dizzy. You pick up the syringe and notice that he has lost consciousness.

Introduction

Syncope is defined as an abrupt, transient loss of consciousness and postural tone with spontaneous recovery, most often caused by loss of cerebral oxygenation and perfusion referred to as cerebral ischemia. Syncope is also referred to as transient loss of consciousness (TLoC). Syncope is a sign rather than a primary disease process and ranges from a benign disorder to a life-threatening situation with the potential for mortality. Many times syncope is a sign of another underlying medical condition. Sixty-six percent of all emergency room visits are attributed to vasovagal syncope. Syncope is often associated with a stressful situation, such as a dental appointment and specifically the administration of local anesthetics.

Syncope is the most common medical emergency in the dental office. It affects individuals of all ages; however, children, pregnant women, and the elderly are particularly susceptible to syncope. In children, most cases of syncope are benign, usually stemming from a particular event, such as a missed meal, heat, dehydration, crying, or exertional activity. Fifteen percent of children have had at least one episode of syncope before adolescence. In the elderly, syncope is often associated with postural changes, defecation, coughing, orthostatic hypotension, and medications. Other diseases or conditions from which the elderly commonly suffer, such as coronary heart disease, **heart failure**, **diabetes mellitus**, renal insufficiency, and chronic obstructive pulmonary disease (COPD), can also lead to syncopal episodes. It has been observed that the mortality from syncope for patients age 60 and older was five times higher than that for patients younger than 60.

A 1992 survey of 4,309 dentists in the United States and Canada found 15,407 syncopal episodes. Syncope was responsible for approximately half of the emergencies experienced by the dental professionals surveyed. A study by Matsuura determined that most emergencies in the dental office occurred during the administration of local anesthetics. Contradicting evidence was provided by Lustig, who administered 2,528 local anesthetic injections to 1,007 consecutive patients and noted only one syncopal occurrence.

Types and Etiologies of Syncope

There are various forms of syncope, and they are generally classified into one of three distinct categories: (1) **neurocardiac syncope**, (2) **noncardiac syncope**, and (3) **cardiac syncope**. Neurocardiac syncope is the most common form of syncope and the type most likely encountered by the dental professional.

Neurocardiac/Vasodepressor Syncope

Neurocardiac syncope, the most common type, is known by various identifiers. **Vasodepressor syncope**, **vasovagal syncope**, **neurocardiogenic syncope**, or **neurally mediated syncope** are all acceptable synonyms for neurocardiac syncope. The exact pathophysiology of this type of syncope is still under investigation; however, most agree that syncope is usually associated with some type of noxious stimuli, such as pain, fear, exhaustion, or acute illness. Noxious stimuli commonly associated with the dental office that may induce a syncopal episode are the sight of blood or the dental anesthetic syringe. Some dental patients are uncomfortable in the dental office atmosphere, so for them the anxiety produced by visiting the office can be extreme and can lead to the physiological responses that produce syncope. The initial response to this stressful situation is activation of the **sympathetic division of the autonomic nervous system**, inciting a fight-or-flight response. A release of the **catecholamines** epinephrine and norepinephrine into the circulatory system produces an increase in the blood flow to many tissues, particularly the peripheral skeletal muscles, in preparation for movement of these muscles. Other signs evident when the sympathetic nervous system is activated are rapid, pounding heart; deep breathing; dry mouth; cold, sweaty skin; and dilated pupils. Figure 5.1 ■ depicts the bodily structures impacted by the sympathetic division of the autonomic nervous system. From the tissues the blood will be pumped back to the heart; however, dental patients do not run from the dental chair. Instead, they remain seated while dental procedures are performed. The blood remains in the peripheral blood vessels or pools in the extremities, causing a hypotensive response, bradycardia, and a decrease in cerebral blood flow, leading to syncope. (See Figure 5.2 ■)

The dental hygiene professional should employ stress reduction protocols for patients with a history of this form of syncope. Examples of stress reduction protocols may include early appointment times, use of oxygen via nasal cannula during the appointment, use of nitrous oxide, and oral sedation with a benzodiazepine prior to the appointment.

Noncardiac Syncope

Noncardiac syncope has a wide scope and includes, but is not limited to, such entities as syncope from **seizures**, orthostatic hypotension, situational occurrences, hyperventilation, and metabolic diseases. In addition, because of the reduction of cerebral oxygenation during a syncopal episode, seizures can result.

There are many physiologic processes that occur when an individual moves from a supine to a standing position in order to adequately perfuse to the body's vital organs. The inability of any of these processes to function properly or in a coordinated manner can lead to a condition called orthostatic hypotension. Orthostatic hypotension, at least a 20-mmHg drop in systolic blood pressure or a 10-mmHg drop in diastolic upon assuming an upright position, can cause a syncopal episode. This

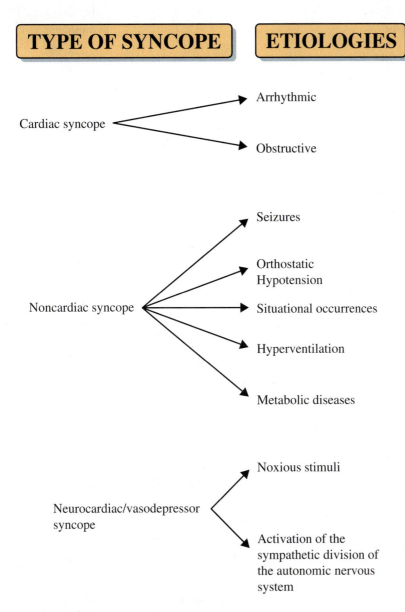

FIGURE 5.1 Types and etiologies of syncope.

form of syncope is common in the dental office when patients are returned to an upright position. Unlike vasodepressor syncope, there are no prodromal symptoms to this condition.

Hyperventilation is a condition whereby excessive breathing causes a disruption in the normal oxygen and carbon dioxide levels in the blood. This condition is often stress induced. Physiologically, hyperventilation may produce sufficient cerebral vasoconstriction to cause syncope.

Situational syncope may result from a number of different circumstances, such as coughing, micturition (urination), defecation, neck stretching, hair grooming, **venipuncture**, or even swallowing. This occurs due to the production of a **Valsalva maneuver**, which is any forced expiratory effort against a closed airway, such as when an individual holds the breath and tightens the muscles in a concerted, strenuous effort.

Metabolic disorders are not common causes of syncope; however, conditions such as **hypoglycemia** or hypoxemia can deprive the brain of essential nutrients and can cause coma or **somnolence** (sleep). When unconsciousness does occur due to hypoglycemia or hypoxemia, it tends not to be an abrupt syncopal episode, which

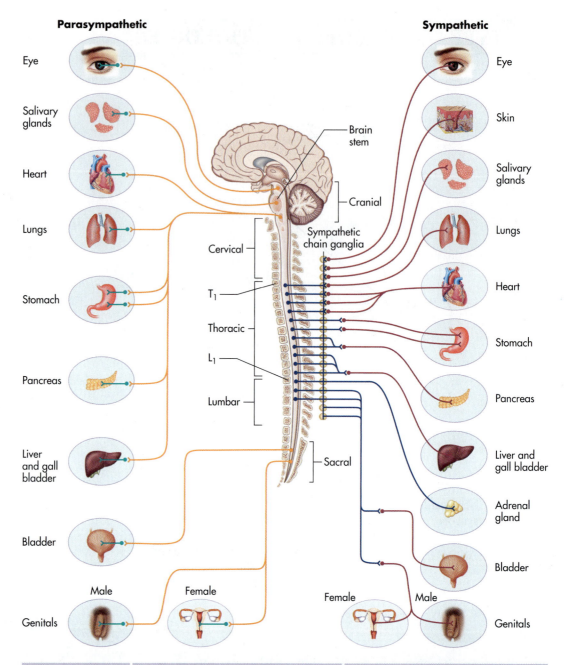

Organ or System	Parasympathetic Effect	Sympathetic Effect
Heart	Decreases rate and contractile force	Increases rate and contractile force and vasodilates coronary arteries
Lungs	Bronchoconstricts	Bronchodilates
Eyes	Pupil constriction	Pupil dilation
Hair muscles	Relaxes	Contracts and causes hair to stand on end (piloerection); produces "goose bumps"
Gastrointestinal	Increases digestion	Decreases digestion
Adrenal gland	No effect	Stimulates medulla to secrete epinephrine and norepinephrine
Urinary	Contracts bladder, relaxes urethral sphincter, and promotes urination (voiding)	Relaxes bladder, constricts urethral sphincter, and inhibits urination

FIGURE 5.2 A comparison of the parasympathetic and sympathetic nervous systems.

aids in distinguishing the two conditions. Another method of distinguishing between syncope and other altered states of consciousness is that the loss of consciousness during syncope is followed by a return to consciousness without disorientation.

Cardiac Syncope

Cardiac syncope results from inadequate cardiac output and usually occurs as a result of serious underlying heart disease. It is the second most common type of syncope. Electrical problems (**arrhythmias**) or mechanical problems (obstructive) within the heart muscle are common etiologies of this type of syncope. Syncope from electrical problems/arrhythmias is commonly caused by **tachyarrhythmia** (rapid, irregular heartbeat), **bradyarrhythmia** (slow, irregular heartbeat), or pacemaker malfunction.

Obstructive/mechanical syncope can be caused by several conditions, such as left ventricular obstruction (most common), right ventricular obstruction, or other myocardial diseases. Cardiac syncope is a serious condition and potentially fatal. Case reports of patients believed to be suffering from psychogenic syncope eventually determined through the use of an implantable loop recorder that the syncopal episodes were actually caused by severe heart block. In these patients once a cardiac pacemaker was implanted, the syncopal episodes were eliminated. Any patient suspected of suffering from cardiac syncope should be carefully evaluated by medical professionals to determine the appropriate course of treatment.

Signs and Symptoms of Syncope

Signs and symptoms of neurocardiac syncope appear several minutes before the actual loss of consciousness. (See Table 5.1 ■) **Presyncopal** or **prodromal** symptoms directly correlate with the sympathetic stimulations and include pupil dilation, **diaphoresis** or a cold sweat, and excitation of the **piloerector muscles**, resulting in goose flesh. Also, patients may complain of weakness, dizziness, vertigo, or nausea. If a decrease in cerebral perfusion exists, yawning and sighing may occur. Also, there may

Table 5.1   Signs and Symptoms of Presyncope and Syncope

Presyncope	Syncope
Pallor	Pallor
Pupil dilation	Unconsciousness
Diaphoresis	Weak, slow pulse
Piloerection	
Weakness	
Dizziness	
Vertigo	
Nausea	
Yawning	
Visual changes	
Blood pressure elevated	
Pulse rate elevated	
Shortness of breath	
Heart palpitation	
Chest pain	

be some visual changes, particularly darkening or blurring of vision or seeing spots. Lastly, the blood pressure and heart rate may be elevated as a result of sympathetic stimulation, and the patient may experience shortness of breath, heart **palpitation**, or chest pain. Onset is generally slow for neurocardiogenic syncope, and the dental professional may see the patient become pale. Once unconsciousness has occurred, syncope is diagnosed, and there will be a decrease in heart rate, resulting in a weak, slow pulse.

Treatment of Syncope

When the presyncopal (prodromal) or syncopal symptoms are recognized, all dental procedures should be suspended and all objects should be removed from the oral cavity. Presyncopal symptoms indicate a 50% to 70% decrease in blood flow to the brain. If consciousness is lost, the patient should be placed in a supine position, with the patient's legs slightly elevated to facilitate blood return. (See Figure 5.3 ■) Additional procedures should include opening the airway and assessing circulation. Tight clothing should be loosened, such as ties or belts that can decrease blood flow to the brain. Oxygen should be administered at 4–6 L/minute. If unconsciousness persists, emergency help should be summoned.

A syncopal episode can last anywhere from a few seconds to several minutes, but is usually very brief. Vital signs should be monitored during the entire episode.

The longer the patient remains in the syncopal episode, the more likely it is that he or she may experience a seizure due to a lack of cerebral oxygenation. If this occurs, the seizure, as well as the syncopal event, need to be treated. EMS needs to be contacted immediately and the patient transported to the emergency department.

Previously, spirits of ammonia or **ammonia inhalants** were recommended for the treatment of syncope, which is the only approved use for ammonia inhalants in the United States. Ammonia inhalants are classified as respiratory and cardiovascular stimulants that act through peripheral irritation of the respiratory system. More recent evidence contraindicates their use as they may cause a withdrawal reaction, with the potential to cause or exacerbate a spine injury, if present. Also, an initial improvement, which healthcare providers may falsely assume to be due to

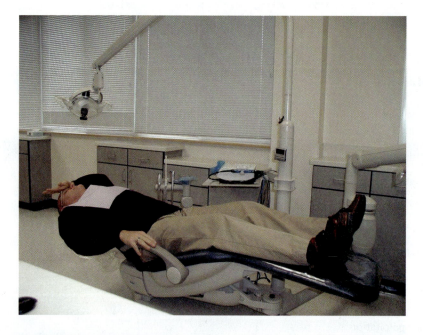

FIGURE 5.3 Patient in appropriate position for treatment of syncope.

the beneficial effects of the ammonia inhalant, may well mask the development of more severe complications. In addition, ammonia inhalant use has been reported to induce allergic reactions, some severe. As ammonia inhalants are an irritant to the respiratory tract, they have the potential to exacerbate underlying asthma and trigger attacks. One death from the use of an ammonia inhalant in a person with the sickle cell trait has been determined. Due to the serious effects of ammonia inhalants, avoidance of their use is recommended.

Following the syncopal episode, patients should remain in a supine position until they feel well enough to be returned to a seated position and their pulse rate returns to a normal baseline reading. Patients should be repositioned slowly to avoid inducing a syncope recurrence. An attempt should be made to determine the cause of the syncopal episode to avoid future episodes. All dental treatment should be suspended for the day, and arrangements should be made to have an emergency contact escort the patient home because syncope can reoccur. Recurrence of another syncopal episode is at a higher risk level for the first 24 hours following the event. Antianxiety medications may be advised for future appointments.

If a condition other than neurocardiac syncope is suspected, patients should be transported via EMS to the nearest emergency facility for a definitive diagnosis. Patients will most likely undergo a complete health history review and physical examination. An account of the syncopal episode, including precipitating conditions prior to the event, the length of the event, a description of the signs and symptoms, vital sign monitoring, and manner of recovery, will be very helpful in making a correct diagnosis. Additional testing may also be needed to determine the exact etiology of the syncopal episode. Typical tests include echocardiography, tilt-table testing, laboratory assessments, neurologic testing, orthostatic blood pressure monitoring, or psychiatric evaluation.

Case Resolution and Conclusion ·····················>

Syncope is the most common medical emergency to occur in the dental office; therefore, it is imperative that the dental professional be familiar with the physiology, types, signs/symptoms, and treatment procedures. Usually syncope is a benign condition and if treated promptly and correctly resolves without further complication. It is apparent that David Michaels, the patient in the case scenario, was experiencing syncope. His symptoms of pallor, diaphoresis, yawning, piloerection, and dizziness were key indicators that his autonomic nervous system had been activated and vasovagal syncope resulted. David was not experiencing any chest pain or severe headache prior to his loss of consciousness (common in MI and CVA), so these two emergencies can most likely be ruled out. The operator placed David in a supine position with his feet elevated and placed a cool cloth on his head. Within a very short period of time David regained consciousness, and he remained in a supine position for 15 minutes. His wife was called to drive him home. Treatment was postponed, and a prescription for lorazepam was provided to David. David will take the lorazepam as directed before his next visit to reduce the likelihood of another syncopal episode.

Review Questions

1. Syncope is the sudden loss of consciousness and postural tone, and is most often caused by a loss of cerebral oxygenation.

    A. The first phrase is true, and the second phrase is false.
    B. The first phrase is false, and the second phrase is true.
    C. Both phrases are true.
    D. Both phrases are false.

2. Which age groups are particularly susceptible to syncope?
    A. infants
    B. adults
    C. middle-age adults
    D. geriatric individuals

3. All of the following are common classifications of syncope *except* one. Which one is the *exception*?

    A. neurocardiac syncope
    B. cardiac syncope
    C. noncardiac syncope
    D. obstructive syncope

4. The most serious form of syncope is

    A. vasodepressor
    B. neurally mediated
    C. cardiac
    D. noncardiac

5. Hyperventilation can cause syncope due to
    A. cerebral vasoconstriction
    B. reduction in blood pressure
    C. inappropriate positioning
    D. reduction in essential nutrients

6. The symptoms associated with syncope stem from the stimulation of the

    A. parasympathetic nervous system
    B. sympathetic nervous system
    C. central nervous system
    D. none of the above

7. All of the following are signs or symptoms associated with syncope *except* one. Which one is the *exception*?

    A. diaphoresis
    B. piloerection
    C. pupil constriction
    D. blurred vision

8. In what position should a patient be placed when suffering from syncope?
    A. trendelenburg
    B. supine with feet elevated
    C. head between the knees
    D. upright

Bibliography

Anderson, D. M., J. Keith, P. D. Novak, and M. A. Elliot (Eds.). *Mosby's Medical, Nursing & Allied Health Dictionary* (6th ed.), 2008. St. Louis, MO: Mosby-Year Book, Inc.

Busschots, G., and B. Milzman. "Dental Patients with Neurologic and Psychiatric Concerns." *Dental Clinics of North America* 43 (1999): 471–83.

Cooper, P. N., M. Westby, D. W. Pitcher, and I. Bullock. "Synopsis of the National Institute for Health and Clinical Excellence Guideline for Management of Transient Loss of Consciousness." *Annals of Internal Medicine* 155 (2011): 543–49.

Duncan, G. W., M. P. Tan, J. L. Newton, P. Reeve, and S. W. Parry. "Vasaovagal Syncope in the Older Person: Differences in Presentation Between Older and Younger Patients." *Age & Ageing* 39 (2010): 465–70.

"Fainting." *Harvard Health Letter* 29 (2004): 4.

Fetzer, S. "Vasodepressor Syncope: The Common Faint." *Journal of PeriAnesthesia Nursing* 14 (1999): 25–30.

Forman, D., and L. Lipsitz. "Syncope in the Elderly." *Cardiology Clinic* 15 (1997): 295–311.

Fragakis, N., S. Papanastasiou, E. Sidopoulos, and G. Katsaris. "Uncommon Cause of Syncope in Patient with Bundle Branch Block and Negative Electrophysiological Study." *Pacing and Clinical Electrophysiology* 29 (2006): 211–12.

Gauer, R. L. "Eavaluation of Syncope." *American Family Physician* 84 (2011): 640–50.

Grubb, B. "Once a Fainter, Always a Fainter?" *Journal of Cardiovascular Electrophysiology* 17 (2006): 55.

Grubb, B. "Pathophysiology and Differential Diagnosis of Neurocardiogenic Syncope." *American Journal of Cardiology* 84 (1999): 3–9.

Haas, D. A. "Emergency Drugs." *Dental Clinics of North America* 46 (2002): 815–30.

Hauer, K. E. "Discovering the Cause of Syncope: A Guide to the Focused Evaluation." *Postgraduate Medicine* 113 (2003): 31–38.

Hayes, O. "Evaluation of Syncope in the Emergency Department." *Emergency Medical Clinics of North America* 16 (1998): 601–15.

Henderson, M., and S. Prabhu. "Syncope: Current Diagnosis and Treatment." *Current Problems in Cardiology* 22 (1997): 242–96.

Kanjwal, K., Y. Kanjwal, B. Karabin, and B. Grubb. "Psychogenic Syncope? A Cautionary Note." *Pacing and Clinical Electrophysiology* 32 (2009): 862–65.

Kapoor, W. "Evaluation of Syncope in the Elderly." *Journal of the American Geriatric Society* 35 (1987): 826.

Kapoor, W. N. "Is There an Effective Treatment for Neurally Mediated Syncope?" *Journal of the American Medical Association* 289 (2003): 2272–75.

Kapoor, W. N. "Syncope." *New England Journal of Medicine* 343 (2000): 1856–63.

Livanis, E. G., D. Leftheriotis, G. N. Theodorakis, P. Flevari, E. Zarvalis, F. Kolokathis, and D. Th. Kremastinos. "Situational Syncope: Response to Head-Up Tilt Testing and Follow-Up: Comparison with Vasovagal Syncope." *Pacing and Clinical Electrophysiology* 27 (2004): 918–23.

Lustig, J., and S. Zusman. "Immediate Complications of Local Anesthetic Administered to 1,007 Consecutive Patients." *Journal of the American Dental Association* 130 (1999): 496–99.

Maatsuura, H. "Analysis of Systemic Complications and Deaths During Treatment in Japan." *Anesthesia Profession* 36 (1990): 219–28.

Maisel, W. H., and W. G. Stevenson. "Syncope—Getting to the Heart of the Matter." *New England Journal of Medicine* 347 (2002): 930–94.

Malamed, S. F. "Managing Medical Emergencies." *Journal of the American Dental Association* 124 (1993): 4–53.

Malamed, S. F. *Medical Emergencies in the Dental Office* (6th ed.), 2007. St. Louis, MO: Mosby Publishing Company.

Marieb, E. N., and K. Hoehn. *Human Anatomy and Physiology* (8th ed.), 2010. Upper Saddle River, NJ: Pearson Publishing Co.

McCrorey, P. "Smelling Salts." *British Journal of Sports Medicine* 40 (2006): 659–60.

Meyer, M., and J. Handler. "Evaluation of the Patient with Syncope: An Evidence Based Approach." *Emergency Medical Clinics of North America* 17 (1999): 189–201.

Miller, T. H., and J. E. Kruse. "Evaluation of Syncope." *American Family Physician* 72 (2005): 1492–500.

Morton, G., and J. Bowes. "Why So Slow?" *Anaesthesia* 58 (2003): 280–300.

Parmet, S. "Fainting." *Journal of the American Medical Association* 292 (2004): 1260.

Pavri, B. B., and R. T. Ho. "Syncope—Identifying Cardiac Causes in Older Patients." *Geriatrics* 58 (2003): 26–31.

Preblik-Salib, C., and A. Jagoda. "Spells: Differential Diagnosis and Management of Strategies." *Emergency Medicine Clinics of North America* 15 (1997): 637–48.

Prodinger, R., and E. Reisdorff. "Syncope in Children." *Emergency Medical Clinics of North America* 16 (1998): 617–26.

Sadovsky, R. "Identifying Short-Term Risk in Patients with Syncope." *American Family Physician* 70 (2004): 1561–64.

Santini, M., F. Ammirati, F. Colivicchi, G. Gentilucci, and V. Guido. "The Effect of Atropine in Vasovagal Syncope Induced by Head-Up Tilt Testing." *European Heart Journal* 20 (1999): 1745–51.

Sheldon, R. S., A. G. Sheldon, S. J. Connolly, C. A. Morillo, T. Klingenheben, A. D. Krahn, M. L. Koshman, and D. Ritchie. "Age of First Faint in Patients with Vasovagal Syncope." *Journal of Cardiovascular Electrophysiology* 17 (2006): 49–54.

Smith, B. K. "The Most Overlooked Emergency—Syncope." *Journal of the Colorado Dental Association* 79 (2000): 16–17.

Smith, B. K. "Treating Syncope in the Dental Office." *Journal of the Indian Dental Association* 80 (2001): 7.

Soteriades, E. S., J. C. Evans, M. G. Larson, M. H. Chen, L. Chen, E. J. Benjamin, and D. Levy. "Incidence and Prognosis of Syncope." *New England Journal of Medicine* 347 (2002): 878–87.

Tan, M. P., and S. W. Parry. "Vasovagal Syncope in the Older Patient." *Journal of the American College of Cardiology* 51 (2008): 599–606.

Tortora, G., and S. Grabowski. *Principles of Anatomy and Physiology* (10th ed.), 2003. New York: HarperCollins.

Valasquez, J. R. "The Use of Ammonia Inhalants Among Athletes." *Strength and Conditioning* 33 (2011): 33–35.

Willis, J. "Syncope." *Pediatrics in Review* 21 (2000): 201–03.

Wynn, R. L., T. M. Meiller, and H. L. Crossley (Eds.). *Drug Information Handbook for Dentistry*, 2010. Hudson, OH: Lexicomp.

Zepf, B. Causes and outcomes in patients with syncope. *American Family Physician* 67 (2003): 414–16.

TREATMENT OF SYNCOPE
R.E.P.A.I.R.

R: Recognize signs and symptoms of the presyncopal or syncopal patient

E: Evaluate level of consciousness

P: Position patient in supine position with feet elevated

A: Activate CABs of CPR—check circulation, airway, breathing, and pulse and blood pressure

I: Implement appropriate emergency protocol for syncope: loosen tight-fitting clothing; administer O_2 4–6 L/min; if consciousness does not return—monitor vital signs; following the syncopal episode keep patient in supine position until feeling well and slowly return to seated position; suspend treatment and contact emergency individual to escort patient home

R: Refer to EMS if a condition other than neurocardiogenic syncope is suspected

6

Shock

LEARNING OBJECTIVES

Upon reading the material in this chapter, the reader will be able to:

- ✓ Define shock.
- ✓ Explain the stages of shock.
- ✓ Discuss various types of shock.
- ✓ Determine specific signs and symptoms associated with the specific types of shock.

- ✓ List suggested treatment modalities for shock.
- ✓ Explain the steps needed to prepare an office for a patient experiencing shock.

Case Study ·······························➤

Scenario

Your first patient after lunch is Beth Crockett, a 21-year-old, normally healthy female who is in your office for her initial examination. While you review the medical history, Beth informs you that yesterday she had an automobile accident in which her airbag deployed. She was sent to the emergency department, where she was treated for minor cuts and abrasions and released. Today she presents with the following symptoms: increased blood pressure of 150/98 mmHg, increased pulse rate of 92 that is weak, and thready, pale skin, and she seems somewhat confused and is becoming less coherent as time goes on. Beth reports that she has had some pain in her abdominal area since the accident. From what condition do you think your patient might be suffering?

Introduction

Shock is the condition produced when the cardiovascular-pulmonary system fails to deliver enough oxygenated blood to body tissues to support the metabolic needs of those tissues and leads to abnormal cellular and tissue function. Because of this oxygen depletion, the body tissues begin to attempt to use anaerobic (not using air or oxygen) metabolic processes, which in turn produces **acidosis** and toxins that cause additional harm to the cardiovascular system.

On rare occasions, dental professionals may experience a patient suffering from some form of shock. This chapter discusses the various types and etiologies of shock. In addition, it focuses on the signs and symptoms and suggested treatment modalities. An emphasis is placed on prevention and adequate preparation for this life-threatening emergency.

Stages and Etiologies of Shock

There are various forms of shock, and they are generally classified into one of four distinct categories: (1) **hypovolemic shock**, (2) **cardiogenic shock**, (3) **distributive shock**, and (4) **obstructive shock**. Each type is associated with a different condition; however, there are four stages a patient will undergo when suffering from any form of shock: (1) **initial stage**, (2) compensatory stage, (3) progressive stage, and (4) refractory stage.

The first stage of shock is appropriately entitled the initial stage. During this phase the cells are deprived of oxygen, which inhibits their ability to produce energy. The cells of the body are not functioning appropriately, which has a major impact on the body systems.

The compensatory stage is characterized by the body performing physiological adaptations in an attempt to overcome the shock. These physiological adaptations include increased respiration rate to help increase oxygen content to the body cells, increased blood pressure to compensate for the hypotension, and reduced blood supply to the peripheral organs to improve blood supply to the brain and therefore to reduce the risk of brain damage. The kidneys are impacted by this reduced blood flow, and as a result urine output is reduced (**oliguria**).

The progressive stage occurs when the compensatory mechanisms that the body has initiated to combat shock begin to fail. If the problem that originally caused the shock is not treated, the condition will worsen. During this stage the vital organs are compromised and will not function appropriately. In addition, there will be systolic hypotension.

The refractory stage is characterized by failure of the vital organs and irreversibility of the shock condition. Cell death and brain damage have occurred, and death will occur within a few hours.

Types of Shock, Signs/Symptoms, and Treatment

Hypovolemic shock is one of the most common forms of shock and is caused by inadequate venous return to the heart. This condition can result from several etiologies, the most common being severe hemorrhage or dehydration. Dehydration can be caused by severe vomiting or diarrhea. Early signs of hypovolemic shock are usually few. Because of the fluid loss, the body initially compensates by increasing the heart rate, resulting in a rapid, thready pulse. In addition, there is peripheral vasoconstriction, which will result in an elevated diastolic blood pressure. The skin will be cool, and urine output will be reduced. In addition, the patient will appear confused. (See Tables 6.1 and 6.2 ■)

Treatment for all forms of shock begins with recognizing the signs and symptoms of the particular type of shock. The patient should be positioned supinely to support the blood supply to the brain. Emergency Medical Services (EMS) should be contacted to transport the patient to the emergency department as soon as possible. Implement the CABs of cardiopulmonary resuscitation training, monitor the patient's vital signs, and ensure adequate oxygenation. Each form of shock has a specific treatment that should be followed. The specific emergency protocol for hypovolemic shock is first to arrest the bleeding, diarrhea, or vomiting that is causing the shock. The blood pressure should be continuously monitored as a narrowed pulse pressure is a sign of a worsening condition. The next step is to provide intravenous

Table 6.1   Signs and Symptoms of Shock

Hypovolemic Shock	Cardiogenic Shock	Distributive Shock	Obstructive Shock
• Dehydration	• Reduction in blood pressure, with systolic below 90 mmHg	• Anaphylactic shock—hypotension and respiratory arrest	• Severe hypotension, dyspnea
• Rapid, thready pulse	• Fast, weak pulse	• Septic shock—fever, increased cardiac output, tissue edema, pink, warm skin, hypotension, anxiety, restlessness, tachycardia, thirst, eventual respiratory failure	
• Cool skin	• Cold, clammy skin	• Neurogenic shock—hypotension, bradycardia, peripheral vasodilation	
• Reduction in urine output, mental confusion	• Cyanosis		
	• Nonspecific chest pain		
	• Shortness of breath		
	• Reduction in urine output, mental confusion		

Table 6.2 Types of Shock

Type of Shock	General Characteristics
Hypovolemic shock	• Most common form of shock • Inadequate venous return to heart • Etiologies: hemorrhage or dehydration
Cardiogenic shock	• Reduction in tissue perfusion due to decrease in cardiac output • Etiologies: MI, cardiac arrhythmias, cardiac dysfunction
Distributive shock	• Also called vasogenic shock • Three types: anaphylactic, septic, neurogenic • Anaphylactic Vasodilation and circulatory collapse caused by an allergen—see Chapter 15 • Neurogenic Loss of sympathetic nerve activity from the brain's vasomotor center Etiologies: emotional trauma, disease, drug, or traumatic injury to brain stem or spinal cord Loss of impulses causes peripheral vascular dilation, leading to reduction in venous return to the heart • Septic Initiation of inflammatory response due to bacterial invasion
Obstructive shock	• Indirect heart pump failure, leading to decreased cardiac function and reduced circulation • Etiologies: arterial stenosis, pulmonary embolism, cardiac tamponade

(IV) fluids to restore circulating blood volume. Types of IV fluids are sodium chloride, Ringer's solution, or an isotonic solution. If the shock is caused by blood loss, the patient will most likely be experiencing internal hemorrhage and will require some form of blood transfusion. These steps will help to restore homeostasis to the patient.

Cardiogenic shock occurs when there is a reduction in tissue perfusion caused by a decrease in cardiac output. Stated simply, the heart fails to pump enough blood to supply oxygen to the peripheral tissues and body organs. Common causes of cardiogenic shock are myocardial infarction (MI), **cardiac arrhythmias**, and cardiac dysfunction. Cardiogenic shock occurs in 7.5% to 7.6% of patients who have experienced an MI. Patients who are most likely to develop cardiogenic shock are the elderly, women, diabetics, and those with anterior infarction, a history of previous infarction, peripheral vascular disease, and/or cerebrovascular accident or large infarcts. Signs and symptoms of this form of shock include reduction in blood pressure, with a systolic reading below 90 mmHg. The patient will also exhibit a fast, weak pulse and cold, clammy, and cyanotic skin. The patient may have nonspecific chest pain and shortness of breath. Urine output will also be reduced, and mental confusion will occur due to poor cerebral perfusion. Treatment of cardiogenic shock includes adequate oxygenation using a non-rebreather mask. The patient needs to be placed on IV fluids and treated pharmacologically in the emergency department with medications to improve the heart rate and blood pressure. Beta blockers, vasodilators, and positive inotropes are often used to improve cardiac output.

Distributive shock, also known as vasogenic shock, is of three types: anaphylactic, septic, and neurogenic. In all three types, shock occurs as a result of vasodilation and abnormal distribution of fluids within the circulatory system.

Anaphylactic shock is characterized by a sudden, massive vasodilation and circulatory collapse caused by the individual being exposed to an allergen for which he or she is extremely sensitive. Treatment for anaphylactic shock includes the use of epinephrine, histamine blockers, and corticosteroids. Anaphylactic shock and its treatment protocol are discussed in detail in Chapter 15.

Septic shock or vasodilatory shock occurs when certain bacteria invade the bloodstream, particularly gram-negative bacilli. This invasion of bacteria causes the body to begin an inflammatory response to try to rid itself of the invader via a cascade of chemical mediators. Signs and symptoms of septic shock include fever, vasodilation, increased cardiac output, and tissue edema. The vasodilation will cause the patient to appear pink and warm, which differs from all other forms of shock. The chemical mediators also cause microthrombi formation, which obstructs blood flow to the tissues, organs, and microvasculature. Septic shock is often fatal and is usually seen in older people, those with poor nutritional status, neonates, critically ill individuals, and immunocompromised patients. Other signs and symptoms include hypotension, restlessness and anxiety, tachycardia, thirst, and eventually respiratory failure. Patients experiencing septic shock need to be treated with aggressive fluid resuscitation and antimicrobial therapy and possibly surgery to reduce or eliminate the infection.

Neurogenic shock is a result of the loss of sympathetic nerve activity from the brain's vasomotor center following an emotional trauma, a disease, a drug, or a traumatic injury to the brain stem or spinal cord. This loss of sympathetic impulses causes major peripheral vascular dilation, which leads to a reduction in venous return to the heart. Moreover, a decrease in cardiac output occurs, with hypotension soon to follow. Signs and symptoms of neurogenic shock include hypotension, bradycardia, and peripheral vasodilation and often take several hours after the injury to develop. The brain, kidneys, and heart will also be at risk because of the body's inability to regulate itself. Specific treatment for neurogenic shock includes using drug therapy, such as phenylephrine or dopamine to promote peripheral vasoconstriction. In addition, epinephrine is recommended to restore systolic blood pressure, stroke volume, and cardiac output.

Obstructive shock results from indirect heart pump failure, leading to decreased cardiac function and reduced circulation. Etiologies of obstructive shock include **arterial stenosis** (narrowing of arterioles), **pulmonary embolism** (blockage of the pulmonary artery located in the lungs), and **cardiac tamponade** (compression of the heart produced by blood accumulating in the pericardial sac). The primary symptoms of obstructive shock are severe hypotension and dyspnea. The key goal in managing obstructive shock is to relieve the source of the obstruction. Surgical intervention is often required. In addition, IV fluids should be administered cautiously by trained professionals.

Case Resolution and Conclusion

Shock can be a very serious condition that requires early intervention. The symptoms our patient Beth Crockett exhibited seemed rather benign; however, when they are coupled with a recent automobile accident and her confused state, the concept of shock should be considered. Also, her weak, thready pulse, pale skin, and reduction in coherence should prompt the clinician to suspect hypovolemic shock due to internal hemorrhage from the accident. Beth was given 6 L oxygen/minute via a non-rebreather mask. EMS was contacted for transport to the emergency department. Her vital signs were monitored until EMS arrived. Once in the emergency department, she was administered IV fluids, and it was determined that Beth had a liver laceration for which she was treated surgically. She recovered fully within two weeks and returned to work.

Review Questions

1. Shock is the condition produced when the cardio-vascular-pulmonary system fails to deliver enough oxygenated blood to body tissues, which results in a reduction of metabolism for those tissues.

    A. The first phrase is true, and the second phrase is false.
    B. The first phrase is false, and the second phrase is true.
    C. Both phrases are true.
    D. Both phrases are false.

2. Which type of shock would you suspect for a patient experiencing a severe infection?

    A. hypovolemic
    B. anaphylactic
    C. cardiogenic
    D. septic

3. Which stage of shock is irreversible and characterized by failure of the vital organs?

    A. initial stage
    B. refractory stage
    C. compensatory stage
    D. progressive stage

4. What is the most important step in the specific emergency treatment for hypovolemic shock?

    A. arrest the fluid loss
    B. administer antimicrobial medication
    C. administer appropriate medication to reduce tachycardia
    D. none of the above

5. All of the following are possible etiologies of neurogenic shock *except* one. Which one is the *exception*?

    A. emotional trauma
    B. a disease of the brain stem
    C. an injury to the spinal cord
    D. myocardial infarction

6. The type of shock that has the symptoms of nonspecific chest pain and shortness of breath would be

    A. hypovolemic
    B. cardiogenic
    C. septic
    D. none of the above

7. All of the following are forms of distributive shock *except* one. Which one is the *exception*?

    A. cardiogenic shock
    B. septic shock
    C. neurogenic shock
    D. anaphylactic shock

8. In what position should a patient be placed when suffering from shock?

    A. supine
    B. head between the knees
    C. upright
    D. on the stomach

Bibliography

Asuncion, N. M., and V. S. Koushik. "Shock State in the Elderly." *Clinical Geriatrics* 8 (2000): 40–48.

Bench, S. "Critical Care, Clinical Skills; Assessing and Treating Shock." *British Journal of Nursing* 13 (2004): 715–21.

Caldwell, J., and M. Ziglar. "Hemorrhagic Shock in Children: Understanding the Underlying Mechanisms of Shock Syndrome." *American Journal of Nursing American Journal of Nursing* 101 (2001): 25–27.

Chavez, J. A., and C. Brewer. "Stopping the Shock Slide." *RN* 65 (2002): 30–35.

Collins, T. "Understanding Shock." *Nursing Standard* 14 (2000): 35–41.

Dickson, E. "The Perfect Solution?" *Journal of Emergency Medical Services* 26 (2001): 40–47.

Fox, A. D. "Shock Sense: Detecting & Correcting Hemorrhagic Shock in Trauma Patients." *Journal of Emergency Medical Services* 36 (2011): 58–65.

Graham, C. A., and T. R. J. Parke. "Critical Care in the Emergency Department: Shock and Circulatory Support." *Emergency Medical Journal* 22 (2005): 17–21.

Guly, H. R., Bouamra, O., and F. E. Lecky. "The Incidence of Neurogenic Shock in Patients with Isolated Spinal Cord Injury in the Emergency Department." *Resuscitation* 76 (2008): 57–62.

Hand, H. "Shock." *Nursing Standard* 15 (2001): 45–52, 54–55.

Holcomb, S. S. "Cardiogenic Shock: A Success Story." *Dimensions of Critical Care Nursing* 21 (2002a): 232–35.

Holcomb, S. S. "Helping Your Patient Conquer Cardiogenic Shock." *Nursing* 32 (2002b), 32cc1–6.

Holmes, C. L., and K. R. Walley. "The Evaluation and Management of Shock." *Clinics in Chest Medicine* 24 (2003): 775–89.

Jordan, K. S. "Fluid Resuscitation in Acutely Injured Patients." *Journal of Intravenous Nursing* 23 (2000): 81–87.

Josephson, L. "Cardiogenic Shock." *Dimensions of Critical Care Nursing* 27 (2008): 160–70.

Khalaf, S., and P. M. C. DeBlieux. "Managing Shock: The Role of Vasoactive Agents, Part 1." *Journal of Critical Illness* 16 (2001): 281–87.

Khalaf, S., and P. M. C. DeBlieux. "Managing Shock: The Role of Vasoactive Agents, Part 2." *Journal of Critical Illness* 16 (2001), 334–38.

Landry, D. W., and J. A. Oliver. "Insights into Shock." *Scientific American* 290 (2004): 36–41.

Landry, D. W., and J. A. Oliver. "Mechanisms of Disease: The Pathogenesis of Vasodilatory Shock." *New England Journal of Medicine* 345 (2001): 588–95.

LeDuc, T. J., and A. J. Heightnan. "Shelter from Shock: Understanding the Body's Shock-Trauma Compensatory Mechanisms." *Journal of Emergency Medical Services* 26(2001): 36–39.

Lee, C. C., K. A. Merrill, W. A. Carter, and R. S. Crupi. "A Current Concept of Trauma-Induced Multiorgan Failure." *Annals of Emergency Medicine* 38 (2001): 170–76.

Liepert, D. J., and M. H. Rosenthal. "Management of Cardiogenic, Hypovolemic and Hyperdynamic Shock." *Current Reviews for PeriAnesthesia Nurses* 22 (2000): 103–13.

Mecham, N. "Early Recognition and Treatment of Shock in the Pediatric Patient." *Journal of Trauma Nursing* 13 (2006): 17–21.

Mower-Wade, D. M., M. K. Bartley, and J. L. Chiari-Allwien. "How to Respond to Shock." *Dimensions of Critical Care Nursing* 20 (2001): 22–27.

Revell, M., I. Greaves, and K. Porter. "Endpoints for Fluid Resuscitation in Hemorrhagic Shock." *Journal of Trauma — Injury, Infection and Critical Care* 54 (2003): 63–67.

Stene, D. O., and M. Smith. "Shock: Inside and Out." *Emergency Medical Services* 30 (2001): 53–54, 56–63.

Young, J. F. "How the Brain Recognizes and Responds to Shock." *AXON* 26 (2004): 20–33.

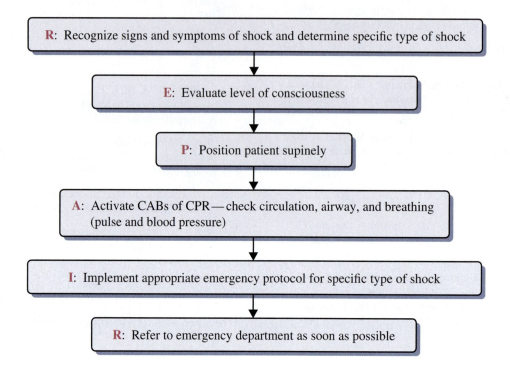

TREATMENT OF SHOCK
R.E.P.A.I.R

R: Recognize signs and symptoms of shock and determine specific type of shock

E: Evaluate level of consciousness

P: Position patient supinely

A: Activate CABs of CPR—check circulation, airway, and breathing (pulse and blood pressure)

I: Implement appropriate emergency protocol for specific type of shock

R: Refer to emergency department as soon as possible

Hyperventilation

Case Study ···➤

Scenario

Your 34-year-old, female patient, Alexandra Harnish, is scheduled for her first periodontal debridement appointment. She is a fairly new patient to your office and was seen last week for her initial examination. She informs you that this is not an experience she enjoys; she has had unpleasant dental experiences in the past. Her medical history is negative, but today she seems unusually anxious and complains of being dizzy and lightheaded. You take her vital signs and find them elevated (pulse 84, respiration 18, blood pressure 120/78 mmHg) but still within the normal range, so you begin treatment. Following the anesthetic injection, you begin the debridement procedure, and Alexandra begins to breathe rapidly and deeply. She cannot seem to catch her breath. She complains of a tingling feeling in her face, particularly around her mouth. You notice that her fingers are beginning to tense and curl. Her skin is pale, moist, and cool. From what emergency do you suspect Alexandra is suffering?

Introduction

Hyperventilation syndrome is a condition in which the patient breathes faster and/or deeper than the metabolic needs of the body, thus eliminating more carbon dioxide (CO_2) than is being produced. The normal respiration rate for an adult is 12–20 respirations/minute and rarely exceeds 22 respirations/minute. A patient who is hyperventilating may experience a respiration rate between 22 and 40 respirations/minute. Hyperventilation syndrome reportedly affects 6% to 15% of the population and is predominantly found in females in the 30–40 age range. This syndrome is common when individuals are exposed to high altitudes, are pregnant, take central nervous system-stimulatory drugs, have aspirin toxicity, and experience anxiety states. Fear and anxiety are common precipitating factors in the dental setting and can cause hyperventilation.

Hyperventilation is characterized by the lack of carbon dioxide (CO_2) in the arterial blood system (**hypocapnia**), resulting in **respiratory alkalosis** and cerebral vasoconstriction. Respiratory alkalosis is an increase in the pH of the circulating blood. The optimal pH for the blood is 7.4, which is slightly alkaline. By increasing respirations, the pH will rise to 7.5 or higher, and the CO_2 level can fall from a normal of 40 mmHg to 30 or 25 mmHg in less than 30 seconds. These minor changes in blood pH can have significant physiological effects and can manifest as the particular symptoms exhibited by the patient.

Signs and Symptoms of Hyperventilation

The most common symptoms of hyperventilation syndrome are abnormally prolonged rapid and deep respirations. This breathing pattern leads to changes in the patient's blood chemistry. The combined high blood pH (alkaline) and low CO_2 leads to certain body changes. The decrease in CO_2 causes vasoconstriction of the arteries and veins in many areas of the body, including the heart and brain. The vasoconstriction of the blood vessels in the heart leads to a decreased **cardiac output** and reduced coronary blood flow, which will give the patient the symptoms of heart palpitations and possibly chest pain.

Hyperventilation has also been shown to impair problem-solving abilities, motor coordination, balance, and perceptual tasks. These symptoms are related to improper cerebral (brain) oxygenation. The vasoconstriction of the blood vessels in the brain can lead to feelings of lightheadedness, dizziness, and impaired vision. In addition, this destabilization of the brain can hasten seizures.

Progressive hyperventilation has been shown to cause **hypocalcemia**, which is a reduction in the calcium levels in the bloodstream. This condition can lead to **tetany**, which manifests clinically as twitching of the muscles or spasms, with sharp flexion of the wrist and ankle joints (also called **carpopedal spasms**). These spasms might also be accompanied by **parasthesia** or numbness in the extremities. Also, as a result of hypocalcemia the patient might experience **Chvostek's sign**, which is an abnormal spasm of the facial muscles elicited by light taps on the facial nerve.

Other symptoms associated with hyperventilation are apprehension and **diaphoresis** (extreme sweating). The patient might also exhibit trembling, fatigue, and **circumoral parasthesia** (numbness or tingling around the oral cavity). Moreover, the patient may experience brief episodes of unconsciousness following stress-induced deep, rapid breathing. (See Table 7.1 ■)

Hyperventilation is frequently a secondary complication to a psychological event, such as a family dispute (anger), death of a family member, pain, or excitement. Patients will begin to have deep, rapid respirations. They will feel they cannot catch their breath and are suffocating (termed **air hunger**). Patients may interpret the sensations as a condition that is more severe than hyperventilation, such as a brain tumor. This will cause further anxiety, which will magnify the symptoms. A vicious cycle occurs, thereby making the condition difficult to control. In addition, often patients are unaware they are overbreathing.

The gravity of hyperventilation is often underestimated. The symptoms of hyperventilation can mimic many respiratory disorders; of particular importance is the condition of pulmonary embolism. A pulmonary embolism is a blockage of the pulmonary artery by some type of obstruction, such as fat, air, a tumor, or **thrombus**. Risk factors for a pulmonary embolus include abdominal/pelvic surgery, immobilization, recent lower limb trauma, pregnancy, and previous deep vein thrombosis. The embolism will lead to reduced arterial carbon dioxide levels, which are also an etiologic factor of hyperventilation. The symptoms between the two conditions are very

Table 7.1 Signs and Symptoms of Hyperventilation

- Abnormally prolonged rapid and deep respirations
- Heart palpitations
- Possible chest pain
- Impairment of problem-solving abilities, motor coordination, balance, perceptual tasks, vision
- Lightheadedness
- Dizziness
- Seizures
- Tetany-twitching of the muscles or spasms with sharp flexion of the wrist and ankle joints (carpopedal spasms)
- Parasthesia or numbness in the extremities
- Chvostek's sign-abnormal spasm of the facial muscles elicited by light taps on the facial nerve
- Apprehension
- Diaphoresis
- Trembling
- Fatigue
- Circumoral parasthesia
- Unconsciousness following stress-induced deep, rapid breathing

similar, yet one is a fairly benign condition and the other is life threatening. Patients suffering from pulmonary embolism will not exhibit spasms of the hands and ankles, nor will they experience tingling in the mouth and fingers. These can be important determining factors during the differential diagnosis of the condition. Two-thirds of all patients with pulmonary embolism die within two hours of onset, so accurate diagnosis and treatment are essential.

Treatment of Hyperventilation

Once a diagnosis of hyperventilation has been determined, therapy is directed at alleviating symptoms. The basic premise for treatment is to increase blood carbon dioxide levels while addressing the psychological factors the patient is experiencing. The practitioner needs to remain calm and keep a nonjudgmental attitude. Breathing into a paper bag was once the well-known cure for hyperventilation. This treatment modality is no longer recommended as breathing into a bag caused suffocation and cardiac arrest. These situations occurred when hyperventilation was mistaken for hypoxemia resulting from myocardial ischemia. In several instances death occurred. Paper bag rebreathing should be implemented only when myocardial ischemia can be ruled out, and the patient's oxygenation has been measured by arterial blood gases or pulse oximetry, which most often does not occur in a dental office. There is some evidence that due to its notoriety the success of the paper bag method is likely the result of expectation versus a physiologic process. The recommended treatment is to place the patient in the position of his or her choice, which is usually sitting upright. In addition, loosen tight clothing around the neck region. The next and most important step is to work with the patient to control the rate of respirations. Having the patient count to 10 in one breath is helpful. Breathing through pursed lips or the nose will help slow breathing, or even having the patient hold his or her breath for as long as possible is beneficial. While attempting to control breathing, the respiratory rate, pulse, and blood pressure should be monitored. If this method is unsuccessful, asking the patient to breathe into his or her cupped hands may be effective. This method serves two purposes. The first is to breathe in CO_2-enriched exhaled air, and the second is to warm the patient's cold hands. Oxygen should *not* be administered to a hyperventilating patient as it can exacerbate the condition.

If the condition does not improve, the healthcare professional may consider intramuscular (IM) or oral administration of a benzodiazepine to help alleviate symptoms. Lorazepam in a dose of 1–2 mg IM or diazepam in a dose of 2-5 mg IM is the recommended medication if symptoms do not subside. (See Figure 7.1 ■) The oral dose of diazepam is 10-15 mg. In addition, patients may require psychological counseling if the hyperventilation episode was stress induced. Transportation by EMS to an emergency department to determine if the patient may be suffering from a more serious condition, such as a pulmonary embolism, may be required.

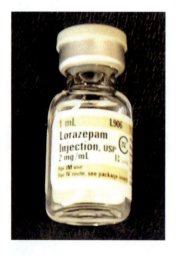

FIGURE 7.1 Lorazepam.

Case Resolution and Conclusion

Hyperventilation is a common emergency seen by the dental professional because for many patients a visit to the dental office can be an anxiety-inducing experience. The patient in the case scenario, Alexandra Harnish, presented to the office with a negative medical history, but today seemed quite anxious. Her vital signs were slightly elevated as compared to her baseline readings. Her sudden onset of tachypnea and a feeling of suffocation

(continued)

are common symptoms of hyperventilation. The circumoral parasthesia that Alexandra exhibited is a result of respiratory alkalosis. The tension in her fingers (carpopedal spasms) is a result of the hypocalcemia accompanying hyperventilation. The clinician placed the patient in an upright position and asked the patient to count to 10 in one breath and to breathe through her nose. The proper method was demonstrated. In addition, the dental practitioner monitored Alexandra's vital signs, which shortly returned to normal, as did her breathing pattern. The clinician and Alexandra discussed her concerns regarding her treatment, and the clinician thoroughly explained the procedure; this seemed to put the patient at ease. The periodontal debridement was performed without further incident.

Review Questions

1. All of the following are symptoms of hyperventilation *except* one. Which one is the *exception*?

   A. circumoral parasthesia
   B. heart palpitations
   C. pulmonary embolism
   D. hyperpnea

2. The chemical lacking in the bloodstream of the hyperventilating patient is

   A. oxygen
   B. hydrogen
   C. iron
   D. carbon dioxide

3. The carpopedal spasms often seen in a patient who is hyperventilating is caused by

   A. the respiratory acidosis
   B. the reduction in calcium in the bloodstream
   C. reduced cerebral oxygenation
   D. none of the above

4. The recommended treatment for a hyperventilating patient is

   A. have him or her breathe into a paper bag
   B. have him or her drink milk to increase calcium levels
   C. administer oxygen at 4 L/minute
   D. work with him or her to control his or her breathing

5. The symptoms of a pulmonary embolism are often similar to the symptoms of hyperventilation, and both conditions are potentially life threatening.

   A. The first phrase is correct, and the second phrase is incorrect.
   B. The first phase is incorrect, and the second phrase is correct.
   C. Both phrases are correct.
   D. Both phrases are incorrect.

6. The respiration rate for a person experiencing hyperventilation is

   A. 12–14 respirations/minute
   B. 14–16 respirations/minute
   C. 16–18 respirations/minute
   D. >22 respirations/minute

7. Abnormal spasm of the facial muscles elicited by light taps on the facial nerve is referred to as

   A. Levine sign
   B. Chvostek's sign
   C. tetany
   D. circumoral parasthesia

8. All of the following are common precipitating factors of hyperventilation *except* one. Which one is the *exception*?

   A. high altitudes
   B. pregnancy
   C. anxiety
   D. hypertension

Bibliography

Anderson, D. M., J. Keith, P. D. Novak, and M. A. Elliot (Eds.). *Mosby's Medical, Nursing & Allied Health Dictionary* (6th ed.), 2008. St. Louis, MO: Mosby-Year Book, Inc.

Balmer, C., and L. Longman. *Management of Medical Emergencies—A Guide for Dental Care Professionals* (1st ed.), 2008. London, EN: Quay Books.

Bennett, J. D., and M. B. Rosenberg. *Medical Emergencies in Dentistry* (1st ed.), 2002. Philadelphia, PA: W. B. Saunders.

Callaham, M. "Hypoxic Hazards of Traditional Paper Bag Rebreathing in Hyperventilating Patients." *Annals of Emergency Medicine* 18 (1989): 622–28.

Callaham, M. "Panic Disorders, Hyperventilation, and the Dreaded Brown Paper Bag." *Annals of Emergency Medicine* 30 (1997): 838.

Dann, K., E. Young, and P. Copp. "How We Would Manage a Patient Who Has Too Much Breathing." *Ontario Dentist* 76 (1999): 41–4.

Folgering, H. "The Pathophysiology of Hyperventilation Syndrome." *Monaldi Archives for Chest Disease* 54 (1999): 365–72.

Foster, G. T., N. D. Vaziri, and C. S. H. Sassoon. "Respiratory Alkalosis." *Respiratory Care* 46 (2001): 384–91.

Gilbert, C. "Hyperventilation and the Body." *Journal of Bodywork and Therapies* 2 (1998): 184–91.

Malamed, S. F. *Medical Emergencies in the Dental Office* (6th ed.), 2007. St. Louis, MO: Mosby Publishing Company.

Mehta, T. A., J. G. Sutherland, and D. W. Hodgkinson. "Hyperventilation: Cause or Effect?" *Journal of Accident & Emergency Medicine* 17 (2000): 376–77.

Professional Guide to Diseases. (7th ed.), 2001. Springhouse, PA: Lippincott Williams & Wilkins.

Professional Guide to Signs and Symptoms. (4th ed.), 2004. Philadelphia, PA: Lippincott Williams & Wilkins.

Schaider, J., S. R. Hayden, R. Wolfe, R. M. Barkin, and P. Rosen (Eds.). *Rosen & Barkin's 5 Minute Emergency Medicine Consult* (2nd ed.), 2003. Philadelphia, PA: Lippincott Williams & Wilkins.

Steinhauer, R. "Acute Hyperventilation Syndrome." *Emergency Medical Services* 30 (2001): 49–52.

Strohl, K. P. In: D. C. Dale, and D. Federman, D (Eds.), *Ventilatory Control During Wakefulness and Sleep. Pulmonary Medicine. WebMD Scientific American Medicine* Section 14, Chap. 6, 2003. New York: WebMD Publishing.

van den Hout, M. A., C. Boek, G. Margo van der Molen, A. Jansen, and E. Griez. "Rebreathing to Cope with Hyperventilation: Experimental Tests of the Paper Bag Method." *Journal of Behavioral Medicine* 11 (1988): 303–9.

Wilson, M. H., N. S. McArdle, J. J. Fitzpatrick, and L. F. A. Stassen. "Medical Emergencies in Dental Practice." *Journal of the Irish Dental Association* 55 (2009): 134–43.

TREATMENT OF HYPERVENTILATION
R.E.P.A.I.R.

R: Recognize signs and symptoms of hyperventilation: prolonged rapid, deep respirations, diaphoresis, trembling, circumoral parasthesia, apprehension, lightheadness, tetany, feeling of suffocation

↓

E: Evaluate respiration rate

↓

P: Position patient comfortably, usually sitting upright

↓

A: Activate CAB's of CPR—check circulation, airway, and breathing (pulse and blood pressure)

↓

I: Implement appropriate emergency protocol for hyperventilation: maintain calm demeanor, attempt to have patient control breathing, loosen tight clothing in neck region, monitor vital signs

↓

R: Refer to appropriate healthcare professional if condition does not improve; may need to be transported to emergency room for administration of other antianxiety drugs, such as benzodiazepine; referral for psychiatric counseling may be required

8

Seizure Disorders

LEARNING OBJECTIVES

Upon reading the material in this chapter, the reader will be able to:

- ✓ Discuss the pathophysiology of seizures.
- ✓ Differentiate between partial and generalized seizures.
- ✓ Discuss the etiologies of seizures.
- ✓ List specific signs and symptoms associated with seizures.
- ✓ Determine suggested treatment modalities for seizures.
- ✓ Explain the steps needed to prepare an office for a patient experiencing a seizure.

Case Study ·····················➤

Scenario

Your patient, Cindy Rainey, a 15-year-old female, comes into the office for her six-month checkup accompanied by several of her friends. From past visits and from the medical history update, you know that she is under treatment for a seizure disorder and that she had a tonic-clonic seizure about a month ago. Cindy informs you that her seizures seem to occur more frequently around her menstrual cycle, which she is experiencing presently. She answers your questions with a somewhat irritable attitude and indicates that she has taken her medication (200 mg topiramate [Topamax] bid). She states that she does not want to discuss her medical problems any further. Her oral hygiene is poor, and you start to reinforce brushing instructions when she states she has a bad headache. Her body becomes rigid, and she starts having convulsions. What do you do?

Introduction

A seizure is a temporary episode of behavior alteration due to massive abnormal electrical discharges in one or more areas of the brain. This electric activity in the brain may be recorded by **electroencephalogram** (EEG) and may be accompanied by convulsions or other neurological, sensory, or emotional changes. Seizures have been illustrated in cave paintings made by prehistoric humans, and Hippocrates wrote of epilepsy and its relationship to the brain. Four-thousand-year-old writings depict epileptics as being possessed by demons, and there are also biblical references to epilepsy.

Any person may experience a seizure if exposed to extreme systemic stress, such as **hypoxia** or rapid drop in blood glucose. Infants and young children may experience febrile seizures if there is a sudden elevation in body temperature. These types of seizure disorders are termed isolated, nonrecurrent attacks. Damage or disease of the brain, such as tumors, trauma, perinatal injuries, toxins, infectious agents, electrolyte imbalance, uremia, withdrawal from long-term use of alcohol or sedative-hypnotics, and vascular disorders may also cause seizures. There appears to be a genetic tendency toward seizure disorders in some families.

Approximately half of all seizures are idiopathic or "without a known cause." Often the terms **epilepsy** or **epileptic** are applied to a group of disorders (epileptic syndrome) that involve chronic, recurrent, attacks of involuntary behavior or changes in neurological function, with each episode classified as a seizure. A seizure or convulsion is a **paroxysmal** disorder of cerebral function characterized by spontaneous, electric discharges from collections of neurons in the cerebral cortex. There is an alteration in the state of consciousness, motor activity, or sensory phenomena, with sudden onset and a brief span of activity. The term **epilepsy** is derived from the Greek word **epilepsia**, which means "to take hold of." Epilepsy refers to a syndrome of associated seizure types and is not a specific disease. The term **ictus** or **ictal** refers to a seizure or to a seizure state.

Epilepsy is a common disorder that affects approximately 3 million persons in the United States. Seizure activity is the most common neurological disorder in pediatrics, and only cerebrovascular disorders account for more neurological problems in adults. Most people experience their first seizure episode before age 20, and initial seizures in adults are usually attributed to structural changes, trauma, disease, or stroke. A seizure is not a disease but a symptom of underlying central nervous system (CNS) dysfunction. Classifications of seizure disorders include causes, symptoms, duration, precipitating factors, and aura. Although witnessing a seizure is quite traumatic, seizures are usually not life threatening. Proper assessment and management of the situation can prevent injury during the seizure and decrease morbidity and mortality. In rare instances when seizures continue without stopping or are repeated without a recovery period (status epilepticus), a true medical emergency exists, and prompt action and appropriate therapy are needed to prevent death or serious postseizure mortality.

Etiology of Seizures

Although many seizures are idiopathic, the abnormal electrical brain activity occurring with the seizure often has an identifiable cause. At the cellular level, seizure activity may be caused by alterations in cell membrane permeability or movement of ions across the cell membrane of the neuron. Other theories about cellular etiology include decreased inhibition of cortical or thalamic neuronal activity or changes in the cell structure that alter cellular excitability. Imbalances of neurotransmitters, such as an excess of the excitatory neurotransmitter acetylcholine or deficiency of the inhibitory neurotransmitter gamma-aminobutyric acid (GABA), have also been theorized to contribute to seizure disorders.

Classification by etiology falls into two broad categories—primary/unprovoked or idiopathic seizures, and secondary/provoked or acute symptomatic seizures. Primary seizures usually occur as part of an epileptic syndrome. Primary epilepsy comprises about 65% of seizure disorders and is believed to have a genetic predisposition. Patients with primary seizures usually require daily antiseizure medication to limit seizure occurrences.

Secondary or provoked seizures account for the remaining 35% of seizure disorders, and a probable cause or causes may be traced to the disorder. Most secondary seizures may be prevented if the underlying cause is treatable. Metabolic disorders, such as electrolyte imbalances, hypoglycemia, hypoxia, hypocalcemia, **uremia**, **alkalosis**, ingestion of toxins, and rapid withdrawal of addictive drugs may induce secondary seizures. Injury to the CNS, such as congenital and perinatal infections, trauma, or hypoxia during delivery, has been linked to seizure disorders. Some medications are known to be **epileptogenic** (seizure provoking), including penicillin, hypoglycemic agents, local anesthetics, and phenothiazines.

Tumors or other space-occupying lesions of the CNS are the most common cause of acquired secondary seizures in the 35- to 50-year age group, and seizures are the initial symptom in 40% of these patients. Any disease that impairs blood flow to the brain can provoke a seizure, and the likelihood of seizures increases with increasing severity of cerebral ischemia. After age 60, vascular diseases become the most common cause of seizures, with atherosclerotic cerebrovascular insufficiency and cerebral infarction the most common vascular disorders provoking seizures.

Infections of the CNS, such as bacterial meningitis, herpetic encephalitis, malaria, neurosyphilis, rabies, tetanus, toxoplasmosis, HIV-associated infections, and brain abscesses, are frequent precipitators of seizures. Infections account for about 3% of acquired epilepsy and 10% to 24% of acute isolated seizures.

One of the most recently reported causes of seizures is a phenomenon called photosensitive epilepsy, which can cause seizures in children and adults exposed to flickering lights or geometric patterns of video games. This concept came to the forefront when thousands of Japanese children experienced seizures when watching a television show with colored, flickering lights.

In the dental setting, there are several potential causes of seizures: hypoglycemia, hypoxia secondary to syncope, local anesthetic toxicity, and epilepsy. The first three causes are totally preventable with appropriate assessment and patient management. Taking a thorough medical history and reducing stress will help prevent seizures caused by epilepsy. (See Table 8.1 ■)

Table 8.1 Seizure Etiologies

Congenital—Developmental malformations of the brain
Genetic—Inherited syndromes, family history
Central nervous system infections—Meningitis, encephalitis, abscesses of the brain, herpetic viruses
Neoplasms—Benign and malignant tumors, primary and metastatic
Trauma—Closed head wounds, perinatal trauma including anoxia, surgery
Metabolic and toxic—Hypoglycemia, pyrexia, hypoxia, alcohol or substance abuse, drug withdrawal
Cerebrovascular and degenerative—Hemorrhage, infarctions, vessel malformation, Alzheimer's disease, prion diseases

Diagnosis and Prognosis

Diagnosis of seizure disorders is based on a thorough history, neurological examination, and description of the seizure. The physical examination, radiographs, and laboratory tests help exclude metabolic or systemic diseases that could precipitate seizures. Fever, stiff neck, and new-onset seizures suggest **meningitis**, **subarachnoid hemorrhage**, or **encephalitis**, and a **lumbar puncture** would be indicated. Skull radiographs and newer, noninvasive techniques like **computerized axial tomography (CT) scans** or **magnetic resonance imaging** (MRI) have greatly improved the detection of lesions and structural defects in patients with seizure disorders. One of the most useful diagnostic tests is the EEG, which is used to record changes in the brain's electrical activity. A negative EEG does not necessarily rule out epilepsy, because the paroxysmal abnormalities occur at irregular intervals. The EEG can help determine the prognosis and help classify the type of seizure disorder. Other tests include serum glucose, complete blood panels, toxicology screening, urinalysis, and calcium and electrolyte studies.

After the underlying disease is treated, the aim of treatment is to control the seizures with the least disruption in the patient's life and the fewest side effects. Since the 1970s the therapy for seizures has greatly improved because of the improved classification system and the availability of more efficacious antiseizure and antiepileptic drugs (AEDs). Drug therapy will completely eliminate seizures in one-third of patients and greatly reduce the frequency of seizures in another third. With proper drug management, 60% to 80% of persons with epilepsy can obtain adequate seizure control. Most patients with epilepsy are neurologically normal between seizures, although anticonvulsants can dull alertness and slow learning in children. Progressive mental deterioration may occur if the neurological disease that caused the seizures is not treated.

Despite the use of long-term anticonvulsant drug therapy, acute seizure activity may still develop. In some cases there is no apparent trigger; in others, factors that increase the likelihood that seizure disorder can occur are present. Children are more susceptible to seizures than adults because of the increased susceptibility to biochemical changes in the immature brain. Seizures due to hypoxia, hypoglycemia, and other metabolic disorders occur much more frequently in younger age groups. Even well-controlled adult patients may have isolated "breakthrough" seizures. Sleep deprivation, extreme stress, and hormonal fluctuations are often correlated with increased seizure activity. Estrogen has been shown to be epileptogenic for persons with seizure disorders, and progesterone seems to have an antiseizure effect. If women with epilepsy become pregnant, about 20% will experience an increase in seizure frequency during pregnancy, with some women experiencing seizures only during birth.

In many cases the triggering event of a seizure is apparent. Triggering factors include flashing lights (especially in generalized absence seizures), fatigue or poor physical health, missed meals, and alcohol ingestion or withdrawal, physical or emotional stress, cerebrovascular insufficiency, or metabolic disturbances may cause seizures in susceptible individuals.

Drug Therapy for Seizure Disorders

Medical management of seizure disorders is usually based on long-term drug therapy. The efficacy of drug therapy varies widely, from complete control to simply reducing the number of seizures. The goal is to control seizures while minimizing adverse reactions (especially important in the long-term use of medications). The choice of AEDs is based on seizure type, EEG pattern, the medication's ability to control seizures, and the patient's tolerance to the medication. Older medications that were used to treat seizures were the barbiturates (phenobarbital and mephobarbital) and hydantoins (phenytoin, ethotoin, and mephenytoin). These medications had many side effects and are now being replaced by drugs that have significantly few side effects; Zarontin (ethosuximide), Lamictal (Iamotrigine), Depacon (valproate) are now commonly used for absence seizures. Topamax (topiramate), Zonegran (zonisamide), and Keppra (leveriracetam) are anticonvulsants used for generalized or partial seizures. Also, a ketogenic diet, one that is high in fat and low in carbohydrates, has been found to be effective for seizures that are difficult to control.

Oral Findings in Patients with Seizure Disorders

Seizure disorders themselves do not produce oral changes, but there may be oral changes associated with adverse effects of antiseizure medications or trauma occurring during the seizure episode. Scars on the oral soft tissues may be noted during the extraoral/intraoral examination, as well as fractured teeth and infections resulting from pulpal exposure during tooth fractures.

Gingival overgrowth associated with phenytoin (Dilantin) treatment occurs in 25% to 50% of persons using this medication, although other AEDs may also induce gingival hyperplasia. Phenytoin may induce fibroblasts and osteoblasts to produce excess extracellular substance, resulting in gingival overgrowth, exacerbated by oral biofilm accumulation or irritation caused by ill-fitting appliances. Meticulous homecare will reduce the severity and occurrence of gingival overgrowth, and the hyperplasia will be reversed if the medication is discontinued.

Other adverse effects associated with AEDs include bone marrow suppression, bleeding problems (including spontaneous hemorrhage and petechiae), and increased risk of infection. There is no contraindication to the use of local anesthetics with vasoconstrictors in proper amounts for seizure patients.

Types of Seizures

Each different type of seizure disorder has a characteristic pattern of events and a specific type of brain wave activity that can be detected on an EEG. Some patients may suffer from more than one type of seizure.

Partial Seizures

PARTIAL (FOCAL/LOCAL) SEIZURES   Partial (focal/local) seizures are the most common type of seizure among newly diagnosed adults. These seizures arise from a localized area in the brain, although the seizure activity may spread to the entire brain, causing a generalized seizure. Signs and symptoms of focal seizures are related to the affected area of the brain. The categories of partial seizures are based on theories related to the spread of the seizure and the extent of brain involvement.

There are two major types of partial seizures: simple and complex partial seizures.

SIMPLE PARTIAL SEIZURES   Simple partial seizures consist of motor, sensory, or psychomotor changes, with no loss of consciousness. Symptoms of sensory seizures include illusions, déjà vu, flashing lights, hallucinations, tingling and creeping sensations, vertigo, sounds, and foul smells or auras. An **aura** consists of subjective sensory symptoms occurring at the onset of a seizure or migraine headache. The aura signals the beginning of abnormal changes within a focal area of the brain. Symptoms may reflect the area of brain activity: visual-occipital lobe, auditory-temporal lobe, or olfactory. Typical auras include strong smells, nausea, mood changes, unusual tastes, or visual disturbances lasting only a few seconds. Patients may not be aware of having an aura, because amnesia often occurs in the prodromal phase. Auras are now considered to be a simple partial seizure, which serve as a warning sign of impending complex or generalized seizures.

COMPLEX PARTIAL SEIZURES Complex partial seizures involve impairment of consciousness and often begin in the temporal lobe, but may rapidly progress to involve both brain hemispheres and thus become generalized. These seizures are also referred to as temporal lobe seizures or psychomotor seizures. Signs and symptoms of complex partial seizures are variable, but usually include losing contact with surroundings for a few seconds to up to 20 minutes. These seizures are often accompanied by **automatisms**: repetitive, nonpurposeful activity, such as lip smacking, grimacing, patting, wandering in circles, or unintelligible speech. Aggressive behavior is not a characteristic of complex partial seizures, but attempting to restrain a patient during the seizure may cause the patient to lash out at the person restraining him or her. At the end of the motor activity, mental confusion may be accompanied with overwhelming fear, which may be mistaken for alcohol or drug intoxication. Up to 33% of persons with temporal lobe seizures have a psychiatric disorder, and 10% may have schizophrenic or depressive psychoses.

GENERALIZED TONIC-CLONIC SEIZURES (GTCS) OR GRAND MAL SEIZURES **Generalized tonic-clonic seizures** are the most common type of seizure disorder, representing about 90% of epileptics and characterizing what most people think of as "epilepsy." About 60% of patients with GTCS suffer from this form by itself, and another 30% may experience additional seizure types. GTCS occurs equally in both sexes and may occur at any age, although over 60% of cases occur by puberty. Tonic-clonic seizures have a specific sequence of events ranging from the warning phase to recovery, although not all seizure patients experience all of these events.

ABSENCE OR PETIT MAL SEIZURES **Absence seizures** are most common in children and often have a genetic tendency. Seizures often occur when the child is sitting quietly, rarely during exercise, and may be precipitated by hyperventilation. The episode usually begins with a brief change in the level of consciousness, signaled by blinking or eye rolling. The child then stops what he or she is doing and has a blank stare. Sometimes the absence seizure is accompanied by minor facial movements (automatisms), such as repetitive blinking or mouth movements. Each episode last from 5 to 30 seconds but may recur up to a hundred times a day and may progress to a generalized tonic-clonic seizure. There are no prodromal or postictal periods, and episodes may stop as suddenly as they began. Once the blank stare has ceased, activity continues, with no memory of the episode. Diagnosis of absence seizures often occurs once the child starts school and teachers advise parents that their child is "off in their own world." Absence seizures are considered idiopathic disorders of early childhood and are rare after age 20. Absence seizures may not readily respond to medications. (See Table 8.2 ■)

Generalized Seizures

Generalized seizures cause an electrical abnormality throughout the brain and involve a loss of consciousness. The motor activity associated with some types of generalized seizures is termed convulsions. These seizures often have a genetic or metabolic cause and are primarily responsible for serious morbidity and mortality associated with seizure disorders. Persons with recurrent generalized seizures may be called epileptics, and although 70% will suffer from only one type of seizure disorder, the remaining 30% suffer from two or more types.

Generalized seizures usually involve the entire body shaking and stiffening, frothing at the mouth, and incontinence. The most common types of generalized seizures are tonic-clonic or grand mal seizures, absence or petit mal seizures, and febrile seizures (as it is unlikely that febrile seizures would occur in the dental office they will not be discussed in this text.)

Table 8.2 Signs and Symptoms of Generalized Absence Seizures

- Brief change in the level of consciousness
- Blinking or eye rolling
- Blank stare
- Automatisms
- Duration of 5 to 30 seconds

Four phases of a GTCS seizure are as follows:

- **Aura or prodromal phase.** Now considered to be a simple partial seizure, an **aura** is a subjective sensation that precedes seizure activity. It may be psychic or sensory, with olfactory, visual, auditory, or taste hallucinations. The patient may hear noise or music, see floating or flashing lights, smell unpleasant odors, and feel an unpleasant sensation in the stomach or twitching in other parts of the body. Some patients experience changes in emotional state, such as extreme anxiety or depression. Most epileptics have the same recurrent aura before each seizure episode, and the aura usually lasts only a few seconds. Not all seizures are preceded by auras, and because of the amnesic effect of seizures the person may not remember experiencing an aura, although he or she may have described the phenomena to a bystander. The changes may not be evident to the dental team, so feedback from family or friends should be noted.
- **Preictal phase.** Soon after the aura, the person will lose consciousness and may fall, if standing. Falling is the most common cause of seizure-related injuries.
- **Ictal phase**
  - **Tonic phase.** Muscles have sustained contraction, so the patient appears stiff and rigid. The sharp, continuous contraction of the chest muscles, the lungs, and vocal cords may produce a loud cry, known as the "epileptic cry." Difficulty in breathing and cyanosis may occur because of the contraction of the airway and respiratory muscles. This period of the seizure usually lasts 10 to 20 seconds.
  - **Hypertonic phase.** The patient experiences extreme muscle rigidity, including hyperextension of the spine.
  - **Clonic phase.** Immediately following the tonic and hypertonic phases, the patient experiences muscular contractions or spasms and relaxation, producing the rhythmic jerking motions associated with convulsions, often accompanied by heavy, labored breathing. The patient's jaw remains clenched, which makes airway management difficult, and the patient may froth at the mouth because air and saliva are mixed. Blood may also appear at the mouth caused by biting of the tongue, and soft tissues and other injuries may occur as result of the violent movement. The **clonic phase** usually lasts two to five minutes and will gradually slow, with the individual exhibiting a final flexor jerk. (See Table 8.3 ■)
- **Postseizure or postictal phase.** Movement has stopped, but the patient remains unconscious. When seizure activity stops, generalized depression occurs in the central nervous, cardiovascular, and respiratory systems, related to the severity of the seizure. The CNS and respiratory depression may be severe enough to lead to airway obstruction, and this is the period of seizure activity most associated with significant morbidity and mortality. In the first several minutes the patient experiences muscle flaccidity, which may lead to urinary and/or fecal incontinence. The patient may awake confused, fatigued, and drowsy, wanting to sleep and not remembering the events preceding the seizure. This phase can last for minutes to several hours. Careful observation of the patient during this phase is critical to protect the airway.

Treatment of Seizures

The primary task of the dental team during a seizure is to try and prevent injury to the patient. Specific steps to follow are described depending on the type of seizure.

Generalized Tonic-Clonic Seizures

Treatment of generalized tonic-clonic seizures is focused on protecting the patient from injury before, during, and after the seizure. Clinicians should be alert for signs of an impending seizure, such as mood changes, reports of auras, or sudden loss of consciousness. At the first indication of a seizure, all dental treatment must stop immediately, and any source of injury (such as dental instruments) must be removed from the mouth and equipment, such as the bracket table should be moved out of the way.

Table 8.3 Signs and Symptoms of Generalized Tonic-Clonic Seizures

- Aura (patients may or may not experience this seizure prior to a GTCS)
- Loss of consciousness
- Total contraction of muscles
- Hyperextension of the spine
- Convulsions
- Heavy, labored breathing
- Clenched jaw
- Froth at the mouth

The time of the initiation of the seizure should be noted. If the patient does not have a history of seizures or is a well-controlled epileptic and is experiencing a seizure, EMS should be contacted. Tight clothing may be loosened to assist breathing, and, if possible, the patient should be placed in a supine position on his or her side to minimize aspirations. If the seizure begins while the patient is still in the dental chair, do not attempt to move the patient; lower the chair and prevent the patient from falling by positioning one person at the head of the chair and one at the foot of the chair. Time the seizure, and if the seizure lasts longer than three minutes or the patient becomes cyanotic from the outset, EMS should be contacted. Oxygen at 6–8 L/minute via non-rebreather mask should be administered if possible. The CABs of life support should be provided if needed, and vital signs should be monitored. The patient should be gently restrained to avoid self-injury, with care to protect injury to the head and body during the seizure. No attempt should be made to place anything in the patient's mouth, and there must not be any forceful attempts to restrain the patient.

POSTICTAL TREATMENT   Patient monitoring during the postictal stage is critical. At the cessation of seizure activity, muscle flaccidity is common, and it is vital that the airway be protected as respiratory arrest is possible. Recovery from a tonic-clonic seizure occurs slowly, with the patient rousing slowly from a sleeplike state to increasing alertness, and may take as long as two hours. Patients recovering from a tonic-clonic seizure may experience significant confusion and disorientation, and reassurance and quiet are helpful. If a family member or friend is available, that person may help reassure the patient. Recovery includes a return to normal vital signs and the patient no longer being disoriented or confused, although the patient may want to fall into a deep sleep and may have headaches and muscle soreness. Patients recovering from a tonic-clonic seizure should never be allowed to drive themselves home and should be released into the care of a responsible adult.

Status Epilepticus

Status epilepticus or grand mal status is a continuous seizure or the repetitive recurrence of any type of seizure without recovery between seizure episodes. Most generally it is a continuation of a tonic-clonic seizure and is a life-threatening situation. Patients experiencing status epilepticus have the same signs and symptoms as in the convulsive phase of the tonic-clonic seizure; the major difference is duration. The normal duration of a tonic-clonic seizure is two to five minutes, while status epilepticus may persist for hours or even days, and is the major cause of mortality related to seizure disorders. Mortality is cited as ranging from 3% to 23% depending on the source. The incidence of grand mal status has decreased since the introduction of effective antiseizure medications, with most cases related to drug (especially barbiturates) or alcohol withdrawal, severe head injury, or metabolic derangements.

The patient is unconscious, cyanotic, and sweating, with generalized clonic contractions and a brief or absent tonic phase. As the seizure continues, the body temperature may rise to 106°F or higher. Tachycardia and **dysrhythmias** occur, and the blood pressure may become elevated to 200/150 mmHg. Uninterrupted grand mal status may continue until death occurs as a result of cardiac arrest, irreversible brain damage occurs due to cerebral hypoxia, a decrease in cerebral blood flow occurs due to increased intracranial pressure, or there is a significant decrease in blood glucose levels as the brain utilizes large quantities for metabolism. Immediate medical intervention is required to prevent any of these consequences. If a tonic-clonic seizure does not stop after five minutes, the use of anticonvulsant drugs may become necessary. All of the steps to manage a tonic-clonic seizure are followed, but then the clinician has two options:

1. Activation of the emergency medical system and continuation of basic life support and patient protection until medical assistance is available.
2. Management of the seizure through intravenous (IV) anticonvulsant drugs. This option should be considered only when both the doctor and the staff are trained in IV drug administration and possess the knowledge, ability, and equipment to perform venipuncture.

Absence or Petit Mal Seizures

Patients experiencing an absence or petit mal seizure do not generally pose problems during dental treatment. If one of these seizures occurs, dental treatment should stop for the duration of the episode and the patient's airway should be protected. All instruments should be removed from the patient's mouth, and the vital signs should be monitored. Treatment can continue at the cessation of the seizure if the patient has no ill effects.

Preventive Strategies for Known Seizure Patients

The major considerations in management of patients with seizure disorders are preventing seizures in the dental setting and preparing for management of a seizure should one occur. Further discussion with patients who respond positively to seizures on their medical history should include

- Recent illnesses, stress, hormonal fluctuations, fatigue, or pain that could precipitate seizure
- Recent history of head trauma
- Recent history of fever, headache, stiff neck
- Alcohol or other substance use or abuse
- General physical condition, including mental states such as depression
- Medications, surgeries, diet alterations, and interactions with dental treatment
- Nonprescription medications and herbal supplement use
- Adherence to prescribed treatment and medications taken on schedule
- Adverse effects of seizure medication
- Information about seizure history

  - Length of time since the last seizure
  - Type of seizures, severity, duration
  - Presence of aura

- Alteration or loss of consciousness
- Postictal symptoms such as confusion or amnesia

Fortunately, most patients with seizure disorders are able to maintain adequate control of their seizures by following their prescribed medications. If a patient's answers indicate that his or her seizures are not well controlled or there are factors that would predispose the patient to a seizure episode (hormonal cycle in females), the clinician may wish to postpone dental treatment until the patient's condition is more stable. Blood glucose levels, fatigue, and anxiety are common triggers for seizures in poorly controlled cases, and consultation with the patient's physician may be indicated. Optimal times are early morning appointments after patients have eaten and within a few hours of taking their antiseizure medication. The clinician should also be aware that irritability is often a symptom that a seizure is imminent. Use of a mouth prop and the removal of dentures and appliances are recommended. In addition, the dental practitioner should discuss with the patient the importance of letting the clinician know immediately if a seizure is impending. If the patient recovers adequately from the seizure, treatment can be continued.

Case Resolution and Conclusion ·····················➤

In the case scenario presented at the beginning of this chapter, Cindy's responses to your questions should have alerted you that she was at high risk for another seizure because of the timing of her menstrual cycle and her last seizure activity. When Cindy complains of a headache and starts becoming

(continued)

rigid, the back of the dental chair should be lowered and assistance should be summoned. All dental equipment is moved out of the way, and Cindy should be positioned on her side. The first operator remains at her head while the second operator stations himself or herself at the foot of the chair. The dental receptionist calls 9-1-1 and Cindy's parents. In this scenario a third operator is responsible for monitoring Cindy's vital signs and timing the seizure. Cindy should not be restrained but should be prevented from falling out of the chair or injuring herself on other dental equipment. Oxygen should be administered at a rate of 6–8 L/minute. After the seizure has ceased, Cindy is very disoriented and embarrassed at having become incontinent. Operator 1 remains with her and allows her to rest quietly. All events should be thoroughly documented in her Emergency Treatment Record. Being prepared allows the dental practitioner to act calmly and quickly and to prevent any serious injury to the seizure patient.

Review Questions

1. All of the following are associated with increased seizure activity *except* one. Which one is the *exception*?

   A. hypoglycemia
   B. hyperglycemia
   C. hypoxia
   D. pyrexia

2. Which of the following are responsibilities of the clinician in treating a patient with seizure disorder?

   A. thoroughly reviewing the medical history and discussing it with the patient
   B. monitoring the patient for signs and symptoms of impending seizures
   C. protecting the patient from harm during the seizure
   D. monitoring the patient's vital signs during recovery and arranging a ride home.
   E. All of the above

3. Generalized tonic-clonic seizures are often preceded by an aura. Patients are always aware that they have had an aura.

   A. Both statements are true.
   B. Both statements are false.
   C. The first statement is true, and the second statement is false.
   D. The first statement is false, and the second statement is true.

4. All of the following are factors used to classify seizure types *except* one. Which one is the *exception*?

   A. signs and symptoms
   B. duration of seizure
   C. age of patient
   D. type of aura
   E. precipitating factors

5. Your patient stiffens and starts to experience a seizure in the middle of periodontal debridement. What is the first thing you should do?

   A. Activate the EMS system.
   B. Stop treatment and remove everything from the patient's mouth.
   C. Administer CPR.
   D. Administer antiepileptic medications.

6. The following oral signs and symptoms are often present in a patient with a history of seizure disorders. Which of the following is an *exception*?

   A. advanced periodontitis
   B. gingival overgrowth
   C. fractured teeth
   D. tongue lacerations and scarring

7. Antiepileptic drugs fall into which of the following pharmaceutical classifications?

   A. muscle relaxants
   B. opioids
   C. central nervous system stimulants
   D. anticonvulsants

8. The most common type of seizure disorder is

   A. absence or petit mal seizures
   B. tonic-clonic or grand mal seizures

9. The injectable drug of choice in the emergency treatment of GTCS or status epilepticus is

   A. phenytoin
   B. carbamazepine
   C. diazepam
   D. codeine

10. Respiratory arrest is most likely to occur during which phase of a generalized tonic-clonic seizure?

    A. aura
    B. preictal
    C. ictal
    D. postictal

Bibliography

Aragon, C. E., and J. Burneo. "Understanding the Patient with Epilepsy and Seizures in the Dental Practice." *Journal of the California Dental Association* 73, no. 1 (2007): 71–76.

Balmer, C., and L. Longman. *The Management of Medical Emergencies: A Guide for Dental Professionals*. 1st ed. London, England: Quay Books, 2008.

Bledsoe, R. E., R. S. Porter, and R. A. Cherry. *Essentials of Paramedic Care*. 2nd ed. Upper Saddle River, NJ: Prentice Hall, 2007.

Chapman, K., and J. M. Rho. "Dietary Therapies for Epilepsy." In *Encyclopedia of Basic Epilepsy Research*, edited by P. Schwartzkroin, 694–701. Waltham, MA: Academic Press, 2009.

Daniel S. J., and S. A. Harfst. *Mosby's Dental Hygiene Concepts, Cases, and Competencies*. 2nd ed. St. Louis, MO: Mosby, 2007.

Darby, M. L. *Mosby's Comprehensive Review of Dental Hygiene*. 6th ed. St. Louis, MO: Mosby, 2006.

Darby, J. L., and M. M. Walsh. (2010). *Dental Hygiene Practice and Theory*. 3rd ed. St. Louis, MO: Saunders, 2010.

Epilepsy Foundation. 2010. "Seizures." http://www.epilepsyfoundation.org

Frazier, M. S., and J. W. Drzymkowski. *Essentials of Human Diseases and Conditions*. 4th ed. St. Louis, MO: Elsevier Saunders, 2009.

Gould, B. E. *Pathophysiology for the Health Professions*. 3rd ed. Philadelphia, PA: Saunders, 2006.

Haller, J. S. "Epilepsy in the Dental Office: Concern, Care and Management." *New York State Dental Journal* 75, no. 3 (2009): 46–47.

Jennings, D., and J. B. Chernega. *Emergency Guide for Dental Auxiliaries*. 4th ed. Albany, NY: Delmar, 2012.

Little, J. W., D. Q. Falace, C. S. Miller, and N. L. Rhodus. *Dental Management of the Medically Compromised Patient*. 7th ed. St. Louis, MO: Saunders, 2008.

Malamed, S. F. *Medical Emergencies in the Dental Office*. 6th ed. St. Louis, MO: Mosby, 2007.

Meiller, T. F., R. L. Wynn, A. M. McMullin, C. Biron, and H. L. Crossley. *Dental Office Medical Emergencies*. 4th ed. Hudson, OH: Lexi-Comp, 2011.

The Merck Manual. "Seizure disorders." http://www.merckmanuals.com/home/brain_spinal_cord_and_nerve_disorders/seizure_disorders/seizure_disorders.html?qt=epilepsy&alt=sh. Accessed October 9, 2001.

Neurology channel. "Epilepsy-seizures." www.neurologychannel.com/seizures. Accessed October 8, 2012.

Pathophysiology Made Incredibly Easy. 4th ed. Philadelphia, PA: Lippincott Williams & Wilkins, 2009.

Pickett, F., and J. Guerenlian. *The Medical History: Clinical Implications and Emergency Prevention in Dental Settings*. Baltimore, MD: Lippincott Williams & Wilkins, 2005.

Porth, C. M. *Pathophysiology*. 8th ed. Baltimore, MD: Lippincott Williams & Wilkins, 2008.

Roach, S. *Pharmacology for Health Professionals*. Baltimore, MD: Lippincott Williams & Wilkins, 2005.

Wilkins, E. M. *Clinical Practice of the Dental Hygienist*. 10th ed. Baltimore, MD: Lippincott Williams, & Wilkins, 2009.

TREATMENT OF THE GENERALIZED TONIC-CLONIC SEIZURE
R.E.P.A.I.R.

R: Recognize signs and symptoms of tonic-clonic seizures: muscles of chest and pharynx may contract producing "epileptic cry"

E: Evaluate level of consciousness: sudden loss of consciousness will occur

P: Position patient supine, turn on left side to minimize aspirations, patient becomes stiff and may fall or slide out of chair, do not try to move patient to floor

A: Activate CAB's of CPR— check circulation, airway, and breathing (pulse and blood pressure) as needed during clonic phase and ensure patent airway

I: Implement appropriate emergency protocol by preventing injury to patient, contact EMS, stop treatment and remove everything from patient's mouth, loosen tight clothing to assist breathing, gently restrain patient and protect head and body from injury during convulsion, do not place anything in the patient's mouth or try to forcibly restrain the patient's extremities, administer O_2 6–8 L/minute
Postictal stage: CNS and respiratory depression require continued monitoring of vitals signs, airway, and level of consciousness

R: Refer to appropriate healthcare professional if indicated or if injury has occurred, reassure patient, and allow patient to recover before discharging to a responsible adult

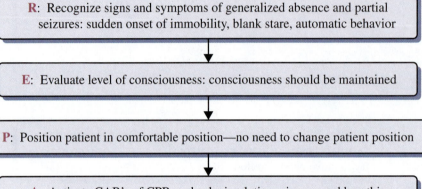

TREATMENT OF GENERALIZED ABSENCE AND PARTIAL SEIZURES
R.E.P.A.I.R.

R: Recognize signs and symptoms of generalized absence and partial seizures: sudden onset of immobility, blank stare, automatic behavior

E: Evaluate level of consciousness: consciousness should be maintained

P: Position patient in comfortable position—no need to change patient position

A: Activate CAB's of CPR—check circulation, airway, and breathing (pulse and blood pressure) if seizure persists more than one minute

I: Implement appropriate emergency protocol if seizure persists; most seizures of this type resolve without incident; reassure patient and determine if seizure was related to dental treatment

R: Refer to appropriate healthcare professional, allow patient to recover before discharging, have emergency contact person drive patient home

9

Cerebrovascular Accident

LEARNING OBJECTIVES

Upon reading the material in this chapter, the reader will be able to:

- ☑ Differentiate the types of cerebrovascular accident (CVA), ischemic versus hemorrhagic.

- ☑ Discuss the concept of TIA and its relation to CVA.

- ☑ Discuss the pathophysiology of both forms of CVA.

- ☑ List specific signs and symptoms associated with CVA.

- ☑ Determine suggested treatment modalities for patients experiencing either type of CVA.

- ☑ Explain the steps needed to prepare an office for a patient experiencing CVA.

- ☑ Discuss precautions to be taken if the patient were to return to the office following a CVA.

Case Study ••➤

Scenario

Your patient Leroy Washington is a 65-year-old black male who is in your office for his four-month dental hygiene recall appointment. Leroy has a history of hypertension, with a baseline blood pressure of 160/110 mmHg. He smokes two packs of cigarettes per day and has a drink or two with dinner to calm his nerves. He takes Cardizem for his hypertension, and his medical history states that he suffers from atrial fibrillation. Leroy informs you that three days ago he was not feeling very well and had some vertigo, mild blurred vision, and some weakness in his right arm. The symptoms lasted about 40 minutes, so he did not call his physician. You take his blood pressure and find that it is 186/124 mmHg, and his pulse rate is 90 beats/minute. Leroy begins to complain of an acute headache, dizziness, loss of vision in one eye, and a tingling feeling on his right side. You notice that his speech is slurred and his breathing is labored at a rate of 12/minute. He remains conscious. From what emergency do you suspect Leory is suffering?

Introduction

A cerebrovascular accident (CVA) or stroke is an abnormal condition of the brain characterized by occlusion or hemorrhage of a blood vessel, resulting in a lack of oxygen to the brain tissues (**ischemia**) that normally receive their blood supply from the damaged vessels. This lack of blood supply to the blood vessels results in a loss of proper oxygenation to the brain cells and eventually cell death. Recently, there has been a move to use the term **brain attack** instead of **stroke** so that the public will become as familiar with CVA's signs and symptoms as they are with a heart attack or myocardial infarction. In so doing, it may be possible to reduce the number of disabilities and deaths resulting from this potentially devastating condition. Moreover, time is of the essence in stroke care so the American Stroke Association (ASA) developed the phrase "Time Is Brain" to stress this concept.

CVAs are the second leading cause of death worldwide, with nearly 4.6 million individuals suffering from the condition annually. In the United States, CVA is ranked as the third leading cause of death and disability, with at least 795,000 new or repeat stroke cases per year. This corresponds to one stroke every minute. It is expected that the number of strokes per year will surpass 1 million in the next few decades. There are several risk factors for CVA. CVA is more often encountered by individuals over 65 years of age, and African Americans seem to be more susceptible than Caucasians. These two groups are more likely to suffer from CVAs as they tend to have a higher incidence of hypertension, which is often a result of **atherosclerosis** (see Chapter 3, Vital Signs). These atherosclerotic plaques on the blood vessel walls in time tend to form thrombi (a blockage composed of various substances, such as platelets, fibrin, and cellular elements at the point of origin) that are the major cause of CVA.

Another group of individuals who are more susceptible to CVAs are those suffering from **atrial fibrillation**, which is a disease that affects approximately 2 million Americans. When a patient is experiencing atrial fibrillation, the two atria of the heart quiver instead of beating properly. This causes the heart to pump blood inefficiently, and the result is pooling of blood with subsequent formation of thrombi.

Atrial fibrillation increases the likelihood of stroke fivefold, and the risk increases as the individual ages or is combined with hypertension, diabetes, or a previous CVA or **transient ischemic attack** (TIA). The annual stroke rate for individuals with atrial fibrillation is about 4.5%.

Younger women who suffer from a CVA often have other risk factors, such as the use of oral contraceptives, headaches, and pregnancy. Older women are at higher risk due to estrogen-associated changes related to menopause.

Diabetic patients also have a higher risk of suffering from CVA as do patients who have previously experienced a CVA or have a familial history of CVA. In addition, individuals who have experienced a TIA are highly susceptible to CVA. TIAs are a "brief episode of neurological dysfunction caused by focal brain ischemia with clinical symptoms typically lasting less than 1 hour without evidence of accompanying infarction on brain imaging." Approximately 200,000–500,000 Americans suffer from TIAs annually. It is estimated that 10% of all strokes are preceded by a TIA. CVA often occurs within the first four days of the TIA, so patients need to be counseled regarding its seriousness.

There is new evidence that there is a relationship between early tooth loss and both ischemic and hemorrhagic CVA. Possible theories for this relationship are the relationship between the microorganisms that cause periodontal disease, a chronic oral infection, producing more inflammatory markers and clotting factors, leading to an increase in platelet aggregation, thus contributing to atherosclerosis and thrombi formation. Another theory suggests that diseases that cause caries and periodontal disease are linked with CVA due to the fact that they share some common lifestyle factors.

Lastly, individuals who suffer from an asymptomatic condition called **carotid bruit** (an abnormal sound in the carotid artery in the neck) have an increased risk of CVA. This condition is highly indicative of atherosclerosis, which has a strong correlation with CVA.

Types of CVA

There are two types of CVA: ischemic or hemorrhagic. (See Table 9.1 ∎) The ischemic type or **occlusive CVA** occurs when there is some form of a blockage in a cerebral blood vessel. The blockage can be either a thrombus or an **embolus** (a foreign object, a quantity of air or gas, or thrombus that originates somewhere in the body and then circulates to another area where it becomes lodged in a blood vessel). The ischemic type of CVA occurs in 85% of patients, with 60% being thrombotic and 40% embolic. The central zone of ischemic tissue is known as the **core** and is deprived of oxygen and glucose, which are critical to the survival of the tissues. The surrounding tissue in the area where the brain tissues receive a diminished blood supply is known as the **penumbra** and is potentially salvageable if arterial blood supply can be restored

Table 9.1   Types of Cerebrovascular Accidents

Hemorrhagic (two types)	Result of a rupture of a blood vessel in the brain; 15% of all CVAs
Intracerebral	Result of a rupture of a blood vessel within the brain tissue; 10% of hemorrhagic CVAs
Subarachnoid	Result of a rupture of a blood vessel on the surface of the brain in the subarachnoid space; 5% of hemorrhagic CVAs
Ischemic (two types)	Result of a blockage of a blood vessel in the brain, causing an oxygen deficiency; 85% of all CVAs
Thrombotic	Blockage composed of various substances, such as platelets, fibrin, and cellular elements at the site of origin; 60% of ischemic CVAs
Embolic	A foreign object, quantity of air, or gas that originates somewhere in the body and then circulates to another area, where it becomes lodged in a blood vessel; 40% of ischemic CVAs

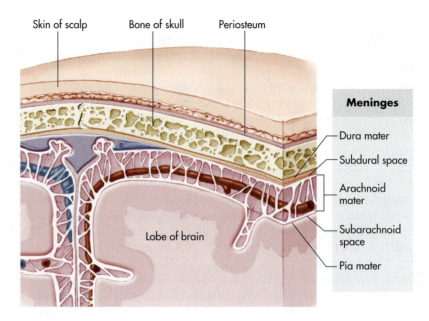

FIGURE 9.1 Layers of the brain.

within several hours of CVA onset; therefore, it is the area that is targeted for therapeutic treatment.

The other type of CVA is hemorrhagic and occurs as a result of the rupture of a blood vessel in the brain. Approximately 15% of all strokes are hemorrhagic, with 10% being the **intracerebral** type and 5% being the subarachnoid type. There are several factors that can lead to a hemorrhagic stroke, such as hypertension, anticoagulation, tumor, or substance abuse (cocaine, amphetamines, or alcohol). In addition, some individuals may have an **aneurysm**, which is a weakening or ballooning of a blood vessel, and with added pressure, such as hypertension, the blood vessel ruptures and causes the stroke.

There are two types of hemorrhagic stroke: intracerebral hemorrhage and subarachnoid hemorrhage. Intracerebral hemorrhagic strokes are twice as common as subarachnoid hemorrhagic strokes. Cerebral hemorrhages occur when a defective artery within the brain bursts and the surrounding tissue fills with blood. The blood places pressure on adjacent brain tissue, which can lead to varying consequences depending on the amount of pressure on the brain tissue. Moreover, because of the ruptured artery, other areas of the brain may be oxygen deprived, leading to damage of those brain cells.

Subarachnoid hemorrhage occurs when a blood vessel on the surface of the brain ruptures and bleeds into the subarachnoid space. The blood places pressure on the cerebellum, which causes pressure damage to the brain cells. (See Figure 9.1 ■)

Hemorrhagic stroke has a much higher mortality rate than occlusive stroke. The size of the initial hemorrhage and hematoma is useful in predicting the patient's outcome, with the larger the area the more serious the consequences. Patients who do survive a hemorrhagic CVA tend to have a better recovery than patients suffering from an ischemic CVA. If the hemorrhagic stroke is treated and the patient survives, the pressure that is causing the damage gradually diminishes and the brain tends to regain some of its former function.

Signs and Symptoms of Ischemic CVA

There are many signs and symptoms associated with an ischemic stroke. The signs and symptoms may stop and start again as the stroke progresses. In addition, the severity and location of the stroke influences the symptoms that are exhibited by

Table 9.2   Signs and Symptoms of Cerebrovascular Accident

Hemorrhagic CVA	Thrombotic CVA	Embolic CVA
• Abrupt onset	• Onset difficult to determine	• Abrupt onset
• Elevated blood pressure	• Total loss of consciousness uncommon	• Total loss of consciousness uncommon
• Altered level of consciousness	• Pupils unequal and dilated	
• Inability to stand or walk	• Confusion	• Confusion
• Pupils unequal and dilated	• Dizziness	• Dizziness
• Pupillary malalignment	• Ataxia	• Ataxia
Subarachnoid hemorrhage	• Vision changes	• Vision changes
• Neck pain or stiffness	• Speech changes	• Speech changes
• Nausea	• Dysphagia	• Dysphagia
• Vomiting	• Deviation of the tongue	• Deviation of the tongue
	• Drooling	• Drooling
Intracerebral hemorrhage	• Hemiparesis	• Hemiparesis
• Nausea	• Nausea	• Nausea
• Vomiting	• Vomiting	• Vomiting

the afflicted individual. The one major difference between the signs and symptoms of embolic and thrombotic strokes is their onset. Embolic strokes tend to have an abrupt onset, whereas the onset of thrombotic strokes is often difficult to determine as the symptoms are often not as severe. As will be discussed later in this chapter, the time of onset is extremely important in determining the appropriate treatment regimen. The signs and symptoms shared by both types of ischemic stroke include the following (See Table 9.2 ■):

1. There is an altered level of consciousness ranging from yawning to coma (however, total loss of consciousness is uncommon). Sudden confusion may also occur.
2. The pupils may be unequal and dilated, confusion and dizziness may be apparent, and there may be a notable change in balance or coordination (**ataxia**). Vision changes, including double vision and blind spots, may occur. **Hemianopia**, the loss of vision in half of the visual field in one or both eyes, may occur.
3. Speech changes are common and can range from poorly articulated speech (dysarthria), impairment of speech (**dysphasia**), to the inability to understand spoken words, to the most severe form, which is the inability to speak at all (**aphasia**).
4. Difficulty swallowing (dysphagia), deviation of the tongue, and drooling are also common symptoms of ischemic stroke.
5. Weakness, numbness, or tingling in the face (usually on only one side and resulting in facial droop) often occurs, as does weakness, numbness, or tingling in an arm or leg (or both) usually on one side of the body (**hemiparesis**).
6. Nausea and vomiting may occur after some time because of increased intracranial pressure.
7. Sudden severe headache may occur with no known cause.

Signs and Symptoms of Hemorrhagic CVA

The signs and symptoms of hemorrhagic stroke have many similarities with those of ischemic stroke, although there are some differences. The onset of symptoms of an individual suffering from an intracerebral hemorrhage will usually be abrupt and rapid. Severe headache is twice as common in hemorrhagic stroke as in ischemic stroke. Two-thirds of all individuals experiencing a hemorrhagic stroke will endure an acute headache commonly occurring in the occipital region. High blood pressure readings are commonly found in hemorrhagic CVA patients. In addition, a specific sign of subarachnoid hemorrhage is neck pain or stiffness. The inability to stand or walk and pupillary malalignment are also signs of hemorrhagic CVA. Nausea and vomiting are commonly seen in intracerebral hemorrhagic and subarachnoid hemorrhagic CVAs. The patient might also experience an altered level of consciousness, ranging from yawning to coma.

Stroke Scales

Early identification of CVA is essential to facilitate prompt treatment of the condition, which is essential to promote an improved prognosis for the patient. There are several scales that can be used to help determine whether a patient is suffering from a CVA. The National Institutes of Health (NIH) developed a rather extensive scale. The Cincinnati Prehospital Stroke Scale (CPSS) is a significantly shortened version of the NIH format and is used by EMS personnel. The survey includes three components that have been consistently identified in individuals with CVA: **facial palsy**, arm motor weakness, and dysarthria. The CPSS is administered as follows:

- The patient is asked to smile while the healthcare provider observes the patient for weakness on one side of the face.
- The patient is asked to hold both arms out with palm up and eyes closed for 10 seconds while the healthcare provider observes for a weakness in one arm. If there is a weakness in both arms or if normal strength is determined, then the patient tests negative for CVA.
- The patient is asked to repeat a simple sentence—"You can't teach an old dog new tricks"—while the healthcare provider observes for difficulty in speech.

If any of the three components are found to be abnormal, then it should be assumed that the patient is experiencing a stroke and proper procedure should ensue.

One other stroke scale that is often used is the Los Angeles Prehospital Stroke Screen (LAPSS). This scale assesses patients on the following variables: age greater than 45 years, prior history of a seizure disorder, time of onset of neurological symptoms less than 24 hours, whether the patient was ambulatory prior to the event, blood glucose level between 60 and 400, facial symmetry, grip strength, and arm weakness determined by drift. Positive responses in all areas indicate the patient is having a CVA. Although this scale provides a better determination of CVA, it takes slightly more time to perform.

Treatment of CVA

The primary goal in CVA treatment is to minimize the cognitive and physical limitations associated with the cerebral ischemia or hemorrhage. If the patient exhibits any signs of CVA, EMS should be contacted immediately and the time of onset of symptoms should be clearly established. The patient should be positioned semisupinely. Basic life support should be initiated by checking the circulation, airway, and breathing (CABs). Fortunately, most patients suffering from CVA and particularly ischemic stroke are able to maintain their CABs during the beginning stages of the event. Oxygen should be administered only if the patient is having dyspnea or shows signs of hypoxia. There is some evidence that additional oxygen may worsen the outcome for the patient. The patient's glucose level should be tested particularly because hypoglycemia may mimic stroke symptoms so it needs to be ruled out as an etiology. Vital signs should be continuously monitored, and the patient should be transported to the emergency department as soon as possible. The importance of transporting the patient to an emergency department that is well equipped to handle CVA patients cannot be overemphasized. Recent studies have indicated that the provision of aspirin for patients with acute ischemic stroke reduced the death and recurrence rates. Surprisingly, patients who were given aspirin and had an intracranial hemorrhage had more favorable outcomes, as well. At the present time, however, it is not recommended for anyone other than the healthcare provider in the emergency department to administer medication to a suspected stroke patient.

Once hospitalized, patients suspected of having some form of CVA need to undergo a CT scan to determine the exact etiology of the symptoms. If the scan indicates a hemorrhagic stroke, the patient will require a consultation with a neurosurgeon, and surgery will be performed. If the scan reveals an ischemic stroke and the onset of the symptoms has been less than three hours, then the current treatment is intravenous thrombolytic therapy with the medication Alteplase. Alteplase is a recombinant tissue plasminogen activator that is often referred to as *r*-tPA. The thrombolytic agent helps to remove the thrombus or embolus in the cerebral blood vessel, thereby restoring blood flow to the area. The use of *r*-tPA after the three-hour window has been shown to be ineffective, and it has been determined that the earlier treatment is begun, the more favorable the outcome; therefore, prompt medical attention is imperative for suspected CVA patients. Some researchers are investigating the use of an intra-arterial thrombolytic agent, particularly in patients with occlusion of a major anterior circulation artery, such as the internal carotid or basilar artery. In these cases, the administration is being studied in patients within 6 to 12 hours of onset of symptoms. The time frame has been extended because of the dire consequences of lack of treatment. Thrombolytic agents are contraindicated for suspected hemorrhagic CVA patients as this will cause additional brain bleeding.

Case Resolution and Conclusion

CVA is a potentially seriously debilitating or fatal condition that can occur in the dental office; therefore, the condition requires swift assessment, diagnosis, and treatment. In the case scenario presented at the beginning of this chapter, Leroy was experiencing a headache, dizziness, loss of vision in one eye, slurred speech, significantly elevated blood pressure, and dyspnea. These signs and symptoms indicate that Leroy is most likely suffering from a thrombotic CVA as he had some symptoms three days ago, but did not pursue treatment. His history of smoking and atrial fibrillation should also alert the clinician that a medical emergency of this type is possible. As soon as the signs and symptoms were recognized, EMS was contacted and Leroy was placed in a semisupine position. Oxygen was administered via non-rebreather mask at 6 L/minute to help relieve his dyspnea. His vital signs were continually monitored; however, there was little improvement to his pulse and blood pressure. The CPSS was administered, and all three components were found to be abnormal, so CVA

(continued)

was verified and glucose monitoring was deemed unnecessary. The individual assisting the clinician noted the time of symptom onset and relayed it to EMS as this would be important to the physician treating the patient in the emergency department. The patient was transported to an emergency department that was specifically equipped to treat CVA patients. Leroy underwent a CT scan, and a thrombotic CVA was diagnosed. He was given *r*-tPA as it had been less than three hours after the initial onset of symptoms. Leroy survived the CVA because of the quick actions of the dental practitioner. After intensive physical therapy, Leroy regained a significant portion of his speech and motor functions. He returned to your office six months later for his oral prophylaxis and was extremely grateful for the swift care he received that led to his full recovery.

Review Questions

1. Which of the following is a condition that often mimics the symptoms of a CVA?

   A. hypoglycemia
   B. hyperventilation
   C. diabetic ketoacidosis
   D. anaphylaxis

2. All of the following are individuals susceptible to CVA *except* one. Which one is the *exception*?

   A. individuals with atrial fibrillation
   B. diabetic patients
   C. young women taking oral contraceptives
   D. males in the 30–40 age range

3. All of the following are symptoms of acute ischemic CVA *except* one. Which one is the *exception*?

   A. vision changes
   B. dysphagia
   C. chest pain
   D. facial droop

4. The preferred treatment for acute ischemic stroke in the emergency department is the administration of intravenous *r*-tPA, and the *r*-tPA needs to be delivered within the first three hours of onset of the CVA symptoms.

   A. The first phrase is true, and the second phrase is false.
   B. The first phrase is false, and the second phrase is true.
   C. Both phrases are true.
   D. Both phrases are false.

5. What can occur in a patient who is experiencing a hemorrhagic CVA and is given *r*-tPA?

   A. formation of a thrombus and worsening symptoms
   B. additional hemorrhage-worsening symptoms
   C. rupturing of an aneurysm and improved symptoms
   D. none of the above

6. Oxygen should be delivered to a patient suspected of a CVA only if

   A. the patient is positioned supinely
   B. the patient is hypoxic
   C. the CVA is hemorrhagic
   D. the blood pressure is below 120/80 mmHg

7. Cerebral hemorrhages occur when a defective artery within the brain bursts and the surrounding tissue fills with blood, whereas subarachnoid hemorrhage strokes occur when a blood vessel on the surface of the brain ruptures and bleeds.

   A. The first phrase is true, and the second phrase is false.
   B. The first phrase is false, and the second phrase is true.
   C. Both phrases are true.
   D. Both phrases are false.

Bibliography

Adeoye, O., and A. Pancioli. "Prehospital and Emergency Department Care of the Patient with Acute Ischemic Stroke." In J. P. Mohr (Ed.), *Stroke: Pathophysiology, Diagnosis, and Management*, 929–44. Philadelphia, PA: Elsevier, Inc., 2004.

Albers, G. W., L. R. Caplan, J. D. Easton, P. B. Fayad, J. P. Mohr, J. L. Saver, and D. G. Sherman. "Transient Ischemic Attack—Proposal for a New Definition." *The New England Journal of Medicine* 342, no. 21 (2002): 1713–16.

American Stroke Association/Ad Council Public Service Announcement. *With a Stroke, Time Lost Is Brain Lost*. http://www.strokeassociation.org/STROKEORG/WarningSigns/Warning-Signs_UCM_308528_SubHomePage.jsp. Accessed November 10, 2011.

Anderson, K. N., L. E. Anderson, and W. D. Glanze, eds. *Mosby's Medical, Nursing & Allied Health Dictionary*. 5th ed. St. Louis, MO: Mosby-Year Book, Inc, 2009.

Benavente, O., and R. G. Hart.. "Stroke: Part II. Management of Acute Ischemic Stroke." *American Family Physician* 59, no. 10 (1999): 2828–34.

Bennett, J. D., and M. B. Rosenberg. *Medical Emergencies in Dentistry*. 1st ed. Philadelphia, PA: W. B. Saunders, 2002.

Bradley, R. N. "Educating the Public about Stroke." *Disease Management Health Outcomes* 11, no. 5 (2003): 321–25.

Flemming, K. D., and R. D. Brown. "Secondary Prevention Strategies in Ischemic Stroke: Identification and Optimal Management of Modifiable Risk Factors." *Mayo Clinic Proceedings* 79, no. 10 (2004): 1330–40.

Fulgham, J. R., T. J. Infall, L. G. Stead, H. J. Cloft, E. F M. Widdicks, and K. D. Flemming. "Management of Acute Ischemic Stroke." *Mayo Clinic Proceedings* 79, no. 11 (2004): 1459–69.

Gorelick, P. B., and S. Rulan. "Diagnosis and Management of Acute Ischemic Stroke." *Disease-a-Month* 56 (2010): 72–100.

Gurenlian, J. R., and C. Kleiman. "Cerebrovascular Accident." *Access* 6, no. 16 (2002): 40–47.

Hart, R. G., and O. Benavente. "Stroke: Part I. A Clinical Update on Prevention." *American Family Physician* 59, no. 9 (1999): 2475–82.

Hines, S. "New Treatments, New Risk Factors for Acute Ischemic Stroke." *Patient Care* 33, no. 6 (1999): 144–56.

Jauch, E. C., B. Cucchiara, O. Adeoye, W. Merurer, J. Brice, Y. Chan, N. Gentile, and F. Hazinski. "Part II: Adult Stroke: 2010 American Heart Association Guidelines for Cardiopulmonary Resuscitation and Emergency Cardiovascular Care." *Circulation* 122 suppl. 3 (2010): S818–28.

Kassner, S. E., and J. C. Grotta. "Emergency Identification and Treatment of Acute Ischemic Stroke." *Annals of Emergency Medicine* 30, no. 5 (1997): 642–53.

Kirschner, H. S. "Medical Prevention of Stroke." *Southern Medical Journal* 96, no. 4 (2003): 354–58.

Murphy, J. "Pharmacological Treatment of Acute Ischemic Stroke." *Critical Care Nursing* 26, no. 4 (2003): 276–82.

Newman, J. "Diagnosis and Treatment of Stroke." *Radiologic Technology* 73, no. 4 (2002): 305–34.

Nunn, T. "Developing a Medical Emergency Protocol." *Access* (2006): 12–15.

O'Rourke, F., H. Dean, N. Akhrar, and A. Shuaib. "Current and Future Concepts in Stroke Prevention." *Canadian Medical Association Journal* 170, no. 7 (2004): 1123–33.

Sayre, M. R. "Damage Control: Past, Present, and Future of Prehospital Stroke Management." *Emergency Medicine Clinics of North America* 20, no. 4 (2002): 877–86.

Schretzman, D. "Acute Ischemic Stroke." *Dimensions of Critical Care Nursing* 20, no. 2 (2001): 14–21.

Smithard, D. G. "Management of Stroke: Acute, Rehabilitation and Long-Term Care." *Hospital Medicine* 64, no. 11 (2003): 666–72.

Solenski, N. J. "Transient Ischemic Attacks: Part I. Diagnosis and Evaluation." *American Family Physician* 69, no. 7 (2004): 1665–78.

Suyama, J., and T. Crocco. "Prehospital Care of the Stroke Patient." *Emergency Medicine Clinics of North America* 20, no. 3 (2002): 537–52.

Swadron, S. P., S. L. Selco, K. A. Kim, G. Fischberg, and G. Sung. "The Acute Cerebrovascular Event: Surgical and Other Interventional Therapies." *Emergency Medical Clinics of North America* 21, no. 4 (2003): 847–72.

Thurman, R. J., and E. C. Jauch. "Acute Ischemic Stroke: Emergent Evaluation and Management." *Emergency Medicine Clinics of North America* 20, no. 3 (2002): 609–30.

Warlow, C., C. Sudlow, M. Dennis, J. Wardlaw, and P. Sandercock. "Stroke." *The Lancet* 362, no. 939 (2003): 1211–24.

Weinberger, J. "Prevention and Management of Cerebrovascular Events in Primary Care." *Geriatrics* 57, no. 1 (2002): 38–43.

Writing Group Members, D. Lloyd-Jones, R. Adams, M. Carnethon, G. DeSimone, T. B. Ferguson, K. Flegal, et al. "Heart Disease and Stroke Statistics–2009 update." *Circulation* 119 (2008): e21-181.

Yoshida, M., and Y. Akagawa. "The Relationship Between Tooth Loss and Cerebral Stroke." *Japanese Dental Science Review* 47 (2011): 157–69.

PEARSON
myhealthprofessionskit™

Use this address to access the Companion Website created for this textbook. Simply select "Dental Hygiene" from the choice of disciplines. Find this book and log in using your username and password to access interactive activities, videos, and much more.

TREATMENT OF CVA
R.E.P.A.I.R.

R: Recognize signs & symptoms of CVA: altered level of consciousness, headache, unequal pupils, confusion, dizziness, lack of coordination or balance, vision changes, impaired speech, difficulty swallowing, weakness, numbness or tingling on ones side of the face or body, possible nausea or vomiting, neck pain or stiffness

E: Evaluate symptoms using stroke scale: 1. Observe patient for weakness on one side of face 2. ask patient to hold arms out with palms up and eyes closed for 10 seconds and observe patient for weakness in one arm 3. ask patient to repeat "the sky is blue in Cincinnati" and observe for difficulty in speech

P: Position patient semi-upright

A: Activate CAB's of CPR—check circulation, airway, and breathing (pulse and blood pressure)

I: Implement appropriate emergency protocol for CVA: contact EMS immediately, administer oxygen 4–6 L/min if the patient is hypoxic, monitor vital signs continuously, check glucose level to rule out hypoglycemia

R: Refer to emergency department as soon as possible as some CVA patients require treatment with a thrombolytic agent within 3 hours of onset

10

Angina Pectoris and Acute Myocardial Infarction

LEARNING OBJECTIVES

Upon reading the material in this chapter, the reader will be able to:

☑ Discuss the factors that increase the risk for development of coronary artery disease (CAD).

☑ Describe the pathophysiology associated with the development of CAD.

☑ Describe the factors that may precipitate an anginal attack or acute myocardial infarction (AMI).

☑ Differentiate among the various forms of angina pectoris (including presentation of symptoms).

☑ Differentiate between cardiac-related and noncardiac-related chest pain.

☑ Describe the procedure for the management of a dental patient experiencing an anginal attack.

☑ Differentiate between the symptoms associated with an anginal attack and an AMI.

☑ Describe the procedure for the management of a dental patient experiencing an AMI.

☑ Describe the procedure for the management of a dental patient experiencing cardiac arrest.

Case Study •••➤

Scenario

Your patient, Manny Rodriquez, is a 55-year-old accountant. Upon completion of his medical/dental history, you note that Mr. Rodriquez presents with the following vital signs: blood pressure of 132/88 mmHg, respiration rate of 20 breaths/minute, and pulse rate of 80 beats/minute. He reports that his present health is "fair." You note that the patient has a heart disorder for which he takes 120 mg of diltiazem daily, 20 mg of atorvastatin calcium daily, 81 mg of aspirin daily, and nitrostat as needed. He smokes 20 cigarettes daily and has done so for 35 years. Upon further questioning, Mr. Rodriquez discloses that he has chest pain about once a week, particularly during physical exertion and periods of stress. He tells you that he is a little tense at the thought of you "scraping" under his gums and he has postponed dental care because of fear of the dentist. Suddenly he has severe, crushing pain in his chest, left arm, and shoulder. He is having difficulty breathing, his skin is pale and clammy, and he is clutching his fist to his chest.

Introduction

The sudden onset of chest pain in a patient receiving dental care is not uncommon. The causes may be cardiac or noncardiac in origin. Chest pain of cardiac origin is most often the result of **coronary artery disease** (CAD; also called coronary heart disease). CAD and its associated complications result in the greatest number of deaths each year in the United States. There are numerous causes of CAD, all of which somehow reduce the flow of oxygenated blood to the heart muscle (**myocardium**). Atherosclerosis of the coronary arteries is the major cause of CAD and results in inadequate oxygenation of the myocardium (**myocardial ischemia**). If left untreated, CAD can result in **angina pectoris** or in severe instances **acute myocardial infarction (AMI)** or heart attack. Dental professionals will undoubtedly treat patients who present with diagnosed or undiagnosed CAD. A thorough evaluation of every patient's medical history is critical prior to the initiation of any dental treatment. The dental clinician must be able to identify factors that may indicate the risk for CAD and/or noncardiac-related chest pain, recognize the clinical signs and symptoms of an ischemic attack, and be prepared to deal with the potentially life-threatening medical emergency that may result. Chances of survival increase significantly if appropriate emergency procedures are activated at the onset of symptoms.

Risk Factors for Coronary Artery Disease

Atherosclerotic heart disease is another common name for CAD. Atherosclerosis is a slow, complex inflammatory arterial disease that typically starts in childhood and often progresses with age. Atherosclerosis of the coronary arteries is a major etiologic factor in the development of all forms of cardiovascular disease and is most likely the cause of myocardial ischemia. There is some evidence that atherosclerosis begins with an injury or damage to the endothelium (inner lining of the artery). Damage to the arterial wall can be caused by elevated blood levels of cholesterol and triglycerides, tobacco smoke, diabetes, high blood pressure, and infectious micro-organisms. Atherosclerosis is characterized by a buildup of yellowish plaques on the inner walls of large and medium-sized elastic and muscular arteries. (See Figure 10.1 ■) Arterial plaque is composed of cholesterol, lipids, platelets, calcium, and cellular debris. As the plaque deposit increases in size, it restricts the opening of the artery, resulting in a decrease in blood/oxygen flow to the heart, brain, and/or extremities. Occlusion of an artery or arteries can result in silent ischemic episodes, angina pectoris, AMI, and stroke.

Based on findings from the Framingham Heart Study, the American Heart Association has identified multiple risk factors associated with the development of CAD. (See Table 10.1 ■) The recognition of these risk factors and their role in the development of cardiovascular disease is critical to prevention and treatment. Some of these factors can be modified, treated, or controlled, whereas others cannot. Major risk factors that cannot be modified include gender, increasing age, and heredity (including race). Risk factors that can be modified, controlled, or treated include obesity, physical inactivity, high blood pressure, high cholesterol, and the use of smoking tobacco.

Gender

Historically, CAD has been considered to predominately affect males. This may be partly because women were less likely to be referred for diagnosis and treatment of possible CAD; however, cardiovascular disease, particularly CAD and stroke, is the leading cause of death among women in the United States and in most developed countries. As a result, more and more research has been directed toward the study of women and cardiovascular disease. Most of the risk factors associated with CAD are the same for women and men; however, the impact of the individual risk factors may be different. For example, there is some evidence that diabetes, elevated high-density lipoproteins (HDLs), and/or triglyceride levels pose an increased risk for CAD in women when compared to men. On the other hand, women have a roughly 10-year

Table 10.1 **Risk Factors for Coronary Artery Disease**

- Gender
- Increasing age
- Heredity (including race)
- Tobacco use
- Hypertension
- Hypercholesterolemia
- Diabetes
- Obesity and lack of physical activity

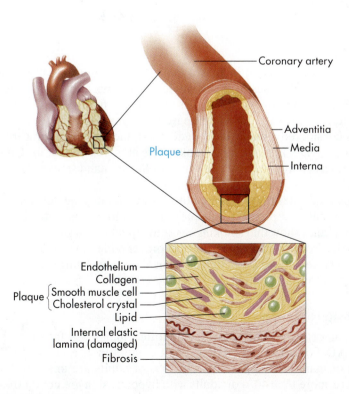

Endothelium
Collagen
Plaque { Smooth muscle cell
Cholesterol crystal
Lipid
Internal elastic lamina (damaged)
Fibrosis

Coronary artery
Adventitia
Media
Interna
Plaque

FIGURE 10.1 Atherosclerosis.

age advantage over men when considering the risk for CAD. This is most likely the result of one factor unique to women: the influence of their hormonal status on CAD. Endogenous estrogens seem to positively affect cardiovascular health; thus the incidence of CAD in premenopausal women is significantly lower when compared to men of the same age. Postmenopausal women are at increased risk for CAD. The use of hormone replacement therapy (HRT) in postmenopausal women may reduce the risk for CAD, but increase the risk for other diseases, including breast cancer. The benefits and risks need to be assessed on an individual basis before HRT is recommended specifically for the prevention of CAD.

Increasing Age

Increasing age increases the risk for CAD in men and women, primarily as a result of progressive atherosclerosis of the coronary arteries associated with aging. Most new-onset CAD occurs after age 65, and primary prevention efforts (modifying risk factors or preventing development of risk factors) should be directed to the "young" elderly (ages 65 to 75).

Heredity (Including Race)

A family history of premature CAD is considered a risk for CAD. Premature CAD is defined as CAD that occurs in a first-degree female relative younger than age 65 or a first-degree male relative younger than age 55. It is often difficult to determine the independent effect of genetics on the development of CAD. Almost always a familial disposition to CAD is mediated by other risk factors, such as high blood pressure and high cholesterol; however, a patient who presents with a family history of premature heart disease should be considered at increased risk.

The mortality rates for CAD differ among the major ethnic groups in the United States. African Americans have the highest CAD mortality rates. When compared to other race/sex groups, middle-aged black men have especially high mortality rates for CAD. Non-Hispanic whites have the second highest mortality rate followed by Hispanics, Native Americans, and Asians. African American women have higher CAD mortality rates when compared to non-Hispanic women.

Tobacco Use

The use of smoking tobacco increases the risk for a multitude of diseases, including cardiovascular diseases. It is the single most important modifiable risk factor for CAD. Smokers are two to four times more likely to develop CAD (particularly angina pectoris and AMI) when compared to nonsmokers. In addition, cigarette smoking is considered a major independent risk factor for sudden cardiac death in patients with CAD. Cigar and pipe smokers are at increased risk for CAD, although the risk is not as great as in cigarette smokers. Secondhand smoke also increases the risk of CAD.

Research indicates that smoking not only accelerates the development of coronary plaques, but also promotes plaque rupture and coronary thrombosis. On the other hand, studies show that smoking cessation quickly and significantly reduces the risk for AMI. Cigarette smoking is the most preventable cause of death in the United States. Tobacco cessation counseling or referral for counseling should be part of the treatment plan for those patients with a tobacco habit.

Hypertension

Hypertension or high blood pressure is another major risk factor in the development of CAD. Fortunately hypertension, if diagnosed, is a risk factor that can be prevented or managed. Approximately 30% of adults are unaware that they are hypertensive, more than 40% of adults with hypertension are not on treatment, and two-thirds of patients receiving treatment for hypertension are not being controlled to blood pressure levels of less than 140/90 mmHg. Current research indicates that in persons over the age of 50, systolic blood pressure greater than 140 mmHg is a more important risk factor in the development of cardiovascular disease than diastolic blood pressure. In addition, persons who have normal blood pressure at age 55 will have a 90% lifetime risk of developing hypertension. It is clear that dental professionals will encounter patients who are at risk for high blood pressure (prehypertension) or who have undiagnosed or diagnosed but uncontrolled blood pressure. A thorough knowledge of the updated guidelines for the classification of blood pressure is critical. (See Table 10.2 ■) A complete medical history, including the taking and recording of blood pressure and vital signs, should be part of every assessment. Referral to a physician is appropriate for patients presenting with undiagnosed or uncontrolled hypertension.

Hypercholesterolemia

Cholesterol is a waxy, fatlike substance made in the liver. It is also found in food derived from animals, including meat and dairy products, such as eggs, cheese, and milk. A small amount of cholesterol is necessary to aid the digestion of fat. Too much cholesterol (hypercholesterolemia) can result in atherosclerosis and CAD. Cholesterol attaches to a protein (lipoprotein) and is carried through the bloodstream. There are several of these lipoproteins, and they are classified based on the proportion of protein to fat. **Low-density lipoprotein** (LDL) can cause atherosclerosis. Optimal serum levels of LDL are less than 100 mg/dL. Levels about 160–189 mg/dL are considered high/very high. **High-density lipoprotein** helps rid the body of LDL. High blood serum levels of HDL help to prevent CAD; levels of 60 mg/dL are desirable. **Triglycerides** are another form of fat found in the bloodstream. Increased serum levels, 150–200 mg/dL or greater, may also increase the risk for CAD. Optimal total serum cholesterol levels are less than 200 mg/dL, although the risk for CAD is lower still at levels less than 160 mg/dL.

Diabetes

One of the most common complications of diabetes (both types) is cardiovascular disease as a result of atherosclerosis and hypertension. Atherosclerosis in diabetics is often accelerated, more severe, and more widespread than in nondiabetics. The term **macroangiopathy** refers to damage done to the large blood vessels in diabetics as a result of atherosclerosis. Hypertension is at least twice as common in diabetics versus nondiabetics. Microvascular damage as a result of hyperglycemia diminishes vascular function, thus making the consequences of atherosclerosis and hypertension more difficult to withstand. Approximately 75% of patients with diabetes die from some form of cardiovascular disease or complication.

Table 10.2 **Blood Pressure Classification for Adults**

	Systolic Blood Pressure (mmHg)	Diastolic Blood Pressure (mmHg)
Normal	<120	and <80
Prehypertension	120–139	or 80–89
Stage 1 hypertension	140–159	or 90–99
Stage 2 hypertension	≥160	or ≥100

Adapted from U.S. Department of Health and Human Services: National Institutes of Health, National Heart, Lung, and Blood Institute (2004). *The Seventh Report of the Joint National Committee on Prevention, Detection, Evaluation, and Treatment of High Blood Pressure.* Retrieved from http://www.nhlbi.nih.gov/guidelines/hypertension/jnc7full.pdf

Obesity and Physical Activity

The American population is becoming increasingly overweight and inactive. Obesity and lack of physical activity negatively impact CAD primarily through their effect on the major risk factors. Obesity is directly related to the increasing rise in the incidence of type 2 diabetes. Weight control, diet, and exercise can positively impact hypertension and hypercholesterolemia.

Angina Pectoris

A patient experiencing chest pain due to angina pectoris is one of the more common medical emergencies encountered in the dental office; thus patients with a history of angina present an increased risk during dental treatment. It is most often the product of an inadequate supply and/or increased demand for oxygen to the myocardium (myocardial ischemia), although rarely it may be associated with valvular heart disease, uncontrolled hypertension, or hypertrophic cardiomyopathy (an abnormality in the structure and function of the heart muscle).

Forms of Angina

CAD, most commonly presenting as angina or AMI, is the leading cause of sudden death in the United States. Three types of angina have been described: stable, unstable, and variant (Prinzmetal's angina).

Stable angina (typical, chronic, classic, or exertional angina) is usually related to CAD and is the most common form of angina. It is usually induced by physical activity and/or stress, and the symptoms are often worse in cold weather or after a large meal. The intensity of a stable anginal attack may vary from mild to severe. The chest pain associated with angina presents as a dull, constant pressure rather than sharp, stabbing, and knifelike pain. There is predictable and reproducible discomfort in the left area of the chest, generally lasting anywhere from 1 to 15 minutes. Stable angina responds positively to rest and/or nitroglycerin, usually within 10 to 15 minutes. Angina is considered stable if the patient has had no changes in the frequency or duration of symptoms within the previous 60 days or there have been no changes in the precipitating causes of the attack.

Patients with stable angina are usually under the care of a physician and are often taking combinations of calcium-channel blockers, beta-adrenergic blocking agents, and nitrates. Regular exercise reduces the frequency of symptoms and increases the functional capacity of the heart muscle. Patients with stable angina can receive dental care, but should be scheduled for short, minimally stressful appointments.

Unstable angina (UA) is also known as preinfarctory angina, coronary insufficiency, crescendo angina, intermediate coronary syndrome, and premature or impending AMI. As these names imply, UA presents as a clinical syndrome that falls between stable angina and AMI and represents an imbalance between myocardial oxygen supply and demand. Of the 8 million patients with chest pain who visit a hospital's emergency department annually, 1.4 million have UA. Up to 50% of patients with UA will develop an AMI within a few hours of arriving at the emergency department.

Five different causes of UA are currently recognized, and these causes are not necessarily mutually exclusive. They are (1) a nonocclusive thrombus on a preexisting plaque, (2) a coronary spasm or vasoconstriction (dynamic obstruction), (3) progressive mechanical obstruction, (4) inflammation and/or infection, and (5) secondary UA caused by other factors. The first four causes are primarily related to coronary plaques that have undergone repeated phases of destruction and repair, ultimately resulting in a reduction in supply of oxygen to the myocardium. Secondary UA is primarily related to an increase in demand for oxygen by the myocardium in the presence of a restricted oxygen supply (i.e., fever, tachycardia, hypotension, and hypoxemia).

Angina pectoris is considered unstable if it presents with at least one of the following three features: (1) the angina occurs at rest or with minimal exertion and lasts more than 20 minutes without the interruption of nitroglycerin; (2) the onset is new, and the pain is severe and definite; (3) the pain is more severe, more frequent, and more prolonged (can last up to 30 minutes) than angina experienced in the past. In addition, UA is classified based on the clinical circumstances of the anginal episode as well as the severity of the ischemic attack.

Patients with UA should receive only minimal or emergency dental care after consultation with a physician. Administration of nitroglycerin may or may not relieve the anginal pain, and patients with UA are at high risk for an AMI. The administration of a vasoconstrictor is contraindicated in patients presenting with UA. Only emergency dental care should be considered for these patients following consultation with their physician. The dental needs of these patients might be best met in a hospital setting.

Variant angina, also known as **Prinzmetal's angina**, atypical, or vasoplastic angina, usually occurs spontaneously. The symptoms are similar to the other forms of angina; however, the majority of these anginal episodes occur while the person is at rest (neither emotional stress nor physical exertion triggers an attack) and at odd hours of the day or night. They are more common in women under 50 and those thought to be at low risk for CAD. A transient spasm of a coronary artery causing a brief occlusion of the vessel is thought to precipitate an attack. Although two-thirds of people who suffer with variant angina have severe coronary atherosclerosis in at least one major artery, Prinzmetal's angina can occur in persons without CAD. An angiogram or cardiac catheterization may be required to identify any underlying CAD before a definitive diagnosis of variant angina can be made. Administration of nitroglycerin generally provides prompt relief of pain. Extreme caution should be used if administering vasoconstrictors to these patients.

Prevention of the Anginal Episode

As with most medical emergencies, assessment of the potential risks and subsequent modification of treatment provided can help to prevent an emergency situation. A complete, comprehensive medical history and thorough evaluation of the history is essential to identify those patients who may be at risk for, or those who present with, CAD. Patients with UA should receive emergency dental treatment only following consultation with a physician. The use of vasoconstrictors in local anesthetic agents is contraindicated, and necessary dental treatment is best provided in a hospital setting.

Patients presenting with stable angina generally can be treated in the dental office. In the dental environment, emotional and physical stresses are often present for the patient. These are both precipitating factors for an anginal episode, so dental treatment should be modified to reduce the stress for the patient. Anginal patients, as all patients, should have their vital signs monitored and recorded at every visit.

Length of appointment time should be adjusted based on the history of the patient's anginal episodes. Generally shorter appointments are preferable, and treatment should end if the patient begins to demonstrate signs of fatigue, stress, or anxiety. Research indicates the endogenous epinephrine levels peak during the morning hours, and the majority of heart attacks occur between 8:00 a.m. and 11:00 a.m.; therefore, late morning and afternoon appointments are recommended.

The use of local anesthetic agents containing a vasoconstrictor on a stable anginal patient (ASA III) is generally not contraindicated; however, the maximum recommended dosage of epinephrine for a cardiac-risk patient is 0.04 mg. This equates to approximately two cartridges (1.7 mL cartridges) of a local anesthetic agent containing a 1:100,000 concentration of epinephrine. Vasoconstrictors should be used with caution on those patients being treated with nonselective β-adrenergic blockers for the management of their angina or other cardiovascular disorders. Patients taking these types of drugs are at increased risk for a hypertensive episode if a vasoconstrictor is administered. UA patients (ASA IV) should not receive local anesthetics with vasoconstrictors.

Anginal patients may benefit from the use of supplemental oxygen at a flow rate of 3 to 5 L/minute via a nasal cannula. (See Figure 10.2 ■) This minimizes the risk of inadequate oxygenation of the myocardium during treatment. It is also suggested

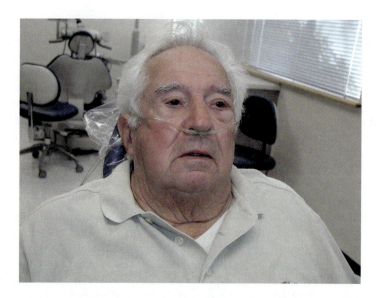

FIGURE 10.2 Anginal patient with nasal cannula to deliver oxygen.

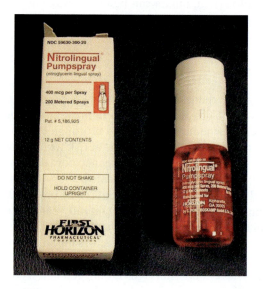

FIGURE 10.3 Nitroglycerin.

that the patient bring his or her nitroglycerin spray or tablets to the appointment and it be readily accessible if needed. (See Figure 10.3 ■) If nitroglycerin is necessary, it is preferable to use the patient's own supply (assuming it has not expired) because the dosage will be correct for that patient. The emergency kit in the dental setting should also be supplied with fresh nitroglycerin (nitrolingual spray is preferred because it is more stable than tablets).

Signs and Symptoms of an Anginal Attack

Stable or typical angina is characterized by generalized chest discomfort rather than frank pain. This discomfort is often described as a pressure, burning, heaviness, squeezing, or choking sensation that often radiates from the thoracic area to a shoulder (usually left), down the arm, and to the neck, lower jaw, or tongue. In many cases diaphoresis, nausea, and pallor are present. The attacks can vary in intensity and last from 1 to 15 minutes. During acute anginal episodes, the patient may be notably apprehensive, may press his or her fist to the sternum (the **Levine sign**), and the heart rate and blood pressure may be significantly elevated. (See Table 10.3 ■) Many predisposing or precipitating factors are associated with angina, including exercise, stress and/or anxiety, use of smoking tobacco, secondhand tobacco smoke, extreme temperatures, a very full stomach, and high altitude.

Unstable angina presents with all of the symptoms of stable angina, but may occur for no apparent reason. The intensity may be more acute, and the episode may last for as long as 30 minutes.

Variant angina has some, but not all, of the symptoms of typical angina. It is more likely to occur at rest and is often associated with dysrhythmias. Additional symptoms can include palpitations, syncope, and dyspnea.

Noncardiac-related chest pain is generally more localized in nature. Patients report a stabbing, knifelike pain that is aggravated by movement and breathing. Chest pain lasting less than 30 seconds is generally not cardiac related.

Treatment of an Anginal Episode

The primary goal in the treatment of an anginal episode is to decrease the myocardium's demand for oxygen. If the patient experiences an anginal episode during treatment, the procedure should be terminated and the patient should be placed in a semisupine or upright position. The circulation, airway, and breathing should be assessed. Oxygen at 100% via a nasal cannula or non-rebreather bag can be administered at any time during the management of this medical emergency. Vital signs should be monitored throughout the treatment of the anginal episode.

Assuming that the patient is conscious, sublingual (e.g., tablet), or transmucosal (e.g., nitrolingual spray), nitroglycerin should be administered immediately. It is preferable to use the patient's own nitroglycerin if possible because the dosage will be accurate for that patient—usually 0.3 to 0.6 mg. If the patient's nitroglycerin is expired or has lost potency due to improper storage, use the fresh nitroglycerin stored in the emergency kit. The drug is still potent if the patient experiences a tingling sensation on the tongue as the tablet dissolves. If sublingual tablets are used, administer one tablet every five minutes, not to exceed three tablets every 15 minutes. If using the nitrolingual spray, one or two metered sprays are recommended initially, with no more than three metered doses within a 15-minute period. Nitroglycerin dilates the blood vessels, resulting in a decrease in cardiac work load. This results in a decrease in the demand for oxygen by the myocardium. The administration of nitroglycerin normally reduces or eliminates anginal pain within two to four minutes. The administration of nitroglycerin is contraindicated in patients with hypotension (SBP < 90 mmHg or ≥ 30 mmHg below baseline), extreme bradycardia (<50 bpm), and tachycardia in the absence of heart failure (>100 bpm), or patients who have recently taken phosphodiesterase-5 (PDE-5) inhibitors (sildenafil, tadalafil, or vardenafil) for erectile dysfunction. Following the administration of the drug, the patient may experience tachycardia, flushing, a pounding or fullness in the head, as well as possible hypotension. Dental treatment may be resumed if the patient feels well enough to continue; however, it may be more prudent to reschedule the patient and complete the treatment at another appointment.

As mentioned previously, nitroglycerin will not be effective if it has expired or lost some of its potency, nor will it be effective if the patient is experiencing an AMI. In patients with known angina pectoris, 9-1-1 should be activated if the chest pain is not relieved by two dosages of nitroglycerin (spray or tablet) over a 10-minute time period. Also, if the patient states that the pain is more severe than previously experienced, then EMS should be contacted immediately. If the patient has no known history of angina pectoris and the chest pain persists for two minutes or longer, 9-1-1 should be activated immediately and then the steps for treating a known anginal attack should be followed.

Table 10.3   Signs and Symptoms of Anginal Attack

- Pressure, burning, heaviness, squeezing in chest
- Pain radiating to shoulders, arms, neck, lower jaw, or tongue
- Diaphoresis
- Nausea
- Pallor
- Apprehension
- Levine sign
- Elevation of pulse
- Elevation of blood pressure
- Attacks lasting from 1 to 15 minutes

Acute Myocardial Infarction

Acute myocardial infarction (AMI) is necrosis of a portion of the myocardium due to total or partial occlusion of a coronary artery. (See Figure 10.4 ■) An occlusion is caused by atherosclerosis, a thrombus, or a coronary spasm; it may form rapidly or occur over a prolonged period of time. Anyone experiencing an AMI is at risk for going into complete cardiac arrest, where the heart fails to beat. In the first couple of hours after the onset of symptoms of an AMI, the development of cardiac dysrhythmia presents the greatest risk for death. Dysrhythmia may present as bradycardia (slow heart rate), ventricular tachycardia (rapid contraction rate with inadequate ventricular filling), **ventricular fibrillation** (VF) (rapid, disorganized, irregular contractions of the ventricle), or **asystole** (complete absence of heart contractions). Since more than half of the deaths from an AMI occur outside of the hospital most within the first few hours after the onset of symptoms, provision of basic life support (BLS) during the time spent waiting for the EMTs (emergency medical technicians) to arrive is critical and could save a life. This means that the entire dental office staff need to be adequately prepared to handle the emergency, including certification in BLS and use of an automated external defibrillator (AED).

Signs and Symptoms of an Acute Myocardial Infarction

Survival from an AMI is dependent on early and appropriate treatment, and it is vital to recognize the signs and symptoms of an AMI. The classic symptom of an AMI is chest pain or discomfort that lasts 20 minutes or longer. Typically victims describe feeling pressure, tightness, heaviness, burning, squeezing, or a crushing sensation in the middle of the chest and/or lower third of the epigastrium. The pain may radiate down the arms, shoulders, neck, jaw, or back. The victim may also experience weakness, dyspnea, diaphoresis, and an irregular pulse. Nausea and vomiting may occur, especially if the pain is intense. In addition, patients experiencing an AMI may seem very apprehensive and express an intense sense of impending doom. They often clutch their fist to their chest (the classic Levine sign). (See Table 10.4 ■)

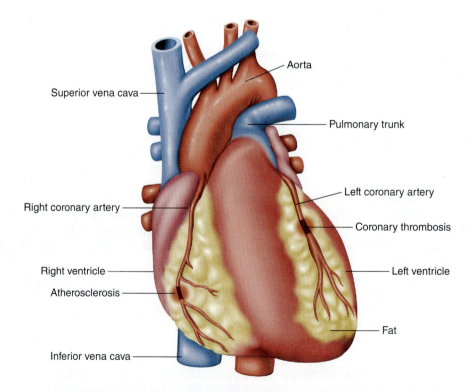

FIGURE 10.4 Blockage of coronary arteries.

TREATMENT OF AN ACUTE MYOCARDIAL INFARCTION **105**

Not all MI victims experience the classic symptoms just described. Women often experience atypical discomfort, upper abdominal pain, shortness of breath, and fatigue. Diabetics are more likely to experience "silent" MI. Elderly persons may exhibit shortness of breath, dizziness, pulmonary edema, altered mental status, or an arrhythmia. It should be noted that many of the symptoms discussed could be related to a noncardiac event. It is important to treat chest pain as cardiac related until a cardiac cause can be ruled out.

Treatment of an Acute Myocardial Infarction

Management of an AMI begins with recognition of the signs and symptoms and initiation of the basic steps for life support. In the dental setting, treatment should be stopped immediately with the onset of chest pain. If the patient has a history of angina, the steps for treatment of an anginal episode should be initiated. If the patient has no history of angina, the situation should be treated as if the pain was cardiac in origin unless another cause can be determined.

If an AMI is suspected to be the cause of the chest pain, position the patient in a comfortable position; assess circulation, airway, and breathing; and activate the EMS system immediately. Oxygen should be administered as soon as possible via a nasal cannula or non-rebreather mask at a flow rate of 2 to 6 L/minute. If the patient has a history of angina, nitroglycerin from the patient's own supply should be administered if possible. If the patient has no history of angina pectoris, nitroglycerin from the emergency kit should be administered. Vital signs should be recorded prior to administering the nitroglycerin. Nitroglycerin should not be administered to patients with a systolic pressure less than 100 mmHg. If the patient is suffering from an anginal attack, the nitroglycerin should act to alleviate the pain within two to four minutes. If the pain continues following the administration of three doses of nitroglycerin over a 15-minute period or if the pain diminishes and then returns, the situation should be managed as a potential AMI.

Fibrinolysis should be initiated as soon as the symptoms are identified as those of an AMI. Aspirin has a proven antithrombotic effect and assists in revascularization of the myocardium during an ischemic attack. (See Figure 10.5 ■) Unless the patient has a significant allergy to aspirin or the possibility of life-threatening hemorrhage exists, a 324-mg dose of aspirin (4 mg × 81 mg of acetylsalicylic acid) should be administered orally, chewed, and swallowed by all patients suspected of experiencing an AMI or UA. Chewing the tablet permits the acetylsalicylic acid to be absorbed through the oral mucous membranes and enter the bloodstream more quickly. When chewed, the clinical effects of the aspirin are realized in about 20 minutes. When swallowed, the clinical effects of the drug are delayed considerably.

Vital signs should continue to be monitored and recorded every five minutes. Management of pain while the patient is waiting for the EMTs to arrive may be required to help prevent cardiogenic shock. Nitroglycerin is usually inadequate for the relief of pain associated with an AMI. Opioid analgesics (morphine or meperidine) are recommended, but are not usually available in the dental setting. The analgesic properties of N_2O combined with O_2 (nitrous oxide and oxygen) provide a good alternative for pain control, with little effect on the blood pressure. If N_2O is available, administer it with O_2 at a concentration approximating 35%. This will usually manage the pain completely or reduce it to a tolerable level.

If the patient goes into full cardiac arrest at any time during the management of an AMI, CPR should begin immediately. Because VF occurs in about 90% of all cardiac arrests, defibrillation may be required. Healthcare providers should be trained in using an AED and be ready to use one if available. According to the American Heart Association, for victims of a witnessed cardiac arrest with VF, the immediate initiation of CPR and use of an AED within the first three to five minutes provide the highest chance for survival.

Table 10.4 Signs and Symptoms of Acute Myocardial Infarction

- Pressure, tightness, heaviness, burning, squeezing, or a crushing sensation in the middle of the chest
- Pain radiating down arms, shoulders, neck, jaw, or back
- Chest pain or discomfort lasting 20 minutes or longer
- Weakness
- Dyspnea
- Diaphoresis
- Irregular pulse
- Nausea and vomiting
- Apprehension
- Levine sign

Women

- Atypical discomfort
- Upper abdominal pain
- Shortness of breath
- Fatigue

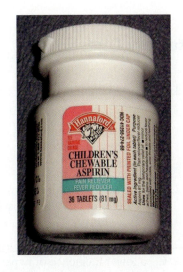

FIGURE 10.5 Baby aspirin for anticoagulation.

Case Resolution and Conclusion ·······························➤

Patients will present to the dental office with known and unknown CAD. A patient may experience an anginal episode or AMI in the dental setting. The dental professional should be prepared to activate the EMS system, initiate BLS, and manage the medical emergency until help arrives. Most deaths from an acute MI occur within the first few hours following the onset of symptoms, before the patient ever reaches the emergency department. It is imperative that the dental professional is prepared to act quickly in the event of such an emergency.

In Mr. Rodriquez's case, the protocol for the management of an AMI was implemented as he was exhibiting crushing pain and the Levine sign, in addition to diaphoresis and nausea, which are usually associated with MI and not angina. The CABs of CPR were initiated, EMS was activated, vital signs were monitored, and oxygen and nitroglycerin were administered. Fibrinolysis using aspirin was initiated following the unsuccessful resolution of the symptoms with nitrate therapy. The patient's vital signs continued to be monitored until EMS arrived to assume management of the emergency and transport the patient to the hospital. Mr. Rodriquez did recover from his acute MI because of the quick recognition of his symptoms and prompt management of the emergency. He returned to the dental office two months post-MI; his physician was consulted to determine if dental hygiene care could be completed, and permission was granted. The six-month waiting period following an MI may still be indicated, particularly if the patient is on anticoagulant therapy; therefore, consultation with a physician is necessary.

Review Questions

1. The most common cause of myocardial ischemia is

 A. obesity
 B. cigarette smoking
 C. atherosclerosis
 D. hypertension

2. The age advantage that women have over men in the development of CAD is most likely related to

 A. better lifestyle habits
 B. the protective effects of estrogen
 C. a lower incidence of hypertension
 D. a lower incidence of diabetes

3. Cigarette smoking contributes to the development of coronary artery disease in all of the following ways *except* one. Which one is the *exception*?

 A. Tobacco use accelerates the development of coronary plaques.
 B. Tobacco use promotes plaque rupture.
 C. Tobacco use promotes coronary thrombosis.
 D. Tobacco use causes vasodilatation and hypotension.

4. In individuals over the age of 50, systolic blood pressure greater than _____ is a more important risk factor than diastolic blood pressure.

    A. 150 mmHg
    B. 130 mmHg
    C. 140 mmHg
    D. 125 mmHg

5. If a patient with angina has had no changes in the cause, frequency, or duration of anginal symptoms in the previous 60 days, he or she is considered to have

    A. unstable angina
    B. stable angina
    C. vasoplastic angina
    D. variant angina

6. A sharp, stabbing chest pain that can be localized and is aggravated by movement or breathing is symptomatic of

    A. variant angina
    B. unstable angina
    C. noncardiac-related chest pain
    D. an acute myocardial infarction

7. Patients who present to the dental office with unstable angina can

    A. be treated in the dental office if their vital signs are monitored throughout the appointment
    B. receive emergency dental treatment after consultation with a physician and preferably in a hospital setting
    C. receive a local anesthetic with epinephrine safely
    D. receive a local anesthetic with epinephrine, but the maximum dose of the vasoconstrictor should not exceed 0.04 mg

8. The protocol for management of a patient with no history of angina and who is experiencing anginal-like chest pain includes

    A. administering three doses of nitroglycerin over 15 minutes prior to activating the EMS system
    B. administering one dose of nitroglycerin and activation of the EMS system if the pain continues for two minutes or longer
    C. immediately administering 81 mg of aspirin
    D. positioning the patient in a trendelenburg position because he or she is probably having an anxiety attack

9. During the first one to two hours following the onset of symptoms of an AMI, the greatest risk for death is the development of

    A. cardiac dysrhythmias
    B. dyspnea
    C. diaphoresis
    D. pulmonary edema

10. It is recommended that out-of-hospital AMI victims begin fibrinolysis as soon as the symptoms are recognized. The recommended drug is

    A. 5 mg of warfarin
    B. 7 mg of Coumadin
    C. 162 to 325 mg of acetylsalicylic acid
    D. 50 mg of chewable aspirin

Bibliography

2011 Writing Committee Members, J. L. Anderson, C. D. Adams, E. M. Antman, C. R. Bridges, R. M. Califf, D. E. Casey, et al. "ACC/AHA 2007 Guidelines for the Management of Patients with Unstable Angina/Non ST-Elevation Myocardial Infarction Executive Summary: A Report of the American College of Cardiology/American Heart Association Task Force on Practice Guidelines (Writing Committee to Revise the 2002 Guidelines for the Management of Patients with Unstable Angina/Non ST-Elevation Myocardial Infarction) Developed in Collaboration with the American College of Emergency Physicians, the Society for Cardiovascular Angiography and Interventions, and the Society of Thoracic Surgeons Endorsed by the American Association of Cardiovascular and Pulmonary Rehabilitation and the Society for Academic Emergency Medicine." *Journal of the American College of Cardiology* 50, no. 7 (2007): 652–731.

Abrams, J. "Chronic Stable Angina." *The New England Journal of Medicine* 352, no. 24 (2005): 2524–33.

American Academy of Periodontology. "Academy Report: Periodontal Management of Patients with Cardiovascular Diseases." *Journal of Periodontology* 73, no. 8 (2002): 954–68.

Anderson, K. N., L. E. Anderson, and W. D. Glanze, eds. *Mosby's Medical, Nursing & Allied Health Dictionary*. 5th ed. St. Louis, MO: Mosby-Year Book, Inc, (1998).

Berg, R. A., R. Hemphill, B. S. Abella, T. P. Aufderheide, D. M. Cave, M. F. Hazinski, E. B. Lerner, et al. "Part 5: Adult Basic Life Support." *Circulation* 122, no. 18, S3 (2010): S685–S705.

Braunwald, E. "Unstable Angina. A Classification." *Circulation* 80 (August, 1989): 410–14.

CDC: National Center for Chronic Disease Prevention and Health Promotion. *Heart Disease Fact Sheet*, 2006a. http://www.cdc.gov/dhdsp/library/pdfs/fs_heart_disease.pdf.

———. *Division for Heart Disease and Stroke Prevention: Heart Attack Fact Sheet*, 2006b. Accessed December 27, 2006. http://apps.nccd.cdc.gov/emailform/print_table.asp.

CDC: National Center for Health Statistics. *Deaths—Leading causes*, 2003. http://www.cdc.gov/nchs/fastats/lcod.htm.

Cooper, R., J. Cutler, P. Desvigne-Nickens, S. Fortmann, L. Friedman, R. Havlik, G. Hogelin, et al. "Trends and Disparities in Coronary Heart Disease, Stroke, and Other Cardiovascular Diseases in the United States: Findings of the National Conference on Cardiovascular Disease Prevention." *Circulation* 102, no. 25 (2000): 3137–47.

Detrano, R. "The Ethnic-Specific Nature of Mechanisms for Coronary Heart Disease." *Journal of the American College of Cardiology* 41, no. 1 (2003): 45–46.

Glick, M. "Screening for Traditional Risk Factors for Cardiovascular Disease: A Review for Oral Health Care Providers." *Journal of the American Dental Association* 133, no. 3 (2002): 291–300.

———. "The New Blood Pressure Guidelines: A Digest." *Journal of the American Dental Association* 135, no. 5 (2004): 585–86.

Glick, M., and B. Greenberg. "The Potential Role of Dentists in Identifying Patients' Risk of Experiencing Coronary Heart Disease Events." *Journal of the American Dental Association* 36, no. 11 (2005): 1541–46.

Granger, B., and C. Miller. "Acute Coronary Syndrome: Putting New Guidelines to Work. *Nursing 2001* 31, no. 11 (2001): 36–43.

Greenwood, M., and J. G. Meechan. "General Medicine and Surgery for Dental Practitioners: Part 1 Cardiovascular System." *British Dental Journal* 194, no. 10 (2003): 537–42.

Grundy, S., G. Balady, M. Criqui, G. Fletcher, P. Greenland, L. Hiratzka, N. Houston-Miller, et al. "AHA Scientific Statements: Primary Prevention of Coronary Heart Disease: Guidance from Framingham: A Statement for Healthcare Professionals from the AHA Task Force on Risk Reduction." *Circulation* 97, no. 18 (1998): 1876–87.

Haas, D. A. "Management of Medical Emergencies in the Dental Office: Conditions in Each Country, the Extent of Treatment by the Dentist." *Anesthesia Progress* 53, no. 1 (2006): 20–24.

Hamm, C., and E. Braunwald. "A Classification of Unstable Angina Revisited." *Circulation* 102, no. 1 (July, 2000): 118–22.

Hennekens, C., M. Dyken, and V. Fuster. "Aspirin as a Therapeutic Agent in Cardiovascular Disease: A Statement for Healthcare Professionals from the American Heart Association." *Circulation* 96, no. 8 (1997): 2751–53.

Herman, W., and J. Konzelman. "Angina: An update for Dentistry." *Journal of the American Dental Association* 127, no. 1 (1996): 98–104.

Herman, W., J. Konzelman, and M. Prisant. (2004). "New National Guidelines on Hypertension: A Summary for Dentistry." *Journal of the American Dental Association* 135, no. 5 (1996): 576–84.

Jowett, N. I., and L. B. Cabot. "Patients with Cardiac Disease: Considerations for the Dental Practitioner." *British Dental Journal* 189, no. 6 (2000): 297–302.

Kahri, J., and J. Rapola. "Cardiovascular Disorders in the Dental Practice." *Den Norske Tannlegeforenings Tidende* 115, no. 2 (2005): 84–90.

Keller, K., L. Lemberg, and C. Lynn. "Cardiology Casebook: Prinzmetal's Angina." *American Journal of Critical Care* 13, no. 4 (2004): 350–54.

Malamed, S. F. "Emergency Medicine: Beyond the Basics." *Journal of the American Dental Association* 128, no. 7 (1997): 843–54.

———. *Medical Emergencies in the Dental Office*. 6th ed. St. Louis, MO: Mosby, Inc, 2007. Original work published 1978.

Mealey, B. L. "Periodontal Implications: Medically Compromised Patients." *Annals of Periodontology* 1, no. 1 (1996): 256–321.

Miracle, V. A. "Coronary Artery Disease in Women: The Myth Still Exists." *Dimensions of Critical Care Nursing* 25, no. 5 (2006): 209–15.

Mosca, L., J. Manson, S. Sutherland, R. Langer, T. Manolio, and E. Barrett-Connor. "Cardiovascular Disease in Women." *Circulation* 96 (1997): 2468–82.

Moskowitz, L. "Cardiac Disease and Hypertension: Considerations for the Dental Office." *Dental Clinics of North America* 43, no. 3 (1999): 495–511.

Nagle, B., and C. Nee. "Recognizing and Responding to Acute Myocardial Infarction." *Nursing* 32, no. 10 (2002): 50–54.

National Institutes of Health. (2004). *The Seventh Report of the Joint National Committee on Prevention, Detection, Evaluation, and Treatment of High Blood Pressure*. NIH Publication No.04-5230.

Nunn, P. "Medical Emergencies in the Oral Health Care Setting." *Journal of Dental Hygiene* 74, no. 11 (2000): 137–51.

Perno, M. "Life-Threatening Emergencies: Are You Ready?" *Access* (January 2002): 30–37.

Ridker, P. M., ed. "Circulation: On Evolutionary Biology, Inflammation, Infection and the Causes of Atherosclerosis." Special issue. *Journal of the American Heart Association* 105, no. 1 (2002): 2–4.

Roeters van Lennep, J., H. T. Westerveld, D. W. Erkelens, and E. van der Wall. "Risk Factors for Coronary Heart Disease: Implications of Gender." *Cardiovascular Research* 53, no. 3 (2002): 538–49.

Rose, L., B. Mealey, L. Minsk, and D. W. Cohen. "Oral Care for Patients with Cardiovascular Disease and Stroke." *Journal of the American Dental Association* 133, no. 1 (2002): 37S–44S.

Ross, R. "Atherosclerosis—An Inflammatory Disease." *The New England Journal of Medicine* 340, no. 2 (1999): 115–216.

Steinhauer, T., S. A. Bsoul, and G. T. Terezhalmy. "Risk Stratification and Dental Management of the Patient with Cardiovascular Disease. Part I: Etiology, Epidemiology, and Principles of Medical Management." *Quintessence International* 36, no. 2 (2005): 119–37.

Thibodeau, G.A., and K. T. Patton. *Anatomy & physiology*. St. Louis, MO: Mosby/Elsevier, 2007.

Writing Group Members, V. L. Roger, A. S. Go, D. M. Lloyd-Jones, E. J. Benjamin, J. D. Berry, W. B. Borden, et al. "Heart Disease and Stroke Statistics—2012 Update." *Circulation* 125, no. 1 (2012): e2 –e220.

Yeghiazarians, Y., J. Braunstein, A. Askari, and P. Stone. "Unstable Angina Pectoris." *New England Journal of Medicine* 342, no. 2 (2000): 101–13.

TREATMENT OF AN ANGINAL ATTACK
R.E.P.A.I.R.

R: Recognize signs and symptoms of an anginal attack: generalized chest discomfort, which is often described as pressure, burning, heaviness, or choking sensation that may radiate down the arm, to the neck, lower jaw, or tongue; diaphoresis, nausea, and pallor; victim may clutch chest

E: Evaluate symptoms to determine if the chest pain is cardiac related: Does the patient have a history of angina? Are there risk factors present in the medical history? Is the pain localized or generalized? Stabbing, knifelike pain that is aggravated by movement and breathing and lasts less than 30 seconds generally is not cardiac related

P: Position patient semi-upright or upright

A: Activate CAB's of CPR—check circulation, airway, and breathing (pulse and blood pressure)

I: Implement appropriate emergency protocol for anginal attack: administer oxygen 4–6 L/minute. At any time, administer nitroglycerin immediately and one tablet every five minutes not to exceed three tablets every 15 minutes or one to two metered spray doses not to exceed three doses over 15 minutes; monitor vital signs continuously

R: Refer to emergency department: Activate 9-1-1 if the chest pain is not relieved by two doses of nitroglycerin over a 10-minute period; if the patient has no history of angina and the chest pain persists for two minutes or longer, activate 9-1-1 immediately and begin to treat the emergency as an AMI

TREATMENT OF AN ACUTE MYOCARDIAL INFARCTION
R.E.P.A.I.R.

R: Recognize signs and symptoms of an acute myocardial infarction: chest pain or discomfort that lasts 20 minutes or longer, feeling of pressure, tightness, heaviness, burning, squeezing, or a crushing sensation in the middle of the chest and/or epigastric pain; pain may radiate down the arms, shoulder, neck, jaw, and back; nausea, weakness, dyspnea, diaphoresis, and an irregular pulse

E: Evaluate symptoms to determine if the chest pain is cardiac related: Does the patient have a history of angina? Are there risk factors present in the medical history? Is the pain localized or generalized? Stabbing, knifelike pain that is aggravated by movement and breathing and lasts less than 30 seconds generally is not cardiac related. Is the pain alleviated or eliminated by the administration of nitroglycerin? Be aware that not all victims experience typical symptoms

P: Position patient semi-upright or upright

A: Activate CAB's of CPR—check circulation, airway, and breathing (pulse and blood pressure)

I: Implement appropriate emergency protocol for acute myocardial infarction: Contact EMS immediately, administer oxygen 4–6 L/minute, monitor vital signs continuously, administer nitroglycerin following the recommended dosage procedure. If nitroglycerin is not successful in eliminating the chest pain, initiate fibrinolysis of 162 to 325 mg of aspirin orally

R: Refer to emergency department: continue to monitor vital signs until EMS arrives; if breathing and/or circulation stops, begin CPR immediately

11

Heart Failure and Acute Pulmonary Edema

LEARNING OBJECTIVES

Upon reading the material in this chapter, the reader will be able to:

- ☑ Discuss the factors that increase the risk for development of heart failure and pulmonary edema.

- ☑ Describe the pathophysiology associated with the development of left ventricular (LV) heart failure.

- ☑ Describe the clinical signs and symptoms associated with LV heart failure.

- ☑ Describe the pathophysiology associated with the development of right ventricular (RV) heart failure.

- ☑ Describe the clinical signs and symptoms associated with RV heart failure.

- ☑ Describe the clinical signs and symptoms associated with late-stage heart failure.

- ☑ Describe the clinical signs and symptoms associated with acute pulmonary edema.

- ☑ Describe the procedure for the management of acute pulmonary edema and heart failure in the dental setting.

Case Study ···➤

Scenario

Your patient, Betty Austin, is a 58-year-old retired nurse. She indicates on her medical history that she suffered an acute myocardial infarction two years ago. She also states that she has swelling in her ankles and feet, especially after being on her feet all day. She has difficulty breathing with physical exertion, and she needs to prop her head up with pillows to sleep at night. She is taking hydrochlorothiazide daily and sublingual nitroglycerin spray as necessary. Mrs. Austin has not had any dental care in 15 years and is very anxious about her dental hygiene appointment today. Shortly after you begin your dental hygiene treatment, Mrs. Austin appears very agitated and is experiencing significant difficulty breathing. She is gasping for air, and her lips are becoming cyanotic. From what emergency do you suspect Mrs. Austin is suffering?

Introduction

Almost 5 million people in the United States are living with heart failure, and half a million new cases are diagnosed every year. These statistics are rising primarily because the population is aging, heart failure mostly affects the elderly, and more people are surviving heart attacks. Heart failure (HF) is a clinical syndrome that occurs when the heart muscle becomes impaired and no longer effectively pumps sufficient volumes of oxygenated blood to the body's tissues and organs. In 2005, the American College of Cardiology and the American Heart Association updated the guidelines for the management of chronic heart failure in an adult. In the guidelines, the term *congestive heart failure* has been changed to *heart failure* to reflect the broad spectrum of the disease. Heart failure can result from any kind of cardiovascular disease. Acute myocardial infarction and hypertension are the most frequent causes, but valvular heart disease, diabetes mellitus, or degenerative conditions of the heart muscle (cardiomyopathies) may also result in heart failure. Heart failure is also associated with noncardiovascular conditions, such as thyroid disease, renal insufficiency, and pulmonary disease. Those at highest risk for heart failure include the elderly and individuals with established coronary heart disease, a history of hypertension—especially uncontrolled hypertension, an abnormal heart rhythm, and a heart valve disorder or a history of rheumatic fever.

The three cardinal symptoms of heart failure are dyspnea, edema, and fatigue; however, these symptoms are seen in many other conditions and are not necessarily diagnostic of heart failure. Most often the symptoms of heart failure initially present during exertion, but as the disease progresses shortness of breath and fatigue are present even at rest. In the dental setting, patients will present with varying levels of heart failure. The physiological and/or psychological stress often associated with dental treatment can exacerbate the symptoms. This could lead to life-threatening **acute pulmonary edema**. The clinician must be able to recognize the varying clinical signs and symptoms of heart failure, appropriately modify and manage the dental treatment of heart failure patients, and be prepared to respond to a medical emergency should it arise.

Signs and Symptoms of Heart Failure

The heart muscle is essentially two pumps functioning together. The left atrium collects the newly oxygenated blood from the lungs, and the left ventricle (LV) pumps the oxygen-rich blood out to the body. The right atrium of the heart collects oxygen-poor blood from the body, and the right ventricle (RV) pumps it to the lungs, where the blood picks up oxygen and gets rid of carbon dioxide. (See Figure 11.1 ■) Heart failure can be classified according to the side of the heart that is affected: right-sided

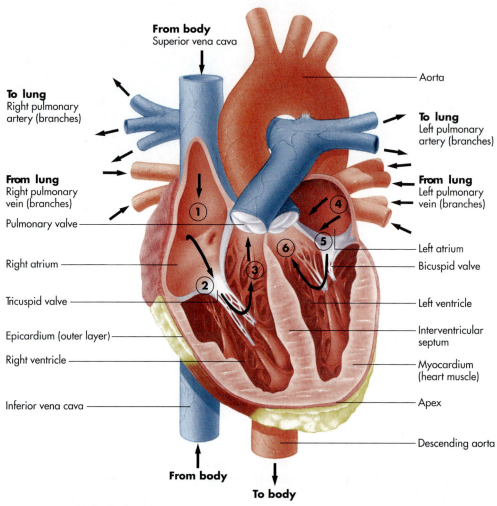

RIGHT HEART PUMP

1. Deoxygenated blood returns from the upper and lower body to fill the right atrium of the heart creating a pressure against the atrioventricular (AV) or tricuspid valve.

2. This pressure of the returning blood forces the AV valve open and begins filling the ventricle. The final filling of the ventricle is achieved by the contracting of the right atrium.

3. The right ventricle contracts increasing the internal pressure. This pressure closes the tricuspid valve and forces open the pulmonary valve thus sending blood toward the lung via the pulmonary artery. This blood will become oxygenated as it travels through the capillary beds of the lung and then return to the left side of the heart.

LEFT HEART PUMP

4. Oxygenated blood returns from the lung via the pulmonary vein and fills the left atrium creating a pressure against the bicuspid valve.

5. This pressure of returning blood forces the bicuspid valve open and begins filling the left ventricle. The final filling of the left ventricle is achieved by the contracting of the left atrium.

6. The left ventricle contracts increasing internal pressure. This pressure closes the bicuspid valve and forces open the aortic valve causing oxygenated blood to flow through the aorta to deliver oxygen throughout the body.

FIGURE 11.1 The functioning of the heart valves and blood flow.

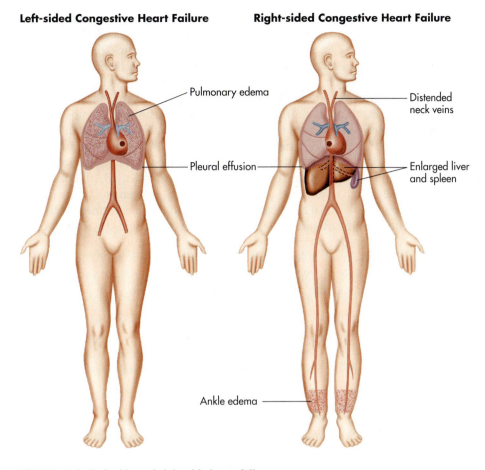

Left-sided Congestive Heart Failure   **Right-sided Congestive Heart Failure**

Pulmonary edema

Distended neck veins

Pleural effusion

Enlarged liver and spleen

Ankle edema

FIGURE 11.2 Left-side and right-side heart failure.

or left-sided failure. The right and left ventricles of the heart must maintain an equal output to function effectively. The initial event that leads to heart failure may be left-sided or right-sided in origin, but most long-term heart failure usually involves both sides. (See Figure 11.2 ■)

Left Ventricular Heart Failure

During the systolic phase of the cardiac cycle, the LV pumps out 60% or more of the blood it holds into systemic circulation. Any condition that causes the LV to lose its ability to contract normally results in a fall in cardiac output. In this situation, the force of the ventricular contraction is inadequate, and not enough oxygenated blood is pumped into circulation. This is known as **left ventricular (LV) heart failure**. Diastolic failure occurs when the LV is unable to relax normally. In this case, the LV cannot fill completely with oxygenated blood during the period between heartbeats. As a result of LV heart failure, blood coming into the LV from the lungs may back up, causing fluid to leak into the lungs, resulting in **pulmonary edema**. LV heart failure usually occurs before **right ventricular (RV) heart failure** and is often the result of an acute myocardial infarction and/or cardiomyopathy. Clinical symptoms become more prominent at night (while the patient is in a supine position) and are primarily related to respiratory distress. In LV heart failure the patient initially notices weakness and fatigue when performing tasks that previously were not tiring. As the severity of the heart failure progresses, the amount of fatigue and weakness increases with little or no exertion.

A cardinal symptom of heart failure is dyspnea (difficulty breathing). Initially this shortness of breath occurs only upon exertion. An increased rate of breathing (tachypnea) as well as an increase in the depth of the breaths may be noted. As the severity of the heart failure progresses, the patient may experience **orthopnea** (difficulty breathing while lying flat), **paroxysmal nocturnal dyspnea** (difficulty breathing during sleep, which causes the patient to awaken gasping for air), and dyspnea at rest. These patients often have to sit or sleep upright or with their heads elevated. Sometimes Cheyne-Stokes respirations will precipitate nocturnal dyspnea and/or contribute to daytime sleepiness. Cheyne-Stokes respirations are characterized by a period of deep breathing when atrial carbon dioxide pressure is high and shallow or no breathing when atrial carbon dioxide pressure is low. In patients with LV heart failure, this type of breathing pattern is thought to be due to the increased time it takes for the blood to be circulated from the heart to the brain. Heart failure patients with moderate to severe breathing difficulty are classified as an ASA III or ASA IV medical risk. They often require the use of supplemental oxygen and may carry portable oxygen containers with a nasal cannula attached. If dental treatment is provided to these patients, modifications must be made, such as shortened appointment times and placing the patient in an upright position during treatment.

Patients with LV heart failure may also exhibit a cough due to congestion in the lungs. This is usually a dry, nonproductive, chronic cough that often occurs in conjunction with dyspnea and under similar conditions (during exertion or lying in a supine position).

Patients with moderate to severe LV heart failure appear pale, sweaty, obviously short of breath, and cool to the touch. The blood pressure is usually elevated, with the diastolic pressure being higher than the systolic pressure. The pulse rate is often rapid and thready. In addition, beats may alternate between strong and weak (**pulsus alternans**).

Right Ventricular Heart Failure

Right ventricular heart failure usually occurs shortly after LV heart failure. The effect of increased fluid pressure ultimately damages the right side of the heart. RV heart failure results in the inability of the heart to pump oxygen-poor blood from the systemic venous circulation into the lungs for oxygenation. The result is congestion of blood in the systemic venous system. Like LV heart failure, patients with RV failure experience fatigue and weakness, but the major clinical symptom is the development of peripheral edema. The lower extremities, especially the legs and ankles, may demonstrate pitting edema. **Pitting edema** is characterized by a depression that remains in the tissue for a few seconds after release of digital pressure to the area. RV heart failure also leads to a reduction in renal blood flow. Decreased renal blood flow results in a decrease in the excretion of sodium, and thus additional retention of fluid. During the day, renal function is especially poor because the patient's activity increases the degree of RV heart failure. This results in less urine production. At night, when the patient is less active and is off his or her feet, renal and cardiac function may improve. In this situation, the patient may experience nocturia (increased frequency of urination at night). Another clinical manifestation of RV failure is the presence of distended external jugular veins while lying or sitting. Normally, the jugular veins are collapsed while standing or when sitting with the head at a 30° angle or higher.

In RV heart failure, engorgement of the liver and spleen occurs. As the disease progresses, edema in the abdomen becomes evident. Congestion in the gastrointestinal (GI) tract can cause nausea, vomiting, and anorexia. Edema in the central nervous system can manifest clinically with the patient experiencing headaches, insomnia, and irritability. (See Table 11.1 ■)

Later Stages of Heart Failure

Patients in the later stages of heart failure often experience mental confusion, anxiety, and restlessness, which are the result of an inadequate supply of oxygenated blood to the brain. Cardiac **cachexia** (malnutrition and wasting of tissues) may be evident in end-stage heart failure. **Cyanosis** of the skin and mucous membranes, especially the nail beds and lips, is also a clinical symptom of late-stage heart failure.

Table 11.1 Signs and Symptoms of Heart Failure

Right Heart Failure	Left Heart Failure
• Weakness	• Weakness
• Fatigue	• Fatigue
• Peripheral edema with pitting	• Dyspnea
• Nocturia	• Tachypnea
• Distended external jugular veins	• Orthopnea
• Abdominal edema	• Paroxysmal nocturnal dyspnea
• Nausea	• Dry, nonproductive, chronic cough
• Vomiting	• Pallor
• Anorexia	• Diaphoresis
• Headaches	• Elevated blood pressure
• Insomnia	• Rapid, thready pulse rate
• Irritability	• *Pulsus alternans*

Treatment of Heart Failure

Changes in lifestyle can often lessen the symptoms of heart failure and prevent the disease from progressing. These changes include smoking cessation, exercise, weight loss (if overweight), a diet low in fat and sodium, limited consumption of caffeine and alcohol, and stress reduction. In addition to lifestyle changes, drug therapy is often indicated. Differentiation between systolic and diastolic dysfunction is essential when treating heart failure. Angiotensin-converting-enzyme inhibitors, digoxin, diuretics, vasodilators, and beta-blockers are used for the treatment of systolic failure. When treating diastolic dysfunction, the underlying cause of impaired diastolic function needs to be determined prior to drug therapy. Beta-blockers and calcium channel blockers are often used when the dysfunction is secondary to ischemic heart disease or hypertension. Many of the drugs used to treat heart failure have potential drug interactions with which the dental clinician must be familiar when evaluating and treating patients with heart failure. The use of local anesthetics containing epinephrine should be considered carefully when treating patients with heart failure. For example, local anesthetic agents containing epinephrine may cause a significant rise in blood pressure in patients taking beta-blockers. This steep rise in blood pressure could result in anginal pain and/or cardiac arrhythmias.

Treatment of the Patient with Heart Failure in the Dental Setting

As is the case with all patients, completion of a comprehensive medical/dental history is essential prior to the initiation of any dental care. The medical history form should include questions that would elicit information indicating that the patient suffers from heart failure or may be at risk for the development of heart failure, for example, "Do you have swelling in your feet or ankles?" and "Do you ever experience shortness of breath?" Heart failure patients who are classified as ASA II (mild dyspnea and fatigue during exertion) can be managed normally in the dental setting provided that the rest of the medical history provides no contraindications to treatment. If physical or psychological stress is anticipated during the provision of dental care, the clinician may consider the use of supplemental oxygen at a flow rate of 3 to 5 L/minute. Placing the patient in an upright or semisupine position in the dental chair will reduce breathing difficulty. Patients who experience dyspnea or fatigue under normal situations fall into the ASA III category. Dental treatment presents an increased risk for these patients. They often experience orthopnea and may experience paroxysmal nocturnal dyspnea. Medical consultation is required prior to any dental treatment. The use of supplemental oxygen and modification of patient positioning must be considered. Cardiac patients who fall into the ASA IV category present a definite risk.

These patients experience fatigue, dyspnea, and orthopnea at all times. Any dental treatment requires consultation with the patient's physician. All elective dental treatment should be postponed until the patient's symptoms are controlled. Emergency dental treatment should be managed with medication if possible. If pharmacologic treatment is ineffective, the patient should be treated in a hospital setting.

The patient's physical characteristics should also be observed. Patients presenting with cyanotic lips and nail beds may be in heart failure. As heart failure worsens, the patient's skin may appear gray and the mucus membranes grayish blue. Prominent jugular veins when the person is sitting upright may also indicate some degree of heart failure.

In the case of patients presenting with varying degrees of heart failure, vital signs should be monitored throughout the appointment. Patients with heart failure may present with an elevated blood pressure, particularly an elevated diastolic pressure.

The patient may also present with an increased rate of respiration, as well as an increased pulse rate. Excessive unexplained weight gain may signal the onset of acute heart failure. Weight gain of more than 3 pounds over seven days, particularly in the presence of edema in the extremities, should raise a red flag for the clinician. Dental treatment should be postponed, and the patient should be referred for a complete medical evaluation.

Acute Pulmonary Edema

The most dramatic and life-threatening symptom of heart failure is acute pulmonary edema. Precipitating events include stress (physiological or psychological), infection, failure to take medications as prescribed, and a meal high in sodium. Acute pulmonary edema is the result of a swift and abrupt accumulation of fluid in the alveolar spaces of the lungs. The pulmonary edema inhibits lung expansion and results in a decreased ability of the lungs to oxygenate the blood. The clinical symptoms are acute and include the following: gasping for air, rapid pulse, cool and moist skin, cyanotic lips and nail beds, and anxiety. Dyspnea may be accompanied by a cough that produces frothy, blood-tinged sputum. The movement of air through the alveolar fluid produces a crackle sound when heard through a stethoscope. As the condition worsens, the lung sounds become louder and coarser. The death rattle indicates the terminal stages of acute pulmonary edema.

Treatment of Patients with Acute Pulmonary Edema in the Dental Setting

Acute pulmonary edema represents a life-threatening situation that requires immediate medical attention. EMS (Emergency Medical Services) should be activated immediately, and management of the medical emergency should continue until EMS arrives. Dental treatment should stop, all instruments and materials should be removed from the mouth, and the patient should be positioned comfortably. A semisupine or upright position is usually the most comfortable for patients suffering from heart failure and acute pulmonary edema. This will ease breathing by allowing the fluid in the alveolar sacs to flow to the base of the lungs. Persons experiencing acute pulmonary edema do not usually lose consciousness, but if loss of consciousness occurs they should be placed in a supine position. As with all medical emergencies, circulation, airway, and breathing need to be assessed, and basic life support need to be started if necessary. Oxygen should be delivered at a rate of 10 L or more/minute via a non-rebreather bag, and vital signs should be monitored and recorded every five minutes. If the patient complains of suffocation, a nasal cannula can be substituted at a rate of 2-5 L/minute.

Maintaining an airway and breathing is of primary concern when managing acute pulmonary edema. Positioning the patient in an upright or semi-upright position often helps to alleviate some of the breathing difficulty these patients experience. In a hospital setting, a phlebotomy may be performed to relieve the congestion in the lungs. In this procedure 350 to 450 mL of blood is removed from the patient, resulting in improvement in air exchange because of a reduction in the return of venous blood to the right side of the heart. It is unlikely that a phlebotomy would be performed in a dental office, but a bloodless phlebotomy is an option. In this case tourniquets or blood pressure cuffs are applied to three extremities at a time. The tourniquets and/or blood pressure cuffs should be placed about 6 inches below the groin and 4 inches below the shoulder. One tourniquet is removed every 5 to 10 minutes and reapplied to the free extremity. The tourniquet or blood pressure cuff should be tight enough to reduce the blood flow but loose enough so that an arterial pulse can be felt distal to each tourniquet or cuff. The pressure applied to the cuff or tourniquet should be less than the systolic pressure, but greater than the diastolic pressure. A bloodless phlebotomy can temporarily remove blood from circulation, thus permitting the heart to pump the remaining blood more effectively. The result is a reduction in pulmonary congestion and improved breathing. (See Figure 11.3 ■)

The use of vasodilators may also be indicated in the management of acute pulmonary edema and heart failure. Nitroglycerin (venodilator) can be administered for the rapid treatment of acute pulmonary edema. The patient should take 0.8 to 1.2 mg every 5 to 10 minutes (two or three tablets or sprays). It takes approximately two minutes for the drug to begin to work, and the effects last about 15 to 30 minutes. The use of nitroglycerin is contraindicated if the systolic blood pressure is below 100 mmHg.

Management of the patient's apprehension and anxiety is essential when dealing with acute pulmonary edema. The resultant increase in cardiac and respiratory work load is absolutely contraindicated in heart failure patients. If all of the previously described steps are ineffective in sufficiently reducing anxiety and respiratory distress, opioid agonists can be administered. Meperidine (IM or IV) or morphine (IM) may be administered with a resulting decrease in anxiety, increase in vasodilation, and decrease in cardiac and respiratory work load. On the other hand, these drugs also depress respiration to some degree. In patients with hypoxia with cyanosis, mental confusion, or delirium, the use of opioids is an absolute contraindication. It is unlikely that these drugs would be available and/or administered in the dental setting. As mentioned previously, administering oxygen and having the patient sit upright to reduce respiratory distress can often help to alleviate the patient's anxiety.

Patients experiencing acute pulmonary edema require hospitalization to manage the emergency. Patients who have recovered from such an event may return to the dental office, and treatment must be considered carefully. If dental care is to be provided, consultation with the patient's physician is essential, and all steps to minimize the risk of a reoccurrence should be implemented.

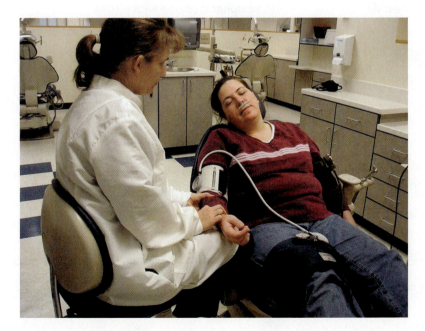

FIGURE 11.3 Bloodless phlebotomy.

Case Resolution and Conclusion ··········➤

As the population ages, the incidence of diagnosed and undiagnosed heart failure is on the rise. This population is also more likely to retain their natural teeth throughout their lifetime. It is likely that the dental practitioner will treat patients with varying forms of heart disease, including heart failure. It is essential that all members of the dental team are familiar with the clinical signs and symptoms associated with acute myocardial infarction, heart failure, and acute pulmonary edema. Based on the clinical signs and symptoms described in the case scenario, it appears that Mrs. Austin is experiencing heart failure and acute pulmonary edema. She is very agitated and was gasping for air. Her lips are cyanotic. Due to your familiarity with these conditions, you immediately contact EMS and position her semisupinely, which is most comfortable for her. You monitor her vital signs and due to her severe dyspnea decide to administer oxygen via a non-rebreather bag at 6 L/minute and initiate a bloodless phlebotomy, which seems to alleviate her symptoms somewhat. You also administer nitroglycerin spray translingually. Betty is transported to the emergency department where she was treated and released after several weeks of intense cardiac therapy.

Review Questions

1. Left ventricular heart failure results in
   A. respiratory distress
   B. peripheral edema
   C. distended jugular veins while lying or sitting
   D. nocturia

2. All of the following symptoms are observed in late-stage heart failure *except* one. Which symptom is the *exception*?
   A. cyanosis of the lips and/or nail beds
   B. cardiac cachexia
   C. mental confusion and anxiety
   D. stabbing chest pain lasting less than 30 seconds

3. Right ventricular heart failure usually develops before left ventricular heart failure. The major clinical symptom of right ventricular heart failure is pulmonary edema.
   A. The first statement is true, and the second statement is false.
   B. The first statement is false, and the second statement is true.
   C. Both statements are true.
   D. Both statements are false.

4. Symptoms of right heart failure include all of the following *except* one. Which one is the *exception*?
   A. distended jugular veins
   B. peripheral edema with pitting
   C. nocturia
   D. carpopedal spasms

5. A bloodless phlebotomy
   A. should be performed in a hospital setting only on patients suffering from heart failure
   B. could be performed in the dental setting to help reduce peripheral edema in heart failure patients
   C. could be performed in a dental setting to help manage lung congestion in patients suffering from acute pulmonary edema
   D. is never a treatment option for patients experiencing acute pulmonary edema

6. The administration of nitroglycerin is indicated in the management of acute pulmonary edema and heart failure. The administration of nitroglycerin is contra-indicated in patients with a systolic pressure lower than 100 mmHg.

   A. The first statement is true, and the second state-ment is false.
   B. The first statement is false, and the second state-ment is true.
   C. Both statements are true.
   D. Both statements are false.

7. Prominent jugular veins while seated in an upright position is indicative of

   A. left heart failure
   B. right heart failure
   C. pulmonary embolism
   D. acute myocardial infarction

8. The most frequent etiology of heart failure is

   A. cerebrovascular accident
   B. diabetes
   C. myocardial infarction
   D. cardiac valve abnormalities

Bibliography

American Academy of Periodontology. "Academy Report: Periodontal Management of Patients with Cardiovascular Diseases." *Journal of Periodontology* 73, no. 8 (2002): 954–68.

Anderson, K. N., L. E. Anderson, and W. D. Glanze, eds. *Mosby's Medical, Nursing & Allied Health Dictionary*. 5th ed. St. Louis, MO: Mosby-Year Book, Inc, 1998.

Bostock, B. "Understanding Heart Failure." *Practice Nurse* 41, no. 4 (2011): 12–16.

Fletcher, L., and D. Thomas. "Congestive Heart Failure: Understanding the Pathophysiology and Management." *Journal of the American Academy of Nurse Practitioners* 13, no. 6 (2001): 249–57.

Herman, W., J. Konzelman, and M. Prisant. "New National Guidelines on Hypertension: A Summary for Dentistry." *Journal of the American Dental Association* 135, no. 5 (2004): 576–84.

Hunt, S., W. Abraham, M. Chin, A. Feldman, G. Francis, G. Ganiats, M. Jessup, et al. "ACC/AHA 2005 Guideline Update for the Diagnosis and Management of Chronic Heart Failure in the Adult: A Report of the American College of Cardiology/American Heart Association Task Force on Practice Guidelines (Writing Committee to Update the 2001 Guidelines for the Evaluation and Management of Heart Failure): Developed in Collaboration With the American College of Chest Physicians and the International Society for Heart and Lung Transplantation: Endorsed by the Heart Rhythm Society." *Circulation* 112 (2005): 154–235.

Jackson, G., C. R. Gibbs, M. K. Davies, and G. Y. H. Lip. "ABC of Heart Failure: Pathophysiology." *British Medical Journal* 320, no. 7228 (2000): 167–70.

Jessup, M., W. T. Abraham, D. E. Casey, A. M. Feldman, G. S. Francis, T. G. Ganiats, M. A. Konstam, et al. "2009 Focused Update: ACCF/AHA Guidelines for the Diagnosis and Management of Heart Failure in Adults: A Report of the American College of Cardiology Foundation/American Heart Association Task Force on Practice Guidelines Developed in Collaboration with the International Society for Heart and Lung Transplantation." *Journal of the American College of Cardiology* 53, no. 15 (2009): 1343–82.

Jowett, N. I., and L. B. Cabot. "Patients with Cardiac Disease: Considerations for the Dental Practitioner." *British Dental Journal* 189, no. 6 (2000): 297–302.

Kahri, J., and J. Rapola. "Cardiovascular Disorders in the Dental Practice." *Den Norske Tannlegeforenings Tidende* 115, no. 2 (2005): 84–90.

Malamed, S. F. "Emergency Medicine: Beyond the Basics." *Journal of the American Dental Association* 128 no. 7 (1997): 843–54.

———. *Medical Emergencies in the Dental Office*. 6th ed. St. Louis, MO: Mosby, Inc, 2007. Original work published 1978.

Mask, A. G. "Medical Management of the Patient with Cardiovascular Disease." *Periodontology* 23, no. 1 (2000): 136–41.

Nunn, P. "Medical Emergencies in the Oral Health Care Setting." *Journal of Dental Hygiene* 74, no. 11 (2000): 137–51.

Porth, C. *Essentials of Pathophysiology: Concepts of Altered Health States*. Philadelphia, PA: Lippincott Williams & Wilkins, 2004.

Shamsham, F., and J. Mitchell. "Essentials of the Diagnosis of Heart Failure." *American Family Physician* 61, no. 5 (2008): 1319–28.

Weaver, T., and J. Eisold. "Congestive Heart Failure and Disorders of the Heart Beat." *Dental Clinics of North America* 40, no. 3 (1996): 543–61.

MANAGEMENT OF HEART FAILURE
R.E.P.A.I.R.

R: Recognize signs and symptoms of heart failure: LVF—dyspnea at rest or upon exertion, tachypnea, orthopnea, nonproductive cough; RFV—pitting edema in the extremities, nocturia, distended jugular veins while lying or sitting. Later stages—symptoms mentioned for LVF and RFV, mental confusion, anxiety, cardiac cachexia, cyanosis of skin and mucous membranes

E: Evaluate symptoms to determine if they are related to heart failure: Does the patient have a history heart failure? Are there risk factors present in the medical history?

P: Position patient semi-upright or upright, terminate dental procedure, and remove materials from the patient's mouth

A: Activate CAB's of CPR—check circulation, airway, and breathing (pulse and blood pressure)

I: Implement appropriate emergency protocol for heart failure: Calm patient, administer oxygen via a nasal cannula at a flow rate of 3 to 5 L per minute, monitor vital signs continuously.

R: Refer to emergency department: activate 9-1-1 if the patient's respiratory distress is not alleviated with the supplemental oxygen and positioning the patient upright; be aware of the symptoms of acute pulmonary edema and prepare to manage that emergency should it occur; perform basic life support if necessary

MANAGEMENT OF ACUTE PULMONARY EDEMA
R.E.P.A.I.R.

R: Recognize signs and symptoms of an acute pulmonary edema: acute onset of dry cough that may progress to a cough that produces blood-tinged sputum, dyspnea (the patient may feel like he or she is suffocating), orthopnea, tachypnea, pallor, sweating, cyanosis, and anxiety

E: Evaluate symptoms to determine if the patient's respiratory distress is related to severe pulmonary congestion as a result of left ventricular failure: Does the patient have a history of heart failure and/or pulmonary edema? Are there risk factors present in the medical history? Is the patient under psychological or physical stress? Has the patient consumed a salty meal recently? Is the patient taking medication as prescribed?

P: Position patient semi-upright or upright, terminate dental procedure, and remove materials from the patient's mouth

A: Activate CAB's of CPR—check circulation, airway, and breathing (pulse and blood pressure)

I: Implement appropriate emergency protocol for acute pulmonary edema: Contact EMS immediately, calm the patient, administer oxygen at a rate of 10 L or more per minute via a non-rebreather bag or 5 L/minute via a nasal cannula, monitor vital signs continuously, perform a bloodless phlebotomy, administer a vasodilator (nitroglycerin should be used only if the systolic pressure is above 100 mmHg)

R: Refer to emergency department: Continue to monitor vital signs until EMS arrives; if breathing and/or circulation stops, begin CPR immediately

12

Cardiac Pacemaker and Implantable Cardioverter Defibrillator Malfunction

LEARNING OBJECTIVES

Upon reading the material in this chapter, the reader will be able to:

☑ Discuss the conditions warranting a pacemaker or an implantable cardioverter defibrillator (ICD).

☑ List specific signs and symptoms associated with pacemaker or ICD malfunction.

☑ Determine suggested treatment modalities for cardiac pacemaker or ICD malfunction.

☑ Explain the special precautions that should be taken to prevent a patient from experiencing a pacemaker or ICD malfunction.

Case Study

Scenario

A 72-year-old male patient, Norman Gilbert, is scheduled for his six-month recall dental hygiene appointment for which he is a year overdue. Norman had a pacemaker placed nine months ago due to consistent bradycardia. He has been coming to your office for a number of years, and you are excited to show him your newly remodeled dental equipment, including the chair with the magnetic headrest. You seat Norman, and he comments on the comfort of the new chair. You are updating his medical history when he begins to complain of chest pain, and dyspnea. You take his pulse, and it is very slow and weak at 50 beats/ minute; his blood pressure is 108/72 mmHg. What is happening to this patient?

Introduction

As our population ages, **cardiac pacemakers** and **internal cardioverter defibrillators** (ICD) have become increasingly more common in dental patients. Estimates state that from 1993 to 2006, 2.4 million new cardiac pacemakers and 800,000 new ICDs were placed in the United States. With 43 million people suffering from cardiovascular disease (CVD) in the United States and more than half the population over the age of 75 affected by CVD, it is reasonable to assume that the number of pacemaker and ICD implants will rise. (See Figure 12.1 ■)

A pacemaker is a device composed of a pulse generator and leads. (See Figure 12.2 ■) The generator contains the electronic circuitry that powers the device and is a small metal box no larger than two stacked silver dollars. The generator is implanted subcutaneously, usually in the clavicle region of the chest wall. The longevity of a generator is approximately 7–10 years.

The leads are the connection between the heart muscle and the generator. They are inserted into the venous system and are maneuvered to the area of the heart

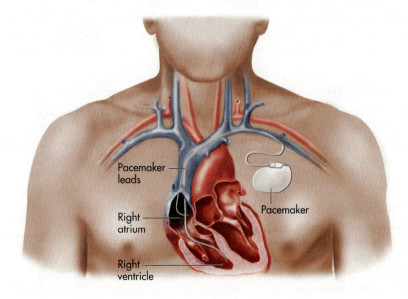

Pacemaker leads

Right atrium

Pacemaker

Right ventricle

FIGURE 12.1 Pacemaker.

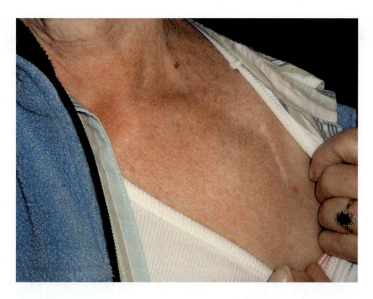

FIGURE 12.2 Area of the pacemaker.

requiring stimulation, usually the right atrium, right ventricle, or both. There are usually one or two leads, but in some instances three leads may be used. The leads monitor the heart rate and provide the pacing impulses when necessary. An ICD is a similar device with the exception that the lead in the ventricle can also provide the cardioversion/defibrillation current.

Pacemakers are often used for the treatment of cardiac arrhythmias or irregular heart rate. Moreover, the most common arrhythmia for which pacemakers are used is severe bradycardia or slow heart rate. If left untreated, the person with bradycardia will have a low cardiac output, which causes symptoms of weakness, dizziness, and syncope. Profound bradycardia can be fatal. The pacemaker monitors the heart rate constantly, and if it observes normal cardiac rhythm, it does nothing. If it observes a slowing of the heart rate below a programmed level, it begins to give electrical impulses to the heart to speed up.

ICDs are used to treat harmful **tachyarrhythmias**. These tachyarrhythmias usually originate in the ventricles whereby the heart rate becomes too fast, over 200 beats/minute. When this occurs cardiac output is diminished, and the patient experiences symptoms of dizziness, palpitations, and syncope. **Ventricular tachycardia** can lead to ventricular fibrillation, a condition in which there is chaotic electrical activation of the ventricles that can be fatal if not treated on time. The ICD continuously monitors the heart for such arrhythmias and, when they occur, delivers an electrical shock called a **cardioversion** or **defibrillation** to return the heart to normal rhythm.

Pacemaker or ICD Malfunction

Patients with cardiac pacemakers or ICDs should have a medical consultation prior to dental treatment. There is small chance of **infective endocarditis** because of the presence of foreign material in the circulatory system. Rarely is prophylactic premedication required; however, the patient's physician should make that determination.

The greater risk of malfunction with pacemakers or ICDs is electromagnetic interference. The electrical interference is interpreted by the pacemaker as cardiac electrical activity and may inhibit pacemaker function. This situation is temporary and does not cause permanent damage to the pacemaker. The extent of the malfunction is dependent upon the strength, duration, and particular type of interference. To reduce the risk of malfunction, pacemakers and ICDs are protected from interference by shielding the circuitry inside a stainless steel or titanium case, signal filtering, interference rejection circuits, noise reversion functions, and programmable parameters.

At the tip of each pacemaker lead is an electrode. Pacemakers can be of the unipolar or bipolar electrode type depending on how many electrodes are on the lead that is located within the heart. Although both types have proven to be reliable, bipolar types are more commonly used because extraneous interference is less likely to occur as both electrodes are in close proximity to each other and are both located within the heart muscle.

There are many causes of pacemaker and ICD malfunction, ranging from cellular phones to magnetic resonance imaging (MRI). Patients should be informed by their physician regarding possible causes of interference, and patients need to take appropriate precautions in their everyday life. In addition, they should carry a card stating that they have a pacemaker or ICD.

The dental office poses only a minimal risk to patients with pacemakers or ICDs as most dental equipment does not involve strong electromagnetic signals. Those procedures performed in the dental office that are considered safe for pacemaker and ICD patients are dental radiographs, dental handpieces, pulp vitality testers, electronic apex locators, and sonic and piezoelectric ultrasonic scalers. Dental devices in which some controversy exists as to their safety with pacemakers and ICDs are older ferromagnetic ultrasonic scalers, magnetostrictive ultrasonic scalers (see Figure 12.3 ■), **transcutaneous electrical nerve stimulators (TENS)**, ultrasonic cleaning baths (see Figure 12.4 ■), select battery-operated composite curing lights, and electrosurgical units. Malfunction was more common in older implant models due to the lack of shielding and with the unipolar pacemaker type. Placement of a lead apron over the pacemaker or ICD reduces the amount of possible electromagnetic interference. (See Figure 12.5 ■)

Magnetic dental headrests also pose a significant risk for pacemaker and ICD malfunction. These strong magnets are found in the pillows of the headrest, and once they are removed from the area, the patient can be treated safely.

Although electric and most battery-operated toothbrushes are safe to use with these patients, sonic toothbrushes with a battery charger need to be used with caution. A distance of 6 inches between the battery and/or charger and the implanted device should be maintained. Moreover, a distance of at least 1 inch should be maintained between the toothbrush itself and the implanted device to ensure safe usage. (See Figure 12.6 ■)

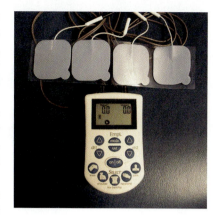

FIGURE 12.3 TENS unit contraindicated in pacemaker and ICD patients.

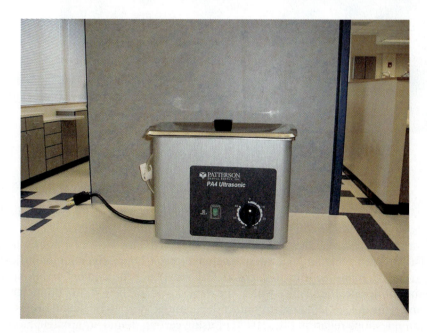

FIGURE 12.4 Ultrasonic bath contraindicated in close proximity to pacemaker and ICD patients.

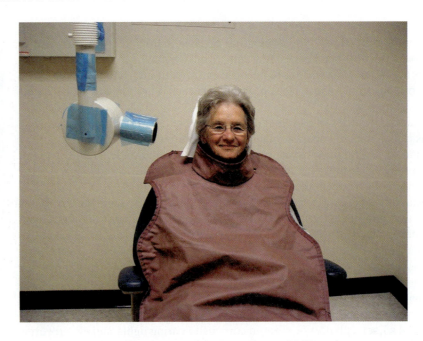

FIGURE 12.5 Use of lead apron with pacemaker and ICD patients.

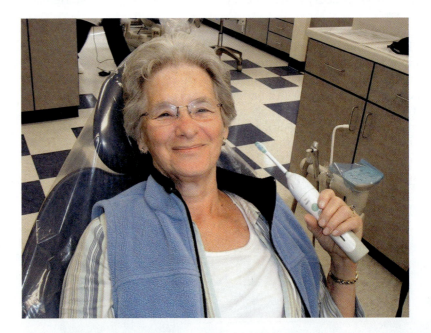

FIGURE 12.6 Appropriate distance of sonic toothbrush with pacemaker and ICD patients.

Although local anesthetics can be used on patients with pacemakers and ICDs, agents with vasoconstrictors should be used with caution. The amount of vasoconstrictor should be carefully monitored to avoid the development of a dysrhythmia.

Patients receiving an implanted pacemaker or ICD are given an identification card from the manufacturer to carry with them. The card includes details such as the kind of device, the facility where the device was implanted, the physician who implanted the device, and how to contact the manufacturer. If the dental professional has any questions regarding the safety of using certain dental equipment, he or she should contact the manufacturer as manufacturers perform continual testing on their products.

Signs and Symptoms of Pacemaker or ICD Malfunction

The symptoms associated with pacemaker malfunction are related to the pacemaker inhibiting itself from giving pacing impulses as it erroneously interprets the external impulses as heartbeats. The symptoms the patient would most likely experience include lightheadedness, dizziness, dyspnea, moist pale skin, weakness, bradycardia or tachycardia, depending on the reason for implantation; chest pain; swelling in extremities; prolonged hiccoughing; muscular twitching; and possibly altered mental status. (See Table 12.1 ■) Once the interference is terminated, the symptoms usually subside, and the pacemaker resumes normal operation. In some more severe cases, syncope may occur and would need to be treated accordingly.

If electromagnetic interference occurs with an ICD, the interference may be erroneously interpreted by the implanted device as a rapid arrhythmia and may cause an inappropriate defibrillation. This may be rather uncomfortable for conscious patients and additionally may cause twitching, biting, or sudden movements. (See Table 12.2 ■)

Treatment of Pacemaker or ICD Malfunction

The first and most important step for the management of pacemaker or ICD malfunction is to turn off all suspected causes of the interference. Then assess the patient's consciousness level. If the patient is conscious, take the vital signs and check pulse rate. The pulse rate should be continuously monitored to determine if it has reverted to normal rhythm, which will more than likely occur. If it has not reverted to normal, EMS (Emergency Medical Services) should be contacted, and the patient should be transported to the nearest emergency department for treatment. If the patient loses consciousness, you should initially treat for syncope, which includes monitoring vital signs. If the patient does not regain consciousness, this should be considered an extremely serious condition, and EMS should be contacted and the patient should be transported to a hospital. Basic life support with appropriate oxygen delivery should be provided until EMS arrives.

Table 12.1 Signs and Symptoms of Pacemaker Malfunction

- Lightheadedness
- Dizziness
- Dyspnea
- Moist, pale skin
- Weakness
- Bradycardia or tachycardia depending on the reason for implantation
- Chest pain
- Swelling in extremities
- Prolonged hiccoughing
- Muscular twitching
- Possible altered mental status

Table 12.2 Signs and Symptoms of ICD Malfunction

- Inappropriate defibrillation
- Chest pain
- Twitching
- Biting
- Sudden movements

Case Resolution and Conclusion ·····················▶

Medical technology has advanced to a point whereby pacemakers and ICDs are becoming more commonplace. At times, however, these devices can malfunction, and although malfunction is unlikely, the appropriate precautions must be taken to eliminate possible causes of interference. In the scenario presented at the beginning of this chapter, the magnetic headrest on the dental chair could be hazardous to Norman. Norman has a pacemaker, so this type of headrest is contraindicated as it can cause interference and pacemaker malfunction. The patient is now exhibiting signs and symptoms of such interference: chest pain, dyspnea, dizziness, and a pulse rate of 50. The clinician realized that the patient's pacemaker was malfunctioning and immediately removed the magnetic headrest, which alleviated the symptoms. She monitored Norman's vital signs, which quickly returned to normal levels. The practitioner continued her treatment and noted in the patient's chart that the headrest could not be used for future appointments.

Review Questions

1. Which of the following should *not* be used on patients with a pacemaker or ICD?

   A. dental handpieces
   B. pulp vitality tester
   C. magnetostrictive ultrasonic scaler
   D. dental radiographs

2. The most common use for an implantable cardio-verter defibrillator is

   A. tachyarrhythmia
   B. syncope
   C. severe hypertension
   D. none of the above

3. The portion of the pacemaker that contains the electronic circuitry and powers the device is the

   A. lead
   B. defibrillator
   C. copper stem
   D. generator

4. All of the following are symptoms of an individual suffering from a pacemaker malfunction *except* one. Which one is the *exception*?

   A. dizziness
   B. hiccoughing
   C. swelling of extremities
   D. wheezing

5. The most important vital sign to monitor on a patient suspected of having a pacemaker malfunction is the

   A. pulse
   B. respiration
   C. blood pressure
   D. temperature

6. Local anesthetics with vasoconstrictors should be used with caution on patients with pacemakers and ICDs.

   A. True
   B. False

7. The factor that causes the greatest risk of malfunction with pacemakers or ICDs is

   A. electromagnetic interference
   B. solar interference
   C. radiation interference
   D. sonar interference

8. The first step in the treatment of suspected pacemaker malfunction is to

   A. remove the cause of the interference
   B. use the AED to regain appropriate heart rate
   C. administer one tablet of nitroglycerin sublingually
   D. contact the manufacturer of the pacemaker for advice

Bibliography

American Academy of Periodontology. "Position Paper: Sonic and Ultrasonic Scalers in Periodontics." *Journal of Periodontology* 71, no. 11 (2000): 1792–1801.

——. "Periodontal Management of Patients with Cardiovascular Diseases." *Journal of Periodontology* 73, no. 8 (2002): 954–68.

Anderson, D. M., J. Keith, P. D. Novak, and M. A. Elliot, eds. *Mosby's Medical, Nursing & Allied Health Dictionary.* 6th ed. St. Louis, MO: Mosby-Year Book, Inc, (2008).

Barold, S. S., B. Herweg, and M. Giudici. "Electrocardiographic Follow-Up of Biventricular Pacemakers." *Annals of Noninvasive Electrocardiology* 10, no. 2 (2005): 231–55.

Bauer, J. "ICD's Malfunction More Than Pacemakers." *RN* 11 no. 68 (2005): 24.

Bendit, J. "Magnets in Dental Chairs." *RDH Magazine* 30, no. 3 (2010): 46.

Bennett, J. D., and M. B. Rosenberg. *Medical Emergencies in Dentistry.* 1st ed. Philadelphia, PA: W. B. Saunders, 2002.

Brand, H. S., M. L. Entjes, A. V. Nieuw Amerongen, E. V. van der Hoeff, and A. M. Schrama. "Interference of Electrical Dental Equipment with Implantable Cardioverter-Defibrillators." *British Dental Journal* 203, no. 10 (2007): 577–79.

College of Dental Hygienists of British Columbia. *Tab 5: Interpretation Guidelines: Implanted Cardiac Devices* (2012): 90–91.

College of Dental Hygienists of Ontario. "Clients with Cardiac Pacemakers." *Milestones* 6 (2005): 1–5.

Conlin, K. "Treating Patients with Implanted Heart Devices." *Dimensions of Dental Hygiene* 6, no. 1 (2008): 14–17.

Crossley, G. H., J. E. Poole, M. A. Rozner, S. J. Asivatham, A. Cheng, M. K. Chung, T. B. Ferguson, et al. "The Heart Rhythm Society (HRS)/American Society of Anesthesiologists (ASA) Expert Consensus Statement on the Perioperative Management of Patients with Implantable Defibrillators, Pacemakers and Arrhythmia Monitors: Facilities and Patient Management." *Heart Rhythm* 8, no. 7 (2011): 1114–54.

Eidelman, R. S., F. J. Dieque, A. Tolentino, and J. Zebede. "Malfunction of a Biventricular Pacing Device?" *Pacing and Clinical Electrophysiology* 27, no. 10 (2004): 1453–54.

Elshershari, H., A. Celiker, S. Ozer, and S. Ozme. "Influence of D-Net (European GSM Standard) Cellular Telephones on Implanted Pacemakers in Children." *Pacing and Clinical Electrophysiology* 25, no. 9 (2002): 1328–30.

Erdogan, O. "Electromagnetic Interference of Pacemakers." *Indian Pacing Electrophysiology Journal* 2, no. 3 (2002): 74–81.

Guidant. *Sources of Electromagnetic Interference (EMI) for Pacemakers, Implantable Cardioverter Defibrillators (ICDs), and Heart Failure Devices*, 1–8, 2005.

Hampton, R. "Cardiac Disease Safety." *Journal of the American Medical Association* 294, no. 20 (2005): 2564.

Hayes, D. D. "Pacemaker Malfunction." *Nursing* 35, no. 7 (2005): 88.

Hayes, D. L. "Electromagnetic Interference with Implantable Cardiac Devices." In Lecture of Arrhythmias and Electrophysiology from the Mayo Clinic Mayo Medical School. Accessed January 30, 2006. http://www.fac.org.ar/tcvc/llave/c016/hayes.htm.

Hayes, D. L., and R. E. Vlietstra "Pacemaker Malfunction." *Annals of Internal Medicine* 119, no. 8 (1993): 828–35.

Jeffries, J. L., G. A. Younis, S. D. Flamm, A. Rasekh, and A. Massumi. "Chest Pain and Diaphragmatic Pacing after Pacemaker Implantation." *Images in Cardiovascular Medicine* 32, 1 (2005): 106–107.

Kahri, J., and J. Rapola "Cardiovascular Disorders in Dental Practice." *Tandlægebladet* 109, no. 2 (2005): 132–40.

Kurtz, S. M., J. A. Ochoa, E. Lau, Y. Shkolnikov, B. B. Pavri, D. Frisch, and A. J. Greenspan. "Implantation Trends and Patient Profiles for Pacemakers and Implantable Cardioverter Defibrillators in the United States: 1993–2006." *Pacing and Clinical Electrophysiology* 33, no. 6 (2010): 705–11.

Maisel, W. H. "Physician Management of Pacemaker and Implantable Cardioverter Defibrillator Advisories. Pacing and Clinical Electrophysiology." *Pacing and Clinical Electrophysiology* 274 (2004): 437–42.

Malamed, S. F. *Medical Emergencies in the Dental Office.* 6th ed. St. Louis, MO: Mosby Publishing Company, 2007.

Medtronic Patient Handbook. Minneapolis, MN: Medtronic, Inc, 2006.

Montejo, M., M. J. Fernandez, C. Grande, and K. Agrirrebengoa. "Pacemaker Endocarditis: Report of 2 Cases." *Scandinavian Journal of Infectious Disease* 33, no. 6 (2001): 470–71.

Paresh, S. M. and K. A. Ellenbogen. "Life after Pacemaker Implantation: Management of Common Problems and Environmental Interactions." *Cardiology in Review* 9, no. 4 (2001): 193–201.

Reynolds, J., and S. Apple. "A Systemic Approach to Pacemaker Assessment. American Association of Critical-Care Nurses." *AACN Clinical Issues* 12, no. 1 (2001): 114–26.

Rickli, H., M. Facchini, H. Brunner, P. Ammann, M. Sagmeister, G. Klaus, W. Angehrn, et al. "Induction Ovens and Electromagnetic Interference: What Is the Risk for Patients with Implanted Pacemakers?" *PACE* 26, no. 7, Part 1 (2003): 1294–497.

Roberts, H. W. "The Effect of Electrical Dental Equipment on Vagus Nerve Stimulator's Function." *Journal of the American Dental Association* 133, no. 42(2002): 1657–64.

Schaider, J., S. R. Hayden, R. Wolfe, R. M. Barkin, and P. Rosen, eds. *Rosen & Barkin's 5 Minute Emergency Medicine Consult.* 4th ed. Philadelphia, PA: Lippincott Williams and Wilkins, 2010.

Sweesy, M. W., J. L. Holland, and K. W. Smith. "Electromagnetic Interference in Cardia Rhythm Management Devices." *AACN Clinical Issues* 15, no. 3 (2004): 391–403.

Wilson, B. L., C. Broberg, J. C. Baumgartner, C. Harris, and J. Kron. "Safetry of Electronic Apex Locators and Pulp Testers in Patients with Implanted Cardiac Pacemakers or Cardioverter/Defibrillators." *Journal of Endodontics* 32, no. 9 (2006): 847–52.

Wolber, T., S. Ryf, C. Binggetli, J. Holzmeister, C. Brunckhorst, R. Luechinger, and R. Duru. "Potential Interference of Small Neodymium Magnets with Cardiac Pacemakers and Implantable Cardioverter Defibrillators." *Heart Rhythm* 4, no. 1 (2007): 1–4.

Young, K. R., and W. M. Bailey "Twiddler's Syndrome: An Unusual Cause of Pacemaker Malfunction." *Journal of the Louisiana State Medical Society* 154, no. 3 (2002): 152–53.

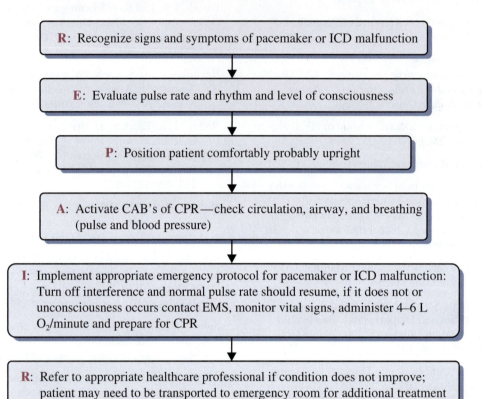

TREATMENT OF PACEMAKER OR ICD MALFUNCTION
R.E.P.A.I.R.

R: Recognize signs and symptoms of pacemaker or ICD malfunction

E: Evaluate pulse rate and rhythm and level of consciousness

P: Position patient comfortably probably upright

A: Activate CAB's of CPR—check circulation, airway, and breathing (pulse and blood pressure)

I: Implement appropriate emergency protocol for pacemaker or ICD malfunction: Turn off interference and normal pulse rate should resume, if it does not or unconsciousness occurs contact EMS, monitor vital signs, administer 4–6 L O_2/minute and prepare for CPR

R: Refer to appropriate healthcare professional if condition does not improve; patient may need to be transported to emergency room for additional treatment

Asthma

LEARNING OBJECTIVES

Upon reading the material in this chapter, the reader will be able to:

☑ Discuss the pathophysiology of asthma.

☑ Identify the specific signs and symptoms associated with asthma.

☑ Describe the different types of asthma.

☑ Explain the treatment modalities for asthma.

☑ Determine appropriate emergency steps for patients experiencing an asthmatic attack.

Case Study ·····················➤

Scenario

Your patient, Pedro Hernandez, is scheduled for a routine examination and prophylaxis. He is seven years old and has been a patient in the practice since age five. There are no significant findings on his medical history; however, he admits to becoming short of breath at times. You notice that Pedro is very apprehensive in the waiting room. He tells his mom that he is afraid to go into the treatment room. After you alleviate his initial fears, Pedro accompanies you into the operatory. Once he is seated, you notice that his breathing is beginning to become labored and a wheezing noise can be heard upon expiration. His respiration rate is 22 breaths/minute. From what condition do you suspect Pedro is suffering?

Introduction

Asthma is a chronic respiratory disorder in which there is increased responsiveness of the trachea, bronchi, and bronchioles to various triggers, resulting in the narrowing of the airways. It is characterized by recurring episodes of dyspnea, wheezing, coughing, and chest tightness.

The disorder has gained world focus because of its rapidly increasing prevalence, affecting up to one in four urban children. In 2010, it was estimated that 25.7 million Americans were asthmatics. Individuals with an increased incidence of asthma are women, children, and African Americans or individuals of Puerto Rican ethnicity. Adults and children with family income below the poverty level also exhibited a higher incidence of asthma. In the United States, deaths resulting from asthma were 3,388 in 2009.

Asthma is a complex disease that is influenced by multiple genetic, developmental, and environmental factors. In the dental office setting, stress-induced asthma or an allergic response to a dental material may result in an asthmatic attack. Although the symptoms of asthma can range from mild to life threatening, they are usually controlled with a combination of medications and lifestyle changes.

More specifically, asthma is the result of an abnormal immune response in the bronchial airways. The airways of asthmatics become hypersensitive to certain triggers known as stimuli. In response to stimuli exposure, the bronchi contract into spasm, resulting in difficulty breathing. Inflammation leads to a further narrowing of the airways and excessive mucus production, which results in coughing and wheezing on expiration and inspiration. (See Figure 13.1 ▪)

The bronchial inflammation in the asthmatic is the result of the body's immune response to an inhaled **allergen**. Typical allergens that are inhaled include waste from common household insects (e.g., dust mites and cockroaches), grass, pollen, mold spores, and pet epithelial cells. These allergens cause the body to initiate the humoral immune response, which produces antibodies in the presence of these inhaled allergens. It has been noted that **Immunoglobulin E (IgE)** is the antibody that is specific for environmental allergens. The overall inflammatory response causes constriction of the bronchioles and increased mucus production, resulting in the clinical manifestations of an asthma attack.

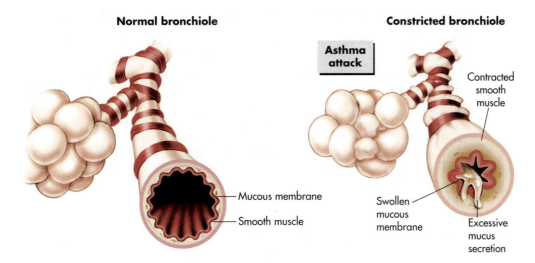

Normal bronchiole

Constricted bronchiole

Asthma attack

Contracted smooth muscle

Mucous membrane

Smooth muscle

Swollen mucous membrane

Excessive mucus secretion

FIGURE 13.1 Bronchioles of normal and asthmatic patient.

Triggers, other than typical allergens, that have been linked to asthma include air pollution, which is thought to be one of the major reasons for the high prevalence of asthma in urban areas. Industrial compounds and other chemicals have been known to induce asthma. In addition, early childhood infections (especially viral respiratory infections), exercise, and emotional stress are common etiologies of an asthma attack.

These triggers are used to classify asthma into five types: extrinsic, intrinsic, drug induced, exercise induced, and infectious. Extrinsic asthma is the most common type, accounting for 50% of asthmatics. Most patients with this form of asthma demonstrate an inherited allergic predisposition. Triggers or stimuli are from outside the body and include such allergens as pollen, dust, mold, air pollutants, and tobacco smoke. In the dental office, dental materials, such as eugenol, impression materials, resins, and latex, can initiate an asthma attack.

Intrinsic asthma is the second major category and typically develops in adults after the age of 35 years, but can be found in children. Episodes are precipitated by nonallergic factors, such as psychological and physiological stress. Dental appointments have been known to create stressful situations for some patients and have been identified as an asthma trigger.

Drug-induced asthma has also been seen in some patients. Nonsteroidal anti-inflammatory drugs (NSAIDs), including ibuprofen and aspirin, are considered triggers along with metabisulfite, which is a preservative found in some foods and local anesthetics containing epinephrine.

In exercise-induced asthma, symptoms typically begin shortly after the start of exercise, resulting in severe bronchospasm. It is believed that the thermal changes during inhalation of cold air may provoke mucosal irritation and airway hypersensitivity. This type of asthma is frequently linked to children and young adults because of their high level of physical activity.

Viral infection of the respiratory tract is the most common cause of infectious asthma. This type of asthma is frequently seen in children and results in increased airway resistance caused by the inflammatory response of the bronchi to infection. Treatment of the infection reduces the asthmatic symptoms.

The use of inhalation analgesia/sedation with nitrous oxide and oxygen is not contraindicated in the asthmatic patient, but prudent judgment based on the patient's respiratory function should be used. Local anesthetics with epinephrine contain sodium bisulfite, which may trigger an asthmatic attack and therefore are not recommended for asthmatic patients.

Signs and Symptoms of Asthma Attacks

In some individuals asthma is characterized by chronic respiratory impairment. Seventy five percent of asthmatics are considered uncontrolled asthmatics, with recurring episodes of asthma attacks. Other asthmatics experience an intermittent illness marked by episodic symptoms that may result from such triggers as upper respiratory infections, airborne allergens, stress, and exercise.

Asthmatic episodes vary in frequency, duration, and the degree of symptoms, ranging from periods of wheezing, mild coughing, and slight dyspnea to severe attacks that can lead to total airway obstruction and respiratory tract failure (known as **status asthmaticus**). In general, episodes caused by infection have a gradual onset and are of long duration, whereas those resulting from allergenic factors are acute and subside quickly if the causative agent is removed.

Signs of an asthma attack can be classified into mild, moderate, and severe depending on the degree of symptoms. In a mild attack there is difficulty in respiration with a slightly elevated respiration rate. Patients will complain of chest tightness and shortness of breath. Some patients will begin coughing and wheezing. A moderate attack increases respiratory distress. Patients tend to speak only in phrases or partial sentences. Their skin color may become pale, and there is a slight to moderate "drawing in" of muscles between the ribs to facilitate breathing. Patients experiencing a severe attack will have a rapid respiration rate. Their speech will be limited to single words. Marked wheezing and coughing will be present along with poor skin color. The patient's level of awareness will decrease as the attack progresses. Table 13.1 ∎ outlines the signs and symptoms of the various classifications of asthma attacks.

Treatment of an Asthma Attack

Once it is determined that a patient has asthma, treatment guidelines focus on maintaining the patient's respiratory status to as close to normal as possible. This includes limiting exposure to known allergens and identified triggers. Current guidelines recommend bronchodilator therapy along with other types of inhaled anti-inflammatory agents, such as corticosteroids, to help in the prevention and treatment of asthmatic attacks.

In the dental office, the treatment goal is to prevent acute episodes of the disease. Patients who have indicated on the medical history that they have asthma

Table 13.1 Signs and Symptoms of Asthma Attack

Mild Asthma Attack	Moderate Asthma Attack	Severe Asthma Attack
• Respiration is difficult • Respiration rate is slightly faster than normal range (14–20 breaths/minute) • Complete sentences can be spoken • Mild complaints of wheezing, cough, shortness of breath, or tightness in the chest • Skin color is good	• Respiration is moderately difficult • Respiration rate is faster than normal range • Only phrases or partial sentences can be spoken • Moderate complaints of wheezing, cough, shortness of breath, or tightness in the chest • Skin color is normal or may be pale • Slight to moderate "drawing in" of muscles between the ribs is necessary to breathe	• Respiration is labored • Respiration rate is very fast or very slow with a lot of distress • Only single words or short sentences are spoken • Severe complaints of wheezing, cough, shortness of breath, or tightness in the chest • Skin color is poor • Level of awareness is decreased

should present for their appointment with their prescribed bronchodilator, and in some instances, particularly for uncontrolled asthmatics, patients should be asked to use their **bronchodilator** prior to their appointment. Access to the bronchodilator during treatment should be made available to the dental practitioner. In the case of an asthmatic attack, it is recommended that treatment be terminated and the patient placed in a seated upright position with arms forward as this position allows more air to enter the lungs. Tight clothing should be loosened to facilitate breathing. (See Figure 13.2 ■) Patients should be given their personal bronchodilator for self-administration and instructed to inhale slowly and exhale through pursed lips. (See Figures 13.3 ■ and 13.4 ■) If patients do not have their inhaler, it is recommended to administer a standard emergency kit inhaler containing albuterol, which takes effect shortly after administration and has a four- to six-hour duration period. Two puffs of the medication is the recommended dosage. The dental professional may provide supplemental oxygen at 4–6 L/minute via a non-rebreather bag and monitor vital signs. If the asthmatic attack does not subside, additional doses of albuterol should be administered at 15-minute intervals and EMS (Emergency Medical Services) should

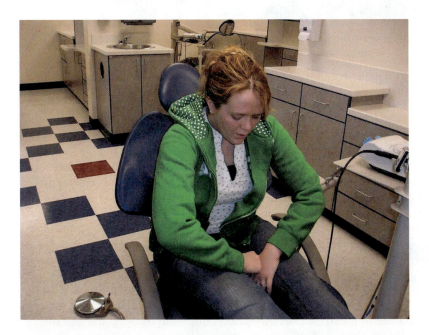

FIGURE 13.2 Patient positioned with arms forward during asthma attack.

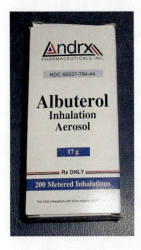
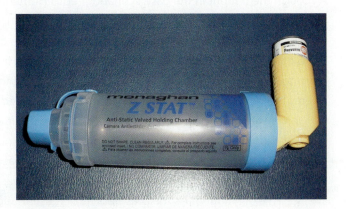

FIGURE 13.3 Albuterol inhaler and spacer device.

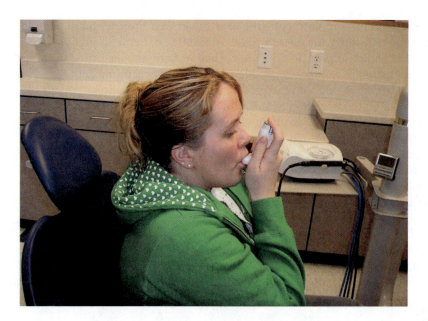

FIGURE 13.4 Patient using inhaler during asthma attack.

be contacted for the prevention of status asthmaticus. It is recommended that the subsequent doses should be administered using a spacer device in conjunction with the inhaler. The spacer device provides more effective distribution of the inhaled drug to the lungs and reduces the need for coordination of inhalation of the drug with activation of the inhaler. The maximum dosage of albuterol is 12 inhalations/day. If the patient's condition worsens they may require subcutaneous epinephrine injection as is used for anaphylaxis and transportation to emergency room for further observation and treatment. Continuation of treatment is determined based on the severity of the attack and speed of recovery.

Case Resolution and Conclusion

Asthma is a disease that can be prevented and controlled through the use of inhalation medication. It is considered a medical emergency when the condition escalates to an asthmatic attack. In the dental office asthmatic attacks are typically triggered by apprehension and anxiety concerning dental treatment. Although the patient in the case scenario, Pedro Hernandez, did not have a history of asthma, his labored breathing and wheezing upon expiration, which were both caused by his apprehension, should alert the clinician to the likelihood of this condition. In addition, his young age and Hispanic nationality are indicators of asthma. Pedro was positioned upright with his arms forward in an attempt to improve his respirations. He was administered a dose of albuterol via inhaler with a spacing device from the emergency kit and directed to inhale slowly through pursed lips. He was also given 4 L O_2/minute via non-rebreathing bag. His symptoms quickly subsided with these measures, and after a discussion with his mother regarding the episode, he was referred to his physician for an examination. As this was Pedro's first asthmatic attack and he was quite upset by the episode, he was reappointed for his prophylaxis.

Review Questions

1. Asthma is a chronic respiratory disease that is increasing in prevalence, and is most commonly seen in children.

    A. The first phrase is correct, and the second phrase is incorrect.
    B. The first phrase is incorrect, and the second phrase is correct.
    C. Both phrases are correct.
    D. Both phrases are incorrect.

2. Asthma is characterized by all of the following *except* one. Which one is the *exception*?

    A. wheezing
    B. coughing
    C. tightness in chest
    D. increased blood pressure

3. The most common type of asthma is

    A. extrinsic asthma
    B. intrinsic asthma
    C. drug-induced asthma
    D. infectious asthma

4. Typical treatment of an asthmatic attack includes all of the following *except* which one. Which one is the *exception*?

    A. use of a bronchodilator inhaler
    B. breathing into a paper bag
    C. upright patient positioning
    D. administration of oxygen

5. An asthmatic condition that is life threatening is termed

    A. severe asthma
    B. asthmatic trauma
    C. status asthmaticus
    D. none of the above

6. What is the appropriate position for a patient having an asthma attack?

    A. supine
    B. semi-supine
    C. upright with arms forward
    D. Trendelenburg

7. The number of metered sprays that should initially be administered to a patient suffering from an asthma attack is

    A. 1
    B. 2
    C. 3
    D. 4

8. An asthma attack in which the patient can speak only in phrases or partial sentences would be considered of _____ severity.

    A. mild
    B. moderate
    C. severe

Bibliography

Akinbami, L. J., J. E. Moorman, and X. Liu. "Asthma Prevalence, Health Care Use, and Mortality: United States, 2005–2009." *National Health Statistics Reports* no. 32 (2011): 1–15.

Anderson, D. M., J. Keith, P. D. Novak, and M. A. Elliot, eds. *Mosby's Medical, Nursing & Allied Health Dictionary*. 6th ed. St. Louis, MO: Mosby-Year Book, Inc., 2008.

Balmer, C., and L. Longman. *The Management of Medical Emergencies: A Guide for Dental Professionals*. 1st ed. London, England: Quay Books, 2008.

Guggenheimer, J., and P. A. Moore. "The Patient with Asthma: Implications for Dental Practice." *Compendium* 30, no. 4 (2009): 200–209.

Institute for Clinical Systems Improvement. *Diagnosis and Outpatient Management of Asthma*. Bloomington, MN: Institute for Clinical Systems Improvement, 2005. http://www.guideline.gov.

Lethbridge-Çejku, M., D. Rose, and J. Vickerie. "Summary Health Statistics for United States: National Health Interview Survey, 2004 National Center for Health Statistics." *Vital Health Statistics* 10, no. 228 (2006): 1–164.

Little, J. W., D. A. Falace, C. S. Miller, and N. L. Rhodus. *Dental Management of the Medically Compromised Patient*. 7th ed. St. Louis, MO: Mosby Publishing Company, 2007.

Loignon, C., C. Bedos, R. Sevigny, and N. Leduc. "Understanding the Self-Care Strategies of Patients with Asthma." *Patient Education and Counseling* 75, no. 2 (2009): 256–62.

Maddox, L., and D. A. Schwartz. "The Pathophysiology of Asthma." *Annual Review Medicine* 53 (2002): 477–98.

Malamed, S. F. *Medical Emergencies in the Dental Office*. 6th ed. St. Louis, MO: Mosby Publishing Company, 2007.

National Asthma Education and Prevention Program. *Guidelines Implementation Panel Report for: Expert Panel*

Report 3: Guidelines for the Diagnosis and Management of Asthma Partners Putting Guidelines into Action. U.S. Department of Health and Human Services, National Institutes of Health, National Heart, Lung, and Blood, 2008. http://www.nhlbi.nih.gov/guidelines/asthma/.

Nunn, T. J. "Developing a Medical Emergency Protocol." *Access* 20, no. 9 (2006): 12–15.

Pickett, F., and J. Gurenlian. *Preventing Medical Emergencies: Use of the Medical History. Philadelphia.* 2nd ed. Philadelphia, PA: Lippincott Williams & Wilkins, 2010.

Rutland, C. "Management of Medical Emergencies in the Dental Practice." *Dental Nursing* 7, no. 5 (2011): 274–77.

Solomon, G., E. Humphreys, and M. D. Miller. "Asthma and the Environment: Connecting the Dots: What Role Do Environmental Exposures Play in the Rising Prevalence and Severity of Asthma?" *Contemporary Pediatrics* 21 (2004): 73–81.

"Vital Signs: Asthma Prevalence, Disease Characteristics, and Self-Management Education—United States, 2001–2009." *Morbidity and Mortality Weekly* 60, no. 17 (2011): 547–52.

Wilson, M. H., N. S. McArdle, J. J. Fitzpatrick, L. F. A. Stassen. "Medical Emergencies in the Dental Practice." *Journal of the Irish Dental Association* 55, no. 3 (2009): 134–43.

Xu, J. Q., K. D. Kochanek, S. L. Murphy, B. Tejada-Vera. "Deaths: Final Data for 2007. National Center for Health Statistics." *Vital Health Statistics* 58, no. 19 (2010): 1–135.

Zhao, J., M. Takamura, A. Yamaoka, Y. Odajima, and Y. Iikura. "Altered Eosinophil Levels as a Result of Viral Infection in Asthma Exacerbation in Childhood." *Journal of Pediatric Allergy Immunology* 13, no. 1 (2002): 47–50.

TREATMENT OF ASTHMA ATTACK
R.E.P.A.I.R.

R: Recognize signs and symptoms of asthma (respiratory distress, increased respiration rate, wheezing, coughing, tightness in the chest, difficulty speaking, pale skin color) and maintain a calm demeanor

E: Evaluate respiration rate

P: Position patient upright with arms forward

A: Activate CAB's of CPR—check circulation, airway, and breathing (pulse and blood pressure)

I: Implement appropriate emergency protocol for asthma: Attempt to have patients use bronchodilator (their own or from the emergency kit), (if first dose in effective use spacer device), administer oxygen 4–6 L/minute, loosen tight clothing in neck region, monitor vital signs

R: Refer to appropriate healthcare professional if condition does not improve; patient may require subcutaneous epinephrine injection and transportation to emergency room for further observation and treatment

Obstructed Airway, Aspiration, or Ingestion of a Foreign Object

LEARNING OBJECTIVES

Upon reading the material in this chapter, the reader will be able to:

- ✓ Discuss the possible etiologies of obstructed airway in the dental office.

- ✓ List specific signs and symptoms associated with obstructed airway.

- ✓ List specific signs and symptoms associated with foreign body aspiration.

- ✓ Determine suggested treatment modalities for obstructed airway.

- ✓ Determine suggested treatment modalities for foreign body aspiration.

Case Study ·····································➤

Scenario

Your 1:00 P.M. patient, Gracey Gatos, is an 80-year-old female. You are attempting to recement a temporary crown that came off over the weekend. The crown slips out of your wet gloves and has entered your patient's throat. She places her hands to her neck, is aggressively coughing, and is having difficulty breathing. What should you do?

Introduction

The nature of the dental profession increases the likelihood that a patient may suffer from an obstructed airway or **aspiration** of a foreign object. The small size of the objects dental professionals place in the mouth and the supine position in which they work increase the likelihood of obstruction or aspiration. The most common item involved in obstruction or aspiration is food; however, dental appliances are a close second. Aspirated or ingested objects often require hospitalization. Ten to twenty percent of ingested foreign bodies require nonsurgical intervention, while approximately 1% require surgery; therefore, it is important that the dental professional understand the signs and symptoms of these emergencies and the appropriate treatment.

Obstructed Airway

An obstructed airway is a common occurrence in the dental office as preventive measures, such as the use of a rubber dam or gauze curtain in the anterior portion of the throat, are not commonly used for this procedure. The patient is still able to cough, so the obstruction would be considered a partial obstruction. Other symptoms of a partially obstructed airway are poor air exchange and a weak cough. If a complete obstruction were to occur, the patient would be unable to speak, cough, or breathe and would be in significant distress.

Another sequelae of this scenario could be that the patient aspirated the temporary crown in the lung tissue and that is why she is still coughing. Aspiration of an object can be extremely serious, and removal of the object is imperative to avoid a major infection or death. The literature is replete with articles regarding foreign body aspiration. Dental objects that have been aspirated include primary and permanent teeth, dental impression material, orthodontic retainers, fixed prosthetics (crowns, bridges, partial dentures), implants, orthodontic wires, orthodontic brackets, anesthetic needles, gauze, a screwdriver used during dental implant placement, ultrasonic scaler tips, and broken instrument tips.

In addition to aspiration, dental objects can be ingested. Ninety percent of these objects usually pass through the digestive tract and are excreted within 2–12 days; however, 10% cause impaction, abscesses, or perforation of the gastrointestinal tract.

Aspiration or ingestion of objects is often associated with children. Children have a tendency to place small objects in their mouths that may become lodged in their throat, ingested, or aspirated into their lungs. In the United States, 500 children per year die because of foreign body aspiration. Other groups for which there are more frequent reports of foreign body aspiration are geriatric patients, psychotics, alcohol and/or drug abusers, developmentally challenged and hyperactive individuals, patients with an excessive gag reflex, and patients with an impaired swallowing reflex. Small, round crunchy foods are commonly associated with aspiration.

Signs and Symptoms of an Obstructed Airway

Partially Obstructed Airway

The signs and symptoms of a partially obstructed airway include coughing, cyanosis from a reduction in the oxygen supply, placing the hands in the area of the throat, wheezing as the person attempts to move air into and out of the lungs, and dyspnea because of the obstruction. Patients will be anxious and fearful as their air supply is reduced.

Completely Obstructed Airway

The signs of a completely obstructed airway are somewhat similar to a partial obstruction in that patients will be in distress, they will grip their throat, and their skin color will be cyanotic. The major difference is that patients will not be able to talk or cough, and there will be an absence of air exchange. The lack of oxygen will eventually cause them to lose consciousness if the obstruction is not removed. Patients experiencing a partial obstruction, but with very poor air exchange, should be treated as if they have a complete airway obstruction. A crowing noise during breathing, also known as a stridor, is an indication of poor air exchange.

Foreign Body Aspiration

The signs and symptoms of foreign body aspiration in the lungs range from nonexistent to severe dyspnea. Symptoms are dependent on the location of the foreign body in the airway. Immediately following the aspiration the patient might present with symptoms of dyspnea, hoarseness, wheezing, coughing, decreased breath sounds, cyanosis, **stupor**, excessive sputum production, and possibly suffocation.

The majority of patients present to an emergency department or physician's office within one week of aspiration of the object. If the aspirated object remains in the lung tissue for some time, the patient will display the following symptoms: fever, pain in the chest and/or lung area, increased respiratory rate (tachypnea), sounds when breathing, and coughing. Other symptoms that may occur with a delay in removal of the aspirated object are **anorexia**, weight loss, and loss of strength. Oftentimes these symptoms may be attributed to other conditions, such as chronic obstructive pulmonary disease, **congestive heart failure**, or pneumonia. If left untreated, death can be the ultimate outcome of an aspirated object. (See Table 14.1 ■)

Foreign Body Ingestion

The signs and symptoms of foreign body ingestion are dependent upon where the object is lodged. Foreign bodies near the oropharyngeal level are the most common. The patient will exhibit symptoms, such as a feeling of something trapped in his or

Table 14.1 Signs and Symptoms of an Obstructed Airway

Partially Obstructed Airway	Completely Obstructed Airway	Aspirated Foreign Body	Ingested foreign body
• Coughing • Cyanosis • Placing hands in throat area • Wheezing • Dyspnea • Anxious • Fear	• Respiratory distress • Place hands in throat area • Cyanosis • Unable to talk or cough and eventual loss of consciousness	• Nonexistent to severe dyspnea depending on the location of the foreign body in the airway • Dyspnea • Hoarseness • Wheezing • Coughing • Decreased breath sounds • Cyanosis • Stupor • Excessive sputum production • Possible suffocation	• Feeling of something trapped in throat • Mild to severe discomfort in throat • Drooling • Dysphagia • Airway compromise • Sensation in chest area • Gagging • Vomiting • Pain in neck or throat • Abdominal distension and discomfort

her throat, mild to severe discomfort, drooling of saliva, **dysphagia** (inability to swallow), possible airway compromise, and possible infection or perforation of anatomic structures. Foreign bodies in the esophagus will cause the patient to feel a sensation in the center of the chest, dysphagia, drooling, gagging, vomiting, or neck or throat pain. Foreign bodies reaching the gastrointestinal tract may lead to abdominal distension and discomfort, fever, vomiting, rectal bleeding, or other symptoms. If the object perforates the surrounding anatomical structures, the symptoms will be more severe and acute.

Treatment of Partially and Completely Obstructed Airways

Treatment for the partially obstructed airway is to position the patient upright and encourage him or her to continue coughing to attempt to expel the object. Applying back blows is no longer recommended as this may cause aspiration of the object. The patient will either expel the object, the object will continue to partially block the airway, or the obstruction can totally block the airway. If the patient ceases coughing and still cannot speak, a total airway obstruction should be suspected, and abdominal thrusts commonly referred to as the **Heimlich maneuver** should be performed. Abdominal thrusts should be continued until the object is expelled, or the patient loses consciousness. Once consciousness is lost, the patient should be placed in a supine position, and the clinician should open the airway and attempt to ventilate the patient. If the breaths do not enter the lungs, the head should be repositioned to ensure that the airway is open, and another attempt to ventilate should ensue. If the breath enters the lungs, then the clinician would continue with the CABs (circulation, airway, and breathing) of cardiopulmonary resuscitation (CPR). If the breath does not enter the lungs, then chest compressions as in CPR should be performed at a rate of 30:2 (compressions to ventilations) for five cycles, inspect the oral cavity for the object, and perform a finger sweep only if the object is apparent. If the object is not visible, then another ventilation attempt should occur. This procedure should be performed until ventilation is successful or until trained medical help arrives. Contacting EMS (Emergency Medical Services) as soon as possible to transport the patient to the emergency department for care is essential particularly in the case of a completely obstructed airway.

Treatment of an Aspirated or Ingested Object

If the aspiration or ingestion of an object is suspected, EMS should be contacted. The patient should be transported to the emergency department where a chest and/or abdominal radiograph will be taken. If the radiograph reveals that an object has been aspirated, doctors will likely perform a **bronchoscopy** to remove the object. A bronchoscopy is a procedure in which a tube with a light is placed in the patient's throat and into the bronchi to view the area and to remove the foreign body. In adults foreign objects usually lodge in the right bronchial tree. If an aspirated object is left untreated, it could cause inflammation, infection, ulceration, and granulation tissue formation in the lungs. Therefore, if aspiration is even the least bit suspected and a foreign body is not recovered, the patient should be referred to the emergency department for a chest X-ray.

If ingestion of the object is suspected and the object is not radio-opaque, an **endoscopy** of the upper gastrointestinal tract may be needed. This procedure uses an endoscope, which is a long, thin tube with a small camera at the end to examine the patient's esophagus and stomach area. CT scanning of the abdomen is also useful for locating ingested objects and is often used if a perforation or abscess formation is suspected. Once located, various procedures are used to remove the object, including surgery.

Thorough documentation of either situation is important. The documentation should include the procedure being performed, precautions that were taken, the patient's condition, actions taken by the clinician, the recommendation for medical evaluation, and how the patient was transported to the medical facility. If the patient refuses further medical treatment, this should be documented.

Prevention of Aspiration or Ingestion of Dental Objects

There are several methods to prevent the aspiration of dental objects. The clinician should use a rubber dam or gauze throat screen whenever possible. For the prevention of aspiration of fixed restorations, a piece of dental floss should be temporarily bonded to the restoration and removed following cementation. Another option is to attach an orthodontic elastic chain to the wax pattern before investment and casting. During the try-in of the restoration, floss can be attached through the loop and knotted securely. The elastic chain loop is easily removed after cementation.

Case Resolution and Conclusion ·····························➤

Aspiration, ingestion, or obstruction of a foreign body can be a serious situation. As in the case scenario, preventive measures should be taken to reduce the risk of this emergency while recementing the patient's crown. Other dental preventive measures include always testing rotary instruments outside of the patient's mouth and never leaving a patient alone in an operatory when dental armamentarium is in his or her mouth. Gracey was obviously experiencing an obstructed airway and was coughing in an attempt to expel the crown. She was experiencing some dyspnea and was allowed to continue to cough. Within a short time, Gracey was able to dislodge the crown from her throat, and after a period of recovery time, the crown was recemented using a gauze curtain in the throat area.

Review Questions

1. If patients are experiencing a partially obstructed airway, they will not exhibit cyanosis, whereas if they are experiencing a completely obstructed airway, they will exhibit cyanosis.

   A. The first phrase is true, and the second phrase is false.
   B. The first phrase is false, and the second phrase is true.
   C. Both phrases are true.
   D. Both phrases are false.

2. The procedure used to remove an aspirated foreign object is

   A. bronchoscopy
   B. Heimlich maneuver
   C. curettage
   D. none of the above

3. You believe your patient is choking on a cotton roll you have placed in her mouth. She is vigorously coughing. What should you do?

   A. Perform the Heimlich maneuver.
   B. Provide four strong back blows.
   C. Call EMS so that the patient can be transported to the emergency department quickly.
   D. Do nothing and let the patient continue coughing.

4. All of the following are symptoms of an untreated aspirated object *except* one. Which one is the *exception*?

   A. weight loss
   B. fever
   C. tachypnea
   D. syncope

5. Treatment for an ingested foreign object is

   A. Heimlich maneuver
   B. bronchoscopy
   C. endoscopy
   D. all of the above

6. All of the following are signs and symptoms of an ingested foreign object *except* one. Which one is the *exception*?

   A. cyanosis
   B. vomiting
   C. rectal bleeding
   D. dysphagia

7. Abdominal thrusts for a conscious patient suffering from a completely obstructed airway should be performed

   A. once every 5 seconds
   B. once every 10 seconds
   C. until the object is dispelled
   D. until the patient turns cyanotic

8. If a victim of a foreign body airway obstruction becomes unconscious, the clinician would then

   A. perform abdominal thrusts
   B. start CPR beginning with chest compressions
   C. begin rescue breathing
   D. use the AED

Bibliography

Al-Rashed, M. A. "A Method to Prevent Aspiration or Ingestion of Cast Post and Core Restorations." *Journal of Prosthetic Dentistry* 91, no. 5 (2004): 501–2.

Anderson, K. N., L. E. Anderson, and W. D. Glanze. *Mosby's Medical, Nursing & Allied Health Dictionary*. 8th ed. St. Louis, MO: Mosby-Year Book, Inc., 2009.

Biron, C. R. "Quick Retrieval of Swallowed Objects Prevent Further Complications of Peritonitis." *RDH* 17, no. 5 (1997): 38–42.

Boyd, M., A. Chatterjee, C. Chiles, and R. Chin. "Tracheobronchial Foreign Body Aspiration in Adults." *Southern Medical Journal* 102, no. 2 (2009): 171–74.

Findlay, C. A., S. Morrissey, and J. Y. Paton. "Subcutaneous Emphysema Secondary to Foreign-Body Aspiration." *Pediatric Pulmonary* 36, no. 1 (2003): 81–82.

Godar, T. "Geriatric Respiratory Emergencies." *Emergency* 24, no. 9 (1992): 30–33, 56.

Gregori, D., L. Salemi, C. Scarinzi, B. Morra, P. Berchialla, S. Snidero, R. Corradetti, and D. Passali. "Foreign Bodies in the Upper Airways Causing Complications and Requiring Hospitalization in Children Aged 0-14: Results from the ESFBI Study." *European Archives of Oto-Rhino-Laryngology* 265, no. 8 (2008): 971–78.

Hill, E. E., and B. Rubel. "A Practical Review of Prevention and Management of Ingested/Aspirated Dental Items." *General Dentistry* 56, no. 7 (2008): 691–94.

Holan, G., and D. Ram. "Aspiration of an Avulsed Primary Incisor. A Case Report." *International Journal of Pediatric Dentistry* 10, no. 2 (2000)" 150–52.

Kimberly, D. R. "Unrecognized Aspiration of Mandibular incisor." *Journal of Oral and Maxillofacial Surgery* 59, no. 3 (2001): 350–52.

Klein, A. M., and S. R. Schoem. "Unrecognized Aspiration of a Dental Retainer: A Case Report." *Otolaryngology—Head and Neck Surgery* 126, no. 4 (2002): 438–39.

Murray, A. D., and D. L. Walner. "Methods in Instrumentation for Removal of Airway Foreign Bodies." *Operative Techniques in Otolaryngology—Head and Neck Surgery* 13, no. 1 (2002): 2–5.

Nakajima, M., and Y. Sato. "A Method for Preventing Aspiration or Ingestion of Fixed Restorations." *Journal of Prosthetic Dentistry* 92, no. 3 (2004): 303.

Parolia, A., M. Kamath, M. Kundubala, T. S. Manuel, and M. Mohan. "Management of Foreign Body Aspiration or Ingestion in Dentistry." *Kathmandu University Medical Journal* 7, no. 2 (2009): 165–71.

Rahulan, V., M. Patel, E. Sy, and L. Menon. "Foreign Body Aspiration in the Elderly: An Occult Cause of Chronic Pulmonary Symptoms and Persistent Infiltrates." *Clinical Geriatrics* 11, no. 11 (2003): 41–43.

Skoulakis, C. E., P. G. Doxas, C. E. Papadakis, E. Proimos, P. Christodoulou, J. G. Bizakis, G. A. Velegrakis, D. Mamoulakis, and E. S. Helidonis, E. S. "Bronchoscopy for Foreign Body Removal in Children. A Review and Analysis of 210 Cases." *International Journal of Pediatric Otorhinolaryngology* 53, no. 2 (2000): 143–48.

Singh, B., M. Kantu, G. Har-El,and F. E. Lucente. "Complications Associated with 327 Foreign Bodies of the Pharynx, Larynx and Esophagus." *Annals of Otology, Rhinology & Laryngology* 106, no. 4 (1997): 301–304.

Sopena, B., L. Garcia-Caballero, P. Diz, J. De la Guente, A. Fernandez, and J. Antonio. "Unsuspected Foreign Body Aspiration." *Quintessence International* 34, no. 10 (2003): 779–81.

Tiwana, K. K., T. Morton, and P. S. Tiwana. "Aspiration and Ingestion in Dental Practice: A 10 year Institutional Review." *Journal of the American Dental Association* 135, no. 9 (2004): 1287–91.

Ulusoy, M., and S. Toksavul. "Preventing Aspiration or Ingestion of Fixed Restorations." *Journal of Prosthetic Dentistry* 89, no. 2 (2003): 223–24.

Villasenor, A. "Aspiration of a Gauze Pressure-Pack Following a Dental Extraction: A Case Report." *Pediatric Dentistry* 21, no. 2 (1999): 135–36.

Wilcox, C. W., and T. M. Wilwerding. "Aid for Preventing Aspiration/Ingestion of Single Crowns." *Journal of Prosthetic Dentistry* 81, no. 3 (1999): 370–71.

Yakamoto, S., K. Suzuki, T. Itaya, E. Yamamoto, and S. Baba. "Foreign Bodies in the Airway: Eighteen-Year Retrospective Study." *Acta Oto-Laryngologica* 525, supplement (1996): 6–8.

Zitzmann, N. U., S. Elsasser, R. Fried, and C. P. Marinello. "Foreign Body Ingestion and Aspiration." *Oral Surgery, Oral Medicine, Oral Pathology* 88, no. 6 (1999): 657–60.

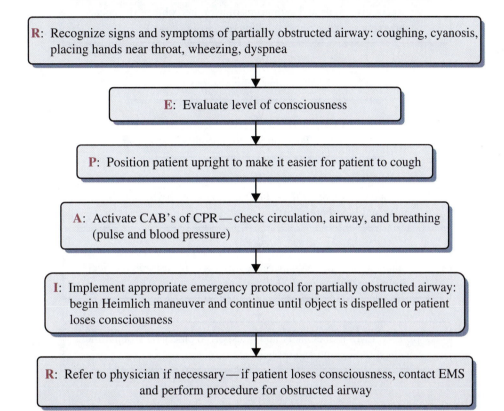

TREATMENT OF A PARTIALLY OBSTRUCTED AIRWAY
R.E.P.A.I.R.

R: Recognize signs and symptoms of partially obstructed airway: coughing, cyanosis, placing hands near throat, wheezing, dyspnea

E: Evaluate level of consciousness

P: Position patient upright to make it easier for patient to cough

A: Activate CAB's of CPR—check circulation, airway, and breathing (pulse and blood pressure)

I: Implement appropriate emergency protocol for partially obstructed airway: begin Heimlich maneuver and continue until object is dispelled or patient loses consciousness

R: Refer to physician if necessary—if patient loses consciousness, contact EMS and perform procedure for obstructed airway

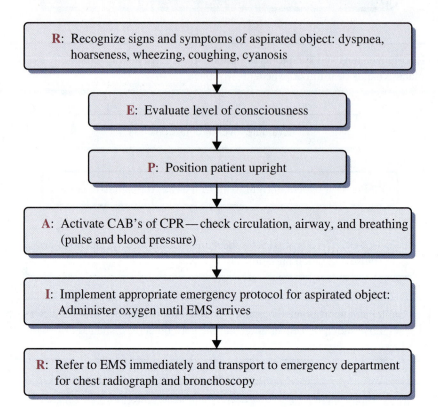

TREATMENT OF ASPIRATED OBJECT
R.E.P.A.I.R.

R: Recognize signs and symptoms of aspirated object: dyspnea, hoarseness, wheezing, coughing, cyanosis

E: Evaluate level of consciousness

P: Position patient upright

A: Activate CAB's of CPR—check circulation, airway, and breathing (pulse and blood pressure)

I: Implement appropriate emergency protocol for aspirated object: Administer oxygen until EMS arrives

R: Refer to EMS immediately and transport to emergency department for chest radiograph and bronchoscopy

Allergic Reactions

LEARNING OBJECTIVES

Upon reading the material in this chapter, the reader will be able to:

- ✓ Discuss the pathophysiology of an allergic reaction.

- ✓ Compare and contrast specific signs and symptoms associated with mild, moderate, and severe allergic reactions.

- ✓ Determine suggested treatment modalities for each type of allergic reaction.

- ✓ Explain the steps needed to prepare an office for a patient experiencing an allergic response.

Case Study ···▶

Scenario

Your patient, Diana Briggs, is a 50-year-old female in good health, except for her prosthetic hip, which was placed one year ago, for which she must be premedicated with 2.0 gm of amoxicillin prior to dental hygiene treatment. She arrives early, stating that she has forgotten to take her antibiotic. You keep a supply of amoxicillin in your office and dispense 2 gm of medication. Diana is sitting in the reception area, waiting the required one hour prior to treatment. About 10 minutes later she begins to complain of a scratchy throat, is beginning to itch all over, and is exhibiting hives on her arms and face. She requests a glass of water and is trying to catch her breath. Her symptoms are worsening. Her lips and eyes are beginning to swell. She is pale and exhibiting severe dyspnea. You take her blood pressure, and it is extremely low—70/40 mmHg—and her pulse is bradypneic at 60 beats/minute. From what emergency do you suspect Diana is suffering?

Introduction

An allergy is a **hypersensitive** reaction to an ordinarily harmless substance, the majority of which are environmental. The most common causes of allergic reactions are exposure to dust, pollen, latex, foods (particularly peanuts, tree nuts, shellfish, milk, eggs, and wheat), insect stings, and medications (particularly aspirin, **NSAIDs**, penicillin, and radiographic contrast media). Common allergens found in the dental office include latex gloves, glutens, pine nuts included in some fluoride varnishes, the sodium bisulfite preservative in local anesthetic agents with vasoconstrictors, and ester-type topical anesthetics. The reaction of the individual to the allergen can vary from mild symptoms, such as a rash, sneezing, watery eyes, runny nose, and/or skin irritation, to severely life-threatening changes, such as severe hypotension and dyspnea. The more severe form of allergy is often referred to as **anaphylaxis** (means the opposite of prophylaxis, which refers to immunologic protection) or anaphylactic shock. The severity of the reaction is often dependent on the amount of allergen to which the individual is exposed, the rate of exposure, and the route of exposure. Generally speaking, the more quickly the reaction occurs, the more life threatening the symptoms. Risk of death is more likely to occur in older individuals and women from **cardiovascular collapse** or respiratory arrest.

Allergies have been estimated to affect more than 15% of the population worldwide. Thirty percent of individuals residing in the United States are believed to have some form of allergy. Due to the variety and variability of symptoms, the exact numbers of allergic reactions are unclear. Severe allergic reactions cause approximately 1,500 deaths annually in the United States.

There are four basic types of allergic reactions: type I, type II, type III, and type IV. A type I reaction is an immediate hypersensitivity caused by immunoglobulin E and is also referred to as a common allergy. Type II reactions are **cytolytic** in nature and cause cell death. Type III reactions are not immunoglobulin E mediated; however, they have anaphylaxis-type symptoms and are often referred to as anaphylactoid reactions. The process that occurs in a type III reaction is as follows: A body is exposed to an **antigen**, and the proteins of the body attack the antigen, causing a cascading effect to help destroy the invading organism. During the process, toxins can be produced and mast cells can become damaged, causing the release of chemicals within the cell. This in turn will result in similar symptoms found in a type I allergic reaction. Type IV hypersensitivity is a delayed allergic response that takes more than 12 hours to develop. Inflammation develops in the affected tissue, and may even result in a chronic inflammatory condition. This type of allergic response often manifests as a **contact dermatitis**, with symptoms of **erythema**, **pruritus**, **eczema**, weeping papules, or vesicles.

Type I allergic reactions tend to follow the same physiological process. The individual must initially be exposed to a particular antigen. This first exposure to the antigen is referred to as the **sensitizing dose** or sensitization and elicits the body's primary immune response. When this occurs, the body stimulates the production of **antibodies** to fight off the antigen. The types of antibodies that are produced in response to an allergic reaction are termed an immunoglobulin E (IgE). The IgE attaches to the **mast cells** and **basophils** and lies dormant until the body encounters that particular antigen again. The mast cells and basophils are primarily found in the lungs, small intestine, intravascularly, and in connective tissue, with mast cells located interstitially. When the body is introduced to the antigen the second time, also known as the **challenge dose**, the antigen is then referred to as an allergen. At this point the IgE recognizes the specific antigen, and the mast cells and basophils undergo **degranulation** (the cell surface ruptures, allowing the cell contents to spill out), releasing chemical mediators in an attempt to destroy the antigen. This release of chemical mediators initiates the allergic reaction. (See Figure 15.1 ■) The major chemical mediator that is released is histamine, which results in smooth muscle contraction, increased vascular permeability, increased gastric acid secretion, systemic vasodilation, and cardiovascular stimulation. These physiological changes will cause the patient to have the following symptoms: flushed skin tone, edema, upset stomach, urticaria (hives), reduced blood pressure, and increased heart rate. (See Figure 15.2 ■)

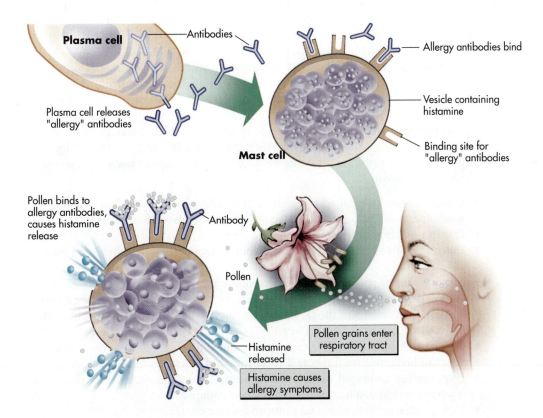

FIGURE 15.1 Allergic rhinitis.

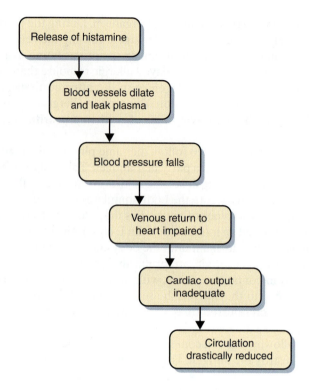

FIGURE 15.2 Sequence of vascular events in anaphylactic shock.

Signs and Symptoms of Allergic Reactions

The symptoms of allergic responses are quite variable and can involve multiple target organs. They tend to develop gradually, usually beginning with pruritus (itching) of the gingiva, throat, palms, or soles of the feet, followed by urticaria or **angioedema** (painless swelling). In some instances, the allergic reaction can begin with cardiovascular, respiratory, or gastrointestinal symptoms. Ultimately, the symptoms are specific to that individual. Patients who experience an allergic reaction to insect stings are more likely to experience cardiovascular symptoms, whereas patients who experience allergic reactions to food exposure or by an oral route are more likely to exhibit respiratory symptoms. In addition, not all signs and symptoms may be present simultaneously or at all. The classic signs and symptoms include the following:

- Urticaria—smooth, raised red lesions or wheals with central blanching due to vasodilation of the capillaries. Also referred to as hives. (See Figure 15.3 ■)
- Pruritus—itching from release of histamine.
- **Conjunctivitis**—inflammation of the conjunctiva of the eye caused by release of histamine.
- Flushed skin or pallor because of vasodilation.
- Angioedema of the lips, eyes, hands, neck, or throat caused by increased tissue fluid. If angioedema of the larynx occurs, airway obstruction can result, leading to asphyxia and respiratory arrest.
- Bronchospasm and dyspnea cause wheezing and chest tightness because of the effect of histamine on the **beta 2 receptors** in the lungs.
- Hypotension and rapid weak pulse because of vasodilation. If the hypotension is very severe, it can lead to cardiovascular collapse.
- Tachycardia, arrhythmias, and reduced cardiac contractility.
- Decreased consciousness and patient responsiveness because of oxygen deficiency.

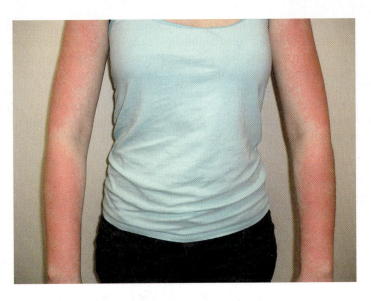

FIGURE 15.3 Urticaria from an allergic response.

Table 15.1   Signs and Symptoms of Allergic Reactions

Mild Allergic Reaction	Moderate Allergic Reaction	Severe Allergic Reaction
• Localized redness • Localized pruritus • Localized urticaria • Edema • Conjunctivitis • Pale or flushed skin • Rhinitis	• Systemic redness • Systemic pruritus • Systemic urticaria • Edema • Rhinitis • Bronchospasm/dyspnea • Abdominal pain • Cramping • Diarrhea	• Systemic redness • Systemic pruritus • Systemic urticaria • Severe hypotension • Dyspnea • Angioedema of the eyes, lips, or larynx

- **Rhinitis**—inflammation of the mucous membranes of the nose because of the effect of histamine on the mucosa of the nasal passages.
- Abdominal pain/cramps, diarrhea, or vomiting caused by circulatory deficiency to the gastrointestinal track. (See Table 15.1 ■)

The early symptoms may be self-limiting or resolve after intervention with some form of histamine blocker, such as chlorpheniramine. On the other hand, the patient can continue to deteriorate along a continuum of symptoms, including abdominal pain, vomiting, and diarrhea.

Allergy symptoms are often classified into one of three categories: mild, moderate, or severe. The symptoms of mild allergy usually include localized redness, pruritus, edema, or urticaria. Rhinitis, pale or flushed skin tone, or conjunctivitis may also be present. A moderate allergic response will exhibit more widespread systemic representation of the redness, pruritus, edema, and urticaria. Moderate rhinitis may be present in addition to bronchospasm and mild dyspnea. Gastrointestinal symptoms, including abdominal pain, cramping, and diarrhea, are common in moderate allergic reactions. The most severe form of allergy is referred to as anaphylaxis, and the patient will exhibit many or all of the signs of moderate allergic reaction; however, the bronchospasm will be severe, and wheezing will be present. In addition, angioedema of the lips, eyes, and larynx may occur. Circulatory symptoms, such as hypotension, tachycardia, or arrhythmias, are often found in the severe allergic response and are life threatening to the patient. Sudden onset with a rapid progression of symptoms over a few minutes is often key feature of anaphylaxis.

Occasionally once the initial allergic symptoms have been resolved, the symptoms may recur; this is referred to as **biphasic** anaphylaxis. The second episode can occur from 1 to 72 hours after successful treatment and resolution of the initial response; however, more commonly it occurs within 3–10 hours. Neither the severity of the initial reaction nor the treatment administered has any bearing on whether a biphasic response occurs; however, ingesting the allergen makes a biphasic response more likely. An insufficient dose of epinephrine and/or a delay in the administration of epinephrine might predispose the individual to a biphasic response.

Treatment of Allergic Reactions

Treatment of the allergic reaction depends on the severity. The first step to take in any allergic response is to attempt to remove the causative agent if possible. For example, if you are wearing latex gloves while treating someone with an unknown allergy to latex, you would remove the gloves immediately. Next, if the reaction is localized to the area of inoculation and appears to be self-limiting (e.g., slight redness and itching of the face after being touched with latex gloves during treatment the day before), then the clinician should treat the patient with an oral histamine blocker first to determine if that alleviates the symptoms. Oral chlorpheniramine (4 mg every four to six hours, as needed) or oral diphenhydramine (25–50 mg every six to eight hours for three days) is recommended; however, chlorpheniramine causes less drowsiness. (See Figure 15.4 ■) Liquid diphenhydramine can also be administered for those patients who are unable to swallow tablets. The adult dosage is 25–50 mg every four to six hours. The pediatric dose for children 6–12 years is 12.5–25 mg every four to six hours. The patient should be placed in a supine position and observed for worsening symptoms.

If symptoms appear to be spreading and becoming more systemic (urticaria on the arms, face, and chest; severe pruritus; some edema of the lips), but the patient's blood pressure, pulse rate, and respirations are still within the normal range, this would exemplify a more moderate allergic response. In this case an injection of diphenhydramine (Benadryl) 50 mg IM (a histamine blocker) (see Figure 15.5 ■) would be beneficial, and provide the patient an oral histamine blocker if this has not already been dispensed. Additionally, vital signs should be monitored, and oxygen should be administered at 4–6 L/minute, if needed. Again, observation of the patient is necessary for at least one hour to ensure the signs and symptoms do not worsen.

If either the signs and symptoms worsen or the allergic response begins with extremely severe symptoms, as in the case presented at the beginning of this chapter, EMS (Emergency Medical Services) should be contacted immediately. This should be followed by an injection of epinephrine after the medical history is reviewed to ensure the patient does not suffer from severe hypertension or ischemic heart disease. Epinephrine is administered intramuscularly in the deltoid or thigh muscle and can be delivered directly through clothing, if necessary. Intramuscular injection into

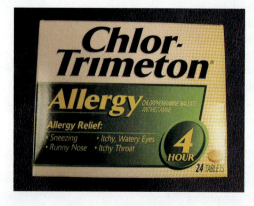

FIGURE 15.4 • Chlorpheniramine.

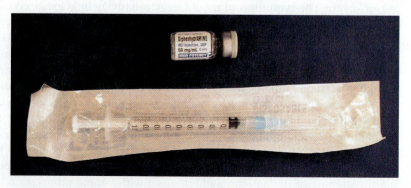

FIGURE 15.5 Diphenhydramine.

the lateral thigh muscle is preferred as it leads to peak plasma concentrations more rapidly than when delivered into the deltoid muscle. The injector should be held in place for 10 seconds to insure complete delivery of the drug, and then the injection site should be gently massaged for 10 seconds to facilitate absorption. Care should be taken by the clinician during the injection to not accidentally inject himself or herself versus the patient as the correct end of the autoinjector may be difficult to determine. The recommended adult epinephrine dosage is 0.2–0.5 mL of 1:1,000 solution, although the autoinjector delivers 0.3 mL of the drug. Epinephrine, a direct-acting sympathomimetic agent, reverses the immediate symptoms of anaphylaxis by its effects on the alpha and beta adrenoreceptors. It reverses the peripheral vasodilation; reduces edema; induces **bronchodilation**; has a positive **inotropic** and **chronotropic** effect on the myocardium; and suppresses the release of chemical mediators, such as histamine, from the cells. The dosage should be repeated after five minutes if there is no improvement or the condition worsens, which is a common occurrence. A maximum of three doses total can be administered. It should be noted that most fatalities occur in cases where injectable epinephrine is given too late.

Epinephrine is available in an autoinjector as a single 0.3-mg dose 1:1,000 concentration. If this is used for an adult, another dose may need to be given after a five-minute period if symptoms persist; therefore, either an additional EpiPen or a vial of epinephrine 1:1,000 with a syringe needs to be included in the medical emergency kit. Children age 6–12 years should receive 0.25 mL of 1:1,000 epinephrine, and children six months to six years should receive 0.012 mL of 1:1,000 epinephrine for a severe allergic reaction. An alternative for children is the pediatric autoinjector or EpiPen Jr., which administers 0.15 mg of epinephrine, and should be used for patients weighing 33 to 66 pounds. All of these doses for adult or child should be reduced if the patient is taking a monoamine oxidase inhibitor (MAOI) or a tricyclic antidepressant or beta blocker as these drugs will increase the patient's susceptibility to arrhythmias and can antagonize the effects of epinephrine. After epinephrine is administered, patients suffering from an allergic reaction should be placed and remain in a supine position, with their legs elevated in an attempt to increase their blood pressure; however, if patients are having severe breathing difficulty, an upright position may be beneficial to aid respiration. There is some evidence that a change in position from supine to sitting or sitting to standing can exacerbate the allergic symptoms and can be fatal because of the change in the blood flow. Positioning the patient supinely with the legs elevated ensures that the vena cava remains the lowest part of the body. Patients experiencing severe cases of allergic response should also be given oxygen at 4–6 L/minute. Vital signs should be continuously monitored, and some form of steroid, such as hydrocortisone 100–500 mg, should be administered intramuscularly; however, its benefit will not be realized until 6–12 hours after administration. If a histamine blocker has not been administered intramuscularly, this should be given to alleviate the symptoms caused by the release of histamine, such as pruritus. The recommended dosage is 10–20 mg. All allergy patients should be monitored for an appropriate length of time and at the very least one hour to ensure that a biphasic reaction does not occur. Referral to the appropriate medical facility is highly recommended. (See Figures 15.6 ■ and 15.7 ■)

Alternative routes of administration for the epinephrine have been studied. Inhaled epinephrine has been tested in clinical trials, but was found to be ineffective as it does not produce high enough blood plasma levels to eradicate the systemic allergic symptoms. A fast-disintegrating, sublingual epinephrine tablet shows promise as it exhibited similar blood plasma concentrations as those achieved via injection in the lateral thigh. In addition, there is a new type of autoinjector that was designed to improve device usability and safety called the Intelliject. The device is the size of a credit card and includes voice prompts to help guide the patient through the process. This injector needs to be held in place only for 5 seconds versus 10 seconds of the EpiPen, which may reduce injection-site reactions, such as pain, bleeding, and bruising. It also includes a retractable needle to prevent exposure incidents.

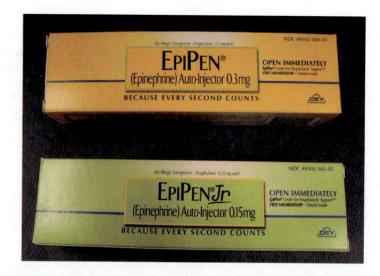

FIGURE 15.6 EpiPens.

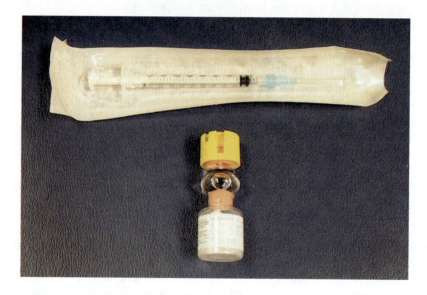

FIGURE 15.7 Injectable Solu-Cortef (hydrocortisone).

Prevention of Allergic Reactions

Avoiding exposure to specific allergens is the best method to prevent an allergic reaction; however, sometimes contact with the allergen is inescapable or even accidental. Contact with allergens may be unavoidable, so allergic individuals should carry an epinephrine autoinjector at all times. If patients are not sure how to operate the device or if they are not familiar with its use, they should contact their dental healthcare professional before using it. Inexpensive training devices are available for this purpose. (See Figure 15.8 ■) This education could be life saving for the patient.

Allergy testing can be performed to determine whether an allergy truly exists. There are three basic methods of allergy testing: skin prick, skin scratch, and radioallergosorbent test (RAST). During the skin prick test, the allergist-immunologist injects the suspected allergen under the skin on the patient's arm or back. If the patient is allergic to the substance, a small, raised, red area will result within 15 minutes of the injection. The skin scratch test is similar to the skin prick test, although instead of injecting the suspected allergen, the allergen is placed on the patient's skin

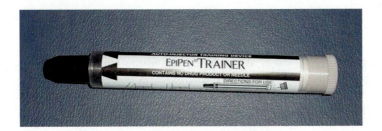

FIGURE 15.8 EpiPen trainer.

and then the skin is scratched. The RAST is a laboratory test performed on blood to test for the amount of specific IgE antibodies in the blood (which are present if there is a true allergic reaction). This is the most reliable test to determine allergy. These tests should be performed only under strict supervision as anaphylaxis can occur and would require immediate treatment.

Case Resolution and Conclusion

Dental professionals may encounter the potentially life-threatening reaction of anaphylaxis in the workplace; therefore, they must be knowledgeable regarding the physiology of allergic reactions, as well as the signs, symptoms, and appropriate treatment. In the case scenario presented, Diana was experiencing the symptoms of a moderate allergic response and was moving toward anaphylaxis. She was exhibiting systemic pruritus and urticaria, as well as the beginning stages of angioedema of her lips, eyes, and larynx. This angioedema of the larynx was contributing to her dyspnea. She was becoming severely hypotensive and bradypneic. Diana was administered 50 mg of diphenhydramine IM and 6 L/minute oxygen via the non-rebreather bag. Her vital signs were continuously monitored, and within a short time her blood pressure began to rise, and her pulse rate increased. She was monitored in the dental office for one hour before being released with directions to take an oral histamine blocker (10 mg for three days). She was also given a prescription for clindamycin (600 mg) to take prior to her next dental visit as it is likely that the amoxicillin was the etiology of her allergic reaction. Quick implementation of the appropriate treatment strategies essentially saved Diana's life.

Review Questions

1. The first time a person is exposed to an allergen, IgE antibodies are produced and attach to basophils and mast cells; upon reexposure the mast cells and basophils degranulate and release chemical mediators, causing the allergic reaction.

   A. The first statement is correct, and the second statement is incorrect.
   B. The first statement is incorrect, and the second statement is correct.
   C. Both statements are correct.
   D. Both statements are incorrect.

2. Which type of allergic reaction is an immediate hypersensitivity caused by immunoglobulin E?

   A. type I
   B. type II
   C. type III
   D. type IV

3. What are the smooth, raised red lesions with central blanching that occur because of vasodilation of the capillaries during an allergic reaction?

   A. pruritus
   B. angioedema
   C. urticaria
   D. none of the above

4. Why should a patient be observed for quite some time even after his or her symptoms have abated following an allergic reaction?

   A. for liability reasons
   B. to administer enough oxygen for the mast cells to regranulate
   C. to ensure a biphasic reaction does not occur
   D. all of the above

5. What should the adult patient suffering from an allergic reaction with severe dyspnea, hypotension, and angioedema of the larynx be administered?

   A. 10 mg of chlorpheniramine orally for three days
   B. 0.3 mg of 1:1,000 epinephrine intramuscularly
   C. 0.5 mg of 1:1,000 epinephrine intravenously
   D. epinephrine by inhalation until symptoms subside

6. All of the following are signs and symptoms of a moderate allergic reaction *except* one. Which one is the *exception*?

   A. localized urticaria
   B. systemic pruritus
   C. bronchospasm
   D. rhinitis

7. What is the appropriate medication to be given to a patient experiencing a mild allergic reaction?

   A. diphenhydramine 50 mg IM
   B. epinephrine 0.3 mg 1:1,000 IM
   C. chlorpheniramine 4 mg every four to six hours
   D. none of the above

8. The test used to determine an allergy whereby the amount of IgE antibodies in the blood is measured is a _____ test.

   A. RAST
   B. skin prick
   C. skin scratch
   D. antigen

Bibliography

Anderson, D. M., J. Keith, J. D. Novak, and M. A. Elliot, eds. *Mosby's Medical, Nursing & Allied Health Dictionary* 6th ed.. St. Louis, MO: Mosby-Year Book, Inc., 2008.

Balmer, C., and L. Longman. *The Management of Medical Emergencies: A Guide for Dental Professionals*. 1st ed. London: Quay Books, 2008.

Bennett, J. D., and M. B. Rosenberg. *Medical Emergencies in Dentistry*. 1st ed. Philadelphia, PA: W. B. Saunders, 2002.

Crusher, R. "Anaphylaxis." *Emergency Nurse* 12, no. 3 (2004): 24–31.

Davis, J. E. "Self-Injectable Epinephrine for Allergic Emergencies." *The Journal of Emergency Medicine* 17, no. 1 (2009): 57–62.

Ellis, A. K., and J. H. Day. "Diagnosis and Management of Anaphylaxis." *Canadian Medical Association Journal* 169, no. 4 (2003): 307–12.

EpiPen® Patient Insert [Brochure]. Columbia, MD: Meridian Medical Technologies, Inc., 2008.

Epipen® Prescribing Information [Brochure]. Columbia, MD: Meridian Medical Technologies, Inc., 2008.

Ferns, T., and I. Chojnacka. "The Causes of Anaphylaxis and Its Management in Adults." *British Journal of Nursing* 12, no. 17 (2003): 1006–12.

Forster, D., and J. Bryant. "Risk of Anaphylaxis: Improving Care at School." *Pediatric Nursing* 16, no. 9 (2004): 29–31.

Guerlain, S., L. Wang, and A. Hugine. "Intelliject's Novel Epinephrine Autoinjector: Sharps Injury Prevention Validation and Comparable Analysis with EpiPen and Twinject." *Annals of Allergy Asthma and Immunology* 105, no. 6 (2010): 480–84.

Homburger, H. A. "Diagnosing Allergic Diseases in Children." *Archives of Pathology and Laboratory Medicine* 128, no. 9 (2004): 1028–31.

Johnston, S. L., J. Unsworth, and M. M. Gompels. "Adrenaline Given Outside the Context of Life Threatening Allergic Reactions." *British Medical Journal* 326, no. 7389 (2003): 589–90.

Jones, G. J. "Anaphylactic Shock." *Emergency Nurse* 9, no. 10 (2002): 29–35.

Kean, T., and M. McNally. "Latex Hypersensitivity: A Closer Look at Considerations for Dentistry." *Journal of the California Dental Association* 75, no. 4 (2009): 279–82.

Kurek, M., and G. Michalska-Krzanowska. "Anaphylaxis During Surgical and Diagnostic Procedures." *Allergy & Clinical Immunology International* 15, no. 4 (2003): 168–74.

Lieberman, P. "Biphasic Anaphylaxis." *Allergy & Clinical Immunology International* 16, no. 6 (2004): 241–48.

Lopes, R. A. M., M. C. C. Benatti, and R. de Lima Zollner. "A Review of Latex Sensitivity Related to the Use of Latex Gloves in Hospitals." *Association of Perioperative Registered Nurses Journal* 80, no. 1 (2004): 64–70.

Malamed, S. F. "Emergency Medicine." *Dental Economics* 100, no. 2 (2010): 38–43.

McLean-Tooke, A., C. A. Bethune, A. C. Fay, and G. P. Spickett. "Adrenaline in the Treatment of Anaphylaxis: What Is the Evidence?" *British Medical Journal* 327, no. 7427 (2003): 1332–35.

Messaad, D., H. Sahla, S. Benahmed, P. Godard, J. Bousquet, and P. Demoly. "Drug Provocation Tests in Patients with a History Suggesting an Immediate Drug Hypersensitivity Reaction." *Annals of Internal Medicine* 140, no. 12 (2004): 1001–1007.

Mills, C. "Type I Latex Allergy Diagnosis Ends Career of Florida Dental Assistant." *The Dental Assistant* 72, no. 6 (2003): 14–16.

Mukai, K., O. Kazushige, Y. Tsujimuar, and H. Karasuyama. "New Insights into the Role for Basophils in Acute and Chronic Allergy." *Allergology International* 58, no. 1 (2009): 11–19.

Mullins, R. J. "Anaphylaxis: Risk Factors for Recurrence." *Clinical and Experimental Allergy* 33, no. 8 (2003): 1033–40.

Pretorius, E. "Basic Principles of Allergic Reactions." *Journal of the South African Dental Association* 57, no. 8 (2002): 332–35.

Rainbow, J., and G. J. Browne. "Fatal Asthma or Anaphylaxis?" *Emergency Medicine Journal* 19, no. 5 (2002): 415–17.

Rea, T. D., C. Edwards, J. A. Murray, D. J. Cloyd, and M. S. Eisenberg. "Epinephrine Use by Emergency Medical Technicians for Presumed Anaphylaxis." *Prehospital Emergency Care* 8, no. 4 (2004): 405–10.

Reading, D. "Managing Anaphylaxis." *Practice Nurse* 28, no. 3 (2004): 28–30.

Reed, K. "Basic Management of Medical Emergencies: Recognizing a Patient's Distress." *Journal of the American Dental Association* 141 (S1, 2010): 205–45.

Resuscitation Council (UK). *Emergency Treatment of Anaphylactic Reactions: Guidelines for Healthcare Providers*, 2008, January. http://www.resus.org.uk/pages/reaction.pdf.

Sicherer, S. H. and E. R. Simons. "Self-Injectable Epinephrine for First-Aid Management for Anaphylaxis." *Pediatrics* 119, no. 3 (2007): 638–46.

Simons, F. E. R., X. Gu, L. M. Johnston, and K. J. Simons. "Can Epinephrine Inhalations Be Substituted for Epinephrine Injection in Children at Risk for Systemic Anaphylaxis?" *Pediatrics* 106, no. 5 (2001): 1040–44.

Tang, A. W. "A Practical Guide to Anaphylaxis." *American Family Physician* 68, no. 7 (2003): 1325–32.

Walker, S., and A. Sheikh. "Managing Anaphylaxis: Effective Emergency and Long-Term Care Are Necessary." *Clinical and Experimental Allergy* 33, no. 8 (2003): 1015–18.

Weiss, M. E. "Recognizing Drug Allergy." *Postgraduate Medicine* 117, no. 5 (2005): 32–39.

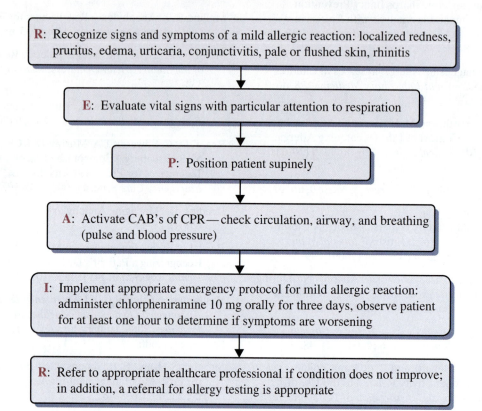

TREATMENT OF A MILD ALLERGIC REACTION
R.E.P.A.I.R.

R: Recognize signs and symptoms of a mild allergic reaction: localized redness, pruritus, edema, urticaria, conjunctivitis, pale or flushed skin, rhinitis

E: Evaluate vital signs with particular attention to respiration

P: Position patient supinely

A: Activate CAB's of CPR—check circulation, airway, and breathing (pulse and blood pressure)

I: Implement appropriate emergency protocol for mild allergic reaction: administer chlorpheniramine 10 mg orally for three days, observe patient for at least one hour to determine if symptoms are worsening

R: Refer to appropriate healthcare professional if condition does not improve; in addition, a referral for allergy testing is appropriate

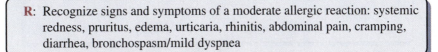

TREATMENT OF THE
MODERATE ALLERGIC REACTION PATIENT
R.E.P.A.I.R.

R: Recognize signs and symptoms of a moderate allergic reaction: systemic redness, pruritus, edema, urticaria, rhinitis, abdominal pain, cramping, diarrhea, bronchospasm/mild dyspnea

E: Evaluate vital signs with particular attention to respiration

P: Position patient supinely

A: Activate CAB's of CPR—check circulation, airway, and breathing (pulse and blood pressure)

I: Implement appropriate emergency protocol for moderate allergic reaction: an injection of diphenhydramine (Benadryl) 50 mg IM, administer an oral histamine blocker if it has not already be administered (chlorpheniramine 10 mg for three days), administer O_2 as needed, monitor vital signs, observe patient for at least one hour to determine if symptoms are worsening

R: Refer to appropriate healthcare professional if condition does not improve; in addition, a referral for allergy testing is appropriate

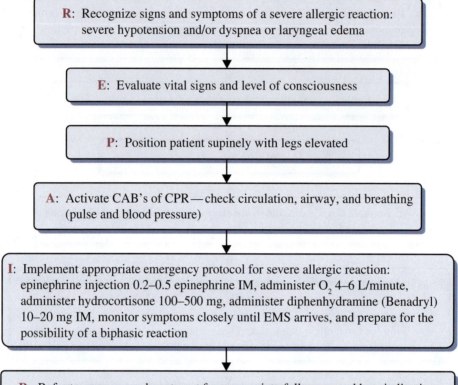

TREATMENT OF THE SEVERE ALLERGIC REACTION PATIENT
R.E.P.A.I.R.

R: Recognize signs and symptoms of a severe allergic reaction: severe hypotension and/or dyspnea or laryngeal edema

E: Evaluate vital signs and level of consciousness

P: Position patient supinely with legs elevated

A: Activate CAB's of CPR—check circulation, airway, and breathing (pulse and blood pressure)

I: Implement appropriate emergency protocol for severe allergic reaction: epinephrine injection 0.2–0.5 epinephrine IM, administer O_2 4–6 L/minute, administer hydrocortisone 100–500 mg, administer diphenhydramine (Benadryl) 10–20 mg IM, monitor symptoms closely until EMS arrives, and prepare for the possibility of a biphasic reaction

R: Refer to emergency department for appropriate follow-up and hospitalization

16

Diabetes-Related Emergencies

LEARNING OBJECTIVES

Upon reading the material in this chapter, the reader will be able to:

☑ State the different classifications of diabetes and their significant characteristics.

☑ Explain the systemic complications of diabetes.

☑ Discuss the oral manifestations of diabetes and appropriate treatment modifications.

☑ State the different treatment options for diabetes.

☑ Discuss the pathophysiology of diabetic ketoacidosis (DKA), hyperosmolar hyperglycemic state, and hypoglycemia.

☑ List specific signs and symptoms associated with DKA and hypoglycemia.

☑ Determine suggested treatment modalities for patients experiencing DKA and hypoglycemia.

☑ Explain the steps needed to prepare an office for a patient experiencing DKA and hypoglycemia.

Case Study ···➤

Scenario

Your patient, Jeff Johnson, is a 29-year-old male disc jockey in good health. His medical history reveals that he is a controlled type 1 diabetic who takes insulin daily. He arrives late for his 8:00 A.M. appointment, stating that he did a gig last, night and overslept. He had just enough time to administer his medication but did not want to be any later for his dental appointment, so he skipped breakfast. You begin the intra/extra oral examination before the oral prophylaxis and notice he is salivating profusely. You ask him where he is, and his response is confused and irrational. You take his vital signs and find a bounding pulse and shallow respirations. He is conscious. From what condition do you suspect Jeff is suffering?

Introduction

Diabetes mellitus (DM) affects approximately 15.7 million people in the United States. More than 90% of these individuals are diagnosed with type 2 diabetes, which often occurs because of obesity, high-fat low-fiber diets, and a sedentary lifestyle. In a dental practice with 2,000 patients, approximately 40 to 70 patients will have diabetes, and one-third will be unaware that they have the condition; therefore, it is vital for the dental professional to obtain an accurate medical history.

Diabetes mellitus is an autoimmune metabolic disorder characterized by **hyperglycemia** (high blood glucose level). The condition is caused by a reduction or an absence of the production of insulin by the beta cells of the pancreas or defects of the insulin receptors. **Insulin** is the hormone that aids in the conversion of sugar and starches to a form that the body can transport to the cells to utilize for energy.

There are three basic forms of diabetes: type 1 (formerly insulin-dependent DM or juvenile), type 2 (formerly non-insulin-dependent DM or adult onset), and gestational diabetes. (See Table 16.1 ■) There is a fourth category, called prediabetes or impaired glucose tolerance, for those individuals not yet diagnosed with full-blown DM.

Table 16.1 **Types of Diabetes Mellitus**

Type 1	Absolute lack of circulating insulin
	Patients dependent on supplemental insulin for survival
	5%–10% of all diabetics are type 1
Type 2	Inability of the body to produce sufficient amount of insulin or to properly use the insulin that is produced
	Managed by diet, oral medications, or injectable medications
	90%–95% of all diabetics are type 2
Gestational diabetes	Occurs in 2%–5% of pregnant women
	Characterized by glucose intolerance, with initial onset during pregnancy
	If left untreated can cause significant developmental disturbances to fetus

Type 1 diabetes is associated with an absolute lack of circulating insulin that results when pancreatic beta cells within the islets of Langerhans have been destroyed because of an immune dysfunction. Patients with type 1 diabetes are dependent on supplemental insulin for survival. Five to ten percent of all diabetics suffer from the type 1 variety.

Type 2 diabetics comprise 90% to 95% of all diabetic patients. Because of an increase in life spans, sedentary lifestyles, and obesity, this figure is increasing. In addition, this form of diabetes is increasing significantly in the adolescent population again because of poor dietary habits and lack of exercise. Type 2 diabetes results from the pancreas's inability to produce a sufficient amount of insulin as the need for insulin increases or to properly use the insulin that is produced.

Gestational diabetes occurs in approximately 2% to 5% of pregnant women. This condition is characterized by glucose intolerance and has an initial onset during pregnancy. It usually disappears after pregnancy; however, in many instances it will return years later. Evidence suggests that presence of an enzyme in the placenta and considerable destruction of insulin by the placenta play a role in the development of gestational diabetes. If left untreated, the infant may suffer from **fetal macrosomia**, hypoglycemia, hypocalcemia, or **hyperbilirubinemia**.

Diabetic Testing

The diagnosis of diabetes is made by a healthcare provider by conducting a fasting plasma glucose test (FPG) or an oral glucose tolerance test (OGTT). With the FPG test, a fasting blood glucose level (taken after a 12–14-hour fast) between 100 and 125 mg/dL signals prediabetes. A person with a fasting blood glucose level of 126 mg/dL or higher has diabetes.

In the OGTT test, a person's blood glucose level is measured after a fast and two hours after drinking a glucose-rich beverage. If the two-hour blood glucose level is between 140 and 199 mg/dL, the person tested has prediabetes. If the two-hour blood glucose level is at 200 mg/dL or higher, the person tested has diabetes.

Systemic Complications

There are many systemic complications associated with diabetes, and many of them are quite debilitating. Nearly every major organ system can be affected. (See Table 16.2 ■)

Diabetic Retinopathy

Diabetic retinopathy is a common sequela of diabetes and one of the leading causes of blindness in individuals age 20–74 years. Diabetic retinopathy progresses from the mild form characterized by increased vascular permeability to a more moderate form characterized by vascular closure. The most severe form results in growth of new blood vessels on the retina and the posterior surface of the vitreous. Macular edema, characterized by retinal thickening from leaky blood vessels, can develop at all stages of retinopathy. Diabetics are also prone to cataracts and glaucoma. Early screening and strict glucose control are essential for preventing diabetic retinopathy.

Diabetic Neuropathy

Mild to severe forms of nervous system damage also referred to as **diabetic neuropathy** affect 60%–70% of diabetics. These conditions are not well understood. Pain in the feet and hands, slowed digestion, and other neurological problems are common.

Macrovascular and Microvascular Complications

Additional complications from diabetes are macrovascular and microvascular complications. They are characterized by **microangiopathic** changes whereby the basement membrane of the capillaries thickens and can cause the formation of thrombi, leading to impairment of normal blood flow. The diminished blood flow causes an increased risk of stroke and myocardial infarction for these patients.

Table 16.2 Systemic Complications of Diabetes Mellitus

Diabetic retinopathy	• Disease of the retina of the eye resulting from changes in the blood vessels • Leading cause of blindness in individuals age 20–74 • Cataracts and glaucoma
Macrovascular and microvascular complications	• Microangiopathic changes in the capillaries, leading to formation of thrombi and impairment of normal blood flow • Can lead to cerebrovascular accident or myocardial infarction • Lack of blood flow to peripheral arteries can lead to gangrene, often resulting in the need for amputation
Diabetic neuropathy	• Impaired sensation in hands or feet, slowed digestion, carpel tunnel syndrome, other neurological problems
Diabetic nephropathy	• Damage to the small blood vessels in the kidneys, leading to impairment in function
Oral complications	• Increased incidence of periodontal disease, abscesses, xerostomia, lichen planus, candidiasis • Impaired wound healing

Individuals with diabetes are two to four times more likely to have heart disease (more than 77,000 deaths from heart disease annually in diabetics in the United States). Moreover, they are five times more likely to suffer a stroke, with more than 11,000 deaths each year. In addition, the lack of blood flow to the nervous tissues results in damage to those nerves. These microangiopathic changes in the peripheral arteries often affect the legs and increase the risk of **gangrene**, with the possible sequela of amputation.

Diabetic Nephropathy

A third complication from diabetes is **diabetic nephropathy**. Diabetes damages the small blood vessels in the kidneys, impairing their ability to filter impurities from blood for excretion in the urine. Persons with kidney failure must have a kidney transplant or undergo dialysis to cleanse their blood. Once diabetic renal failure has occurred, there is nearly 100% morbidity within 10 years.

Oral Manifestations

The various oral manifestations of DM may include an increased incidence and severity of periodontal disease, oral abscesses, xerostomia, caries, lichen planus, and candidiasis. Diabetics may suffer from delayed wound healing, and their risk of secondary oral and systemic infections is increased.

Although there are numerous complications from which diabetics may suffer, the best method to avoid these problems is by maintaining optimal glucose levels. Diabetics should test their blood levels several times during the day to determine if their medication levels are appropriate. The process for testing one's own blood sugar level involves using a small lancet to gain a drop or two of blood from the pad or side of a fingertip. The blood drop is then placed on a test strip, and the strip is inserted into a calibrated **glucometer**. A few seconds later the glucometer will display the patient's blood glucose reading. A normal blood glucose reading is between 50 and 150 mg/dL. A reading below 50 indicates the patient is hypoglycemic, and a reading

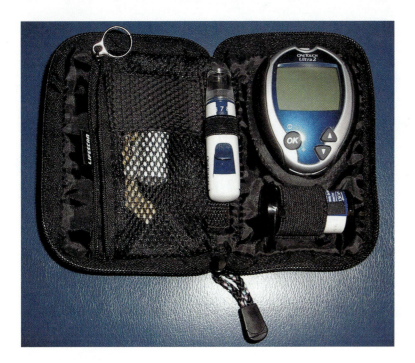

FIGURE 16.1 Glucometer.

above 150 indicates the patient is hyperglycemic. Either of these conditions requires medical intervention by a healthcare professional. (See Figure 16.1 ■)

Daily blood glucose testing tells patients what their blood sugar level is at the time of the test; an additional test called the **glycated hemoglobin test (HbA1c)** is important. This test reveals the patient's "average" blood sugar level over the past two to three months. Home testing methods for HbA1c levels are now available, making it easier for patients to monitor their levels. Both tests are very important in protecting patients' long-term health. Maintaining optimal HbA1c levels will help reduce the risk of diabetes complications such as blindness, kidney disease, nerve damage, stroke, and heart failure.

Medications/Treatments for Diabetics

There are a wide variety of medications or treatments that may be prescribed for a diabetic patient. Type 1 diabetics ordinarily will be taking some type of insulin, such as Humalog or Novolog; however, there are a number of different insulin types. They vary by time of onset, peak effectiveness, effective duration, and maximal duration. It is recommended that these medications be kept refrigerated to lengthen effectiveness.

There are a number of different oral agents used to treat type 2 diabetes. Some of the more common medications are metformin (Glucophage), tolbutamide (Orinase), and glyburide (Micronase, Diabeta, Glynase). The type of medication is prescribed based on the cause of the diabetes, as well as the severity of the condition.

In addition to medications, there are now some more recent advances in the treatment of type 1 diabetes. Insulin pumps or continuous infusion therapy were introduced in the 1970s as a replacement for daily injections. They are compact devices with an insulin-filled syringe or cartridge that is attached to a subcutaneously inserted catheter. The catheter is usually changed every four to six days. Patients with insulin pumps still need to measure their glucose levels and adhere to a proper nutritional regimen. Data suggest that patients with insulin pumps have better glycemic and metabolic control. (See Figures 16.2 and 16.3 ■)

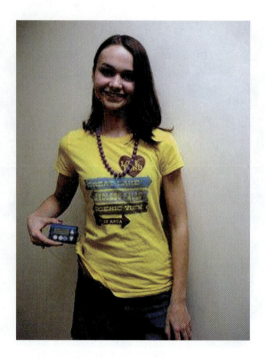

FIGURE 16.2 Twelve-year-old type 1 patient with insulin pump.

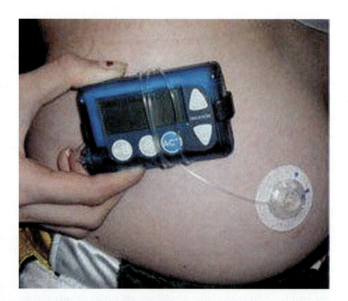

FIGURE 16.3 Insulin pump in place.

Pancreas or pancreatic islet cell transplantation is another option for some diabetic patients to aid in controlling blood glucose levels. Although there has been some success with this treatment option, there are some concerns, such as the need for continuous immunosuppression to prevent rejection of the islet cells or pancreas.

The delivery of insulin via an inhalation device is the latest advance in diabetes treatment. The system uses a modified nebulizer connected to a special holding chamber that allows a specific number of measured puffs to deliver the appropriate amount of insulin. The medication is more rapidly absorbed than injected insulin and avoids the use of needles, which are objectionable to most patients. There are two major concerns with this treatment method: There is a risk of sensitivity using the inhalation route, and some of the insulin may be deposited in the mouth and throat rather than the lungs, which reduces the amount of medication delivered to the patient.

Role of the Dental Professional

The dental professional is in a key position to aid diabetic patients. Several questions should be asked of all diabetic patients prior to dental treatment, including

- Do you monitor your blood sugar levels? If so, how often?
- What were your most recent blood sugar values?
- How are you feeling?
- Do you take medication for your diabetes? If so, did you take it today?
- Have you eaten today? If so, when?
- Are you having problems with your eyes, feet, or legs?
- Do you see your physician regularly?
- Do you see an eye doctor yearly?
- Do you know your average hemoglobin value?

Other strategies that should be employed when treating a diabetic patient in the dental office include the following:

- Scheduling appointments in the early to mid-morning hours
- Keeping appointments short
- Instructing the patient to continue normal dietary intake before the appointment
- Checking patient's blood glucose prior to any invasive procedure or if patient complains of feeling unwell
- Scheduling frequent recall examinations and prophylaxis
- Using topical fluoride when patients are at risk for caries
- Recommending saliva substitutes for xerostomia

Medical Emergencies

Essentially, there are three medical emergencies from which a diabetic patient may suffer in the dental office: severe hyperglycemia or **diabetic ketoacidosis (DKA)**, **hyperosmolar hyperglycemic state**, and hypoglycemia.

Signs and Symptoms of DKA

DKA is not an emergency that a dental professional would likely encounter; however, there is a chance that it could occur. Twenty-five percent of all cases of DKA occur in newly presenting type 1 diabetics. The condition can also occur in any diabetic who is not medicating or eating appropriately; that is why older adults and teenagers, particularly girls who have negative attitudes toward eating, often suffer from this disorder. Brittle diabetics or poorly controlled diabetics are also at risk for this condition. DKA is also common in children on insulin pump therapy since only the short-acting type of insulin is used in those pumps. In addition, individuals suffering from an infection are prone to DKA as their bodies may require additional insulin. Alcohol and cocaine have also been implicated in the formation of DKA in diabetics.

DKA is potentially life threatening, with a 5%–10% average mortality rate. This rate is even higher for elderly patients. The condition is caused by insufficient insulin levels in the blood. Because of these low levels of insulin, glucose metabolism is an insufficient energy source, and the body shifts to metabolizing fatty acids for energy. The by-products of fatty acids when metabolized are ketone bodies, which cause the blood to become more acidic than usual. In an attempt to reverse the acidosis, the body begins to exhale excess carbon dioxide, which results in tachypnea

Table 16.3 Signs and Symptoms of DKA

- Tachypnea accompanied by an increased depth in respiration—Kussmaul respirations
- Alteration in mental status—drowsiness to coma
- Dehydration
- Poor skin turgor
- Warm, dry skin and mucous membranes
- Increased thirst
- Muscle weakness
- Severe fatigue
- Nausea
- Vomiting
- Blurred vision
- Fruity odor on breath
- Hypotension
- Tachycardia

accompanied by an increased depth in respiration (known as Kussmaul respirations or air hunger). These ketones are excreted in the urine along with sodium and potassium, resulting in a more severe electrolyte disturbance. Even though some ketones are eliminated, more are produced than are excreted, and therefore the acidosis increases, causing various signs and symptoms. DKA signs and symptoms may be mild at first, but as time passes and the ketones accumulate, the patient's state will worsen.

Ten to twenty percent of patients suffering from DKA will often have some alteration in mental status ranging from drowsiness to coma. Most patients will be dehydrated, which will lead to poor skin turgor. In addition, the skin will be warm and dry, as will the mucous membranes. Patients will complain of increased thirst. DKA patients may complain of muscle weakness and severe fatigue and have difficulty walking. Nausea and vomiting are also common. Blurred vision occurs because of fluid accumulation in the lens of the eye. Tachypnea and Kussmaul breathing are common, and the patient's breath may have a characteristic fruity odor resulting from the exhalation of ketones. The odor has been described as smelling like "nail varnish" or "musty apples." The patient's pulse and blood pressure will indicate hypotension and tachycardia. (See Table 16.3 ■) In children, a common complication of DKA is **cerebral edema** which has a high mortality and morbidity rate; therefore, appropriate and swift treatment of the condition is essential.

Treatment of DKA

The first step in treating this patient is to determine an accurate blood glucose level; therefore, each dental office should have a glucometer and all personnel should be familiar with its use. The necessary treatment for this patient is to lower blood glucose levels by providing insulin; however, the provision of insulin should be performed by a medical professional as the appropriate dosage is essential to insure the patient does not become hypoglycemic. If the clinician is unsure as to which diabetic emergency the patient is experiencing, then it is best to provide some form of glucose as it will not significantly harm a patient experiencing DKA and it will benefit a patient suffering from severe hypoglycemia. In addition, fluid therapy is needed to reverse dehydration. Vital signs should be monitored to determine the severity of the DKA.

Hyperosmolar Hyperglycemic State

A second emergency that can occur in diabetic patients is **hyperosmolar hyperglycemic state** (formerly known as hyperosmolar nonketotic syndrome). In this condition patients will be hyperglycemic and dehydrated; however, they will not be acidotic. Hyperosmolar hyperglycemic state usually occurs in the elderly, infirm, neglected, institutionalized, or mentally challenged diabetic patients who cannot recognize their thirst or express their need for water; therefore, it is uncommon, but not impossible, for this condition to be seen in a dental office.

Table 16.4 Signs and Symptoms of Hypoglycemia

- Confusion
- Seizures
- Coma
- Dizziness
- Weakness
- Syncope
- Headache
- Intense hunger
- Cold, clammy skin
- Profuse perspiration
- Irritability or aggressive behavior

Signs and Symptoms of Hypoglycemia

The third emergency that can occur in diabetic patients is hypoglycemia. This condition used to be referred to as insulin shock, which essentially was severe hypoglycemia with a blood glucose level lower than 40–50 mg/dL. Mild episodes of hypoglycemia in diabetics occur frequently, whereas severe hypoglycemia affects approximately 30% of diabetics. Hypoglycemia usually occurs because of a missed meal or irregular eating, consumption of alcoholic beverages, or increased exercise without adjusting the insulin dosage. The brain is dependent on a continuous supply of glucose, so brain function is affected when glucose levels fall below a critical level. Hypoglycemia can lead to confusion, seizures, and eventually coma. Symptoms of acute hypoglycemia include dizziness or fainting, weakness, intense hunger, cold, clammy skin, profuse perspiration, shakiness, nausea, vomiting, and tachycardia. If the episode is prolonged, additional symptoms of lethargy, irritability, confusion, slurred speech, headache, and aggressive or bizarre behaviors may occur. (See Table 16.4 ■) This condition may be mistaken for an acute central nervous system event, sepsis, or psychiatric disease. This emergency is much more likely to occur in the dental office setting than DKA or hyperosmolar hyperglycemic state.

Treatment of Hypoglycemia

Treatment for the conscious patient suffering from hypoglycemia is to provide 15–20 gm of some form of sugar, such as table sugar, soda, honey, candy, orange juice, or glucose tablets (two to six)/paste. The airway should be secured, and vital signs should be monitored. Once the glucose has been administered, a positive response should occur within 10–15 minutes. For unconscious patients who are not able to take an oral carbohydrate, the treatment of choice is Glucagon (1 mg administered subcutaneously, intramuscularly, or intravenously), which is effective at stimulating hepatic glycogenolysis. (See Figures 16.4 and 16.5 ■)

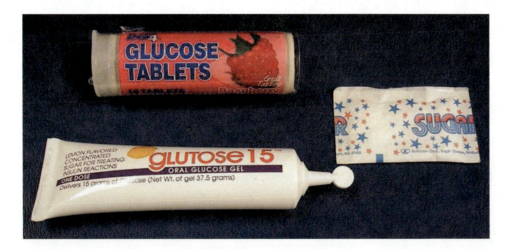

FIGURE 16.4 Oral glucose tablets, paste, sugar packets.

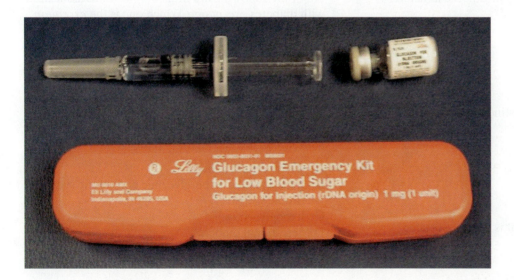

FIGURE 16.5 Injectable glucagon.

Case Resolution and Conclusion ·····················➤

The diabetic patient requires special attention. The patient in the case scenario, Jeff, chose to take his medication but did not eat breakfast (he was trying to get to his dental appointment on time). The signs and symptoms he is experiencing (profuse salivation, confusion, irrationality, bounding pulse) are those of severe hypoglycemia. This indicates that he has too much insulin and not enough glucose to take to the body cells. Jeff was administered six glucose tablets, which quickly reversed the symptoms of hypoglycemia. He was monitored in the office for about 30 minutes and was given information about the necessity of properly managing his glucose levels. Jeff was very grateful for the information and rescheduled his appointment immediately after lunch at 1:00 the next day.

Building a relationship with diabetic patients is essential to discern important information regarding their glucose levels, nutritional status, medication regimens, and physical condition. The dental professional is in an ideal position to help diabetic patients manage their disease and thus avoid or minimize the unfortunate sequelae of their condition.

Review Questions

1. An absolute lack of circulating insulin is characteristic of which condition?

   A. hypoglycemia
   B. type 1 diabetes
   C. type 2 diabetes
   D. none of the above

2. A result of 115 mg/dL on a fasting plasma glucose test would indicate

   A. prediabetes
   B. type 1 diabetes
   C. type 2 diabetes
   D. hypoglycemia

3. What causes the gangrene that is often associated with diabetic patients?

   A. diabetic retinopathy
   B. diabetic nephropathy
   C. microangiopathic changes
   D. none of the above

4. All of the following are oral complications associated with diabetes *except* one. Which one is the *exception*?

   A. periodontal disease
   B. xerostomia
   C. candidiasis
   D. squamous cell carcinoma

5. Which diabetic emergency is associated with the following symptoms: tachypnea, Kussmaul's breathing, nausea, blurred vision, fruity odor on the breath?

   A. diabetic ketoacidosis
   B. hyperosmolar hyperglycemic nonketotic syndrome
   C. hypoglycemia
   D. gestational diabetes

6. What is the needed treatment for the emergency in the condition cited in question 5?

   A. administration of insulin
   B. administration of oral glucose
   C. immediate surgery to repair the patient's defective pancreas
   D. reduction in the amount of insulin the patient is using

7. The test used to measure a diabetic's average glucose level over the past three months is

   A. fasting plasma glucose test
   B. oral glucose tolerance test
   C. HbA1c test
   D. none of the above

8. All of the following are symptoms of hypoglycemia in a diabetic patient *except* one. Which one is the *exception*?

   A. confusion
   B. profuse sweating
   C. aggressive behavior
   D. cyanosis

9. What is the diabetic emergency that is often seen in institutionalized individuals?

   A. hyperosmolar hyperglycemic state
   B. diabetic ketoacidosis
   C. diabetic nephropathy
   D. gestational diabetes

10. All of the following are medications often prescribed for type 2 diabetics *except* one. Which one is the *exception*?

    A. glucagon (Glucagon)
    B. metformin (Glucophage)
    C. glyburide (Diabeta)
    D. tolbutamide (Orinase)

Bibliography

Alexander, R. E. "Portable Blood Glucose Testing Meters in Dental Practice: A Valuable Medical Emergencies Adjunct." *Texas Dental Journal* 121, no. 12 (2004): 1158–63.

American Diabetes Association. 2012a. Symptoms. Accessed January 2, 2012. http://www.diabetes.org.

American Diabetes Association. 2012b. *Complications of Diabetes in the United States*, Accessed January 7, 2012. www.diabetes.org.

Anderson, D. M., J. Keith, P. D. Novak, and M. A. Elliot, eds. *Mosby's Medical, Nursing & Allied Health Dictionary*. 6th ed. St. Louis, MO: Mosby-Year Book, Inc., 2008.

Balmer, C., and L. Longman. *The Management of Medical Emergencies: A Guide for Dental Professionals*. 1st ed. London: Quay Books, 2008.

Bennett, J. D., and M. B. Rosenberg. *Medical Emergencies in Dentistry*. 1st ed. Philadelphia, PA: W. B. Saunders, 2002.

Birrer, R. B. "Hyperglycemic Emergencies: What You Need to Know." *Emergency Medicine* 32, no. 10 (2000): 24–31.

Boyd, R. "Towards Evidence Based Emergency Medicine: Best BETs from the Manchester Royal Infirmary. Glucose or Glucagons for Hypoglycemia." *Journal of Accident and Emergency Medicine* 17, no. 4 (2000): 287.

Brink, S. J. "Diabetic Ketoacidosis." *Acta Paediatric Supplement*, Supplement 427 (1999): 14–24.

Carlton, F. B. "Recent Advances in the Pharmacologic Management of Diabetes Mellitus." *Emergency Medicine Clinics of North America* 18, no. 4 (2000): 745–53.

Carroll, M. F., M. R. Burge, and D. S. Schade. "Severe Hypoglycemia in Adults." *Reviews in Endocrine & Metabolic Disorders* 4, no. 2 (2003): 149–57.

Curtis, J. A., and D. Hagerty. "Managing Diabetes in Childhood and Adolescence." *Canadian Family Physician* 48 (2002): 499–509.

Egede, L. E. "Patterns and Correlates of Emergency Department Use by Individuals with Diabetes." *Diabetes Care* 27, no. 7 (2004): 1748–50.

Fincher, A. L. "Managing Diabetic Emergencies." *Athletic Therapy Today* 4, no. 4 (1999): 45–46.

Fogel, M., and D. Zimmerman. "Management of Diabetic Ketoacidosis in the Emergency Department." *Clinical Pediatric Emergency Medicine* 10, no. 4 (2009): 246–51.

Glaser, N., and N. Kupperman. "The Evaluation and Management of Children with Diabetic Ketoacidosis in the Emergency Department." *Pediatric Emergency Care* 20, no. 7 (2004): 477–84.

Golla, K., J. B. Epstein, R. E. Rada, R. Sanai, Z. Messieha, and R. J. Cabay. "Diabetes Mellitus: An Updated Overview of Medical Management and Dental Implications." *General Dentistry* 52, no. 6 (2004): 528–29.

Grinsdale, S., and E. A. Buck. "Diabetic Ketoacidosis: Implications for the Medical-Surgical Nurse." *MedSurg Nursing* 8, no. 1 (1999): 37–45.

Harden, R. D., and N. D. Quinn. "Emergency Management of Diabetic Ketoacidosis in Adults." *Emergency Medicine Journal* 20, no. 3 (2003): 210–14.

Hess-Fischl, A. "Practical Management of Patient with Diabetes in Critical Care." *Critical Care Nursing Quarterly* 27, no. 2 (2004): 189–200.

Hurlock-Chorostecki, C. "Managing Diabetic Ketoacidosis: The Role of the ICU Nurse in Endocrine Emergency." *Dynamics* 15, no. 1 (2004): 18–22.

Jimenez, C. C. "Recognizing and Managing Diabetes-Related Emergencies." *Athletic Therapy Today* 9, no. 2 (2004): 6–10.

Josefson, J., and D. Zimmerman. "Hypoglycemia in the Emergency Department." *Clinical Pediatric Emergency Medicine* 10, no. 4 (2009): 285–91.

Kearney, T., and C. Dang. "Diabetic and Endocrine Emergencies." *Postgraduate Medical Journal* 83 (2007): 79–86.

Konick-McMahan, J. "Riding Out a Diabetic Emergency." *Nursing 99* 29, no. 9 (1999): 34–39.

Leese, G. P., J. Wang, J. Broomhall, P. Kelly, A. Marsden, W. Morrison, B. M. Frier, and A. D. Morris, "Frequency of Severe Hypoglycemia Requiring Emergency Treatment in Type 1 and Type 2 Diabetes: A Population-Based Study of Health Service Resource Use." *Diabetes Care* 26, no. 4 (2003): 1176–81.

Lewis, R. "Diabetic Emergencies: Part 2. Hyperglycemia." *Accident & Emergency Nursing* 8, no. 1 (2000): 24–30.

Malamed, S. F. *Medical Emergencies in the Dental Office.* 6th ed. St. Louis, MO: Mosby Publishing Company, 2007.

Mattera, C. "Glucose Gone Wild. Part 2. Common Diabetic Emergencies: The EMS Assessment & Treatment of Diabetic Ketoacidosis & Hyperosmolar Nonketotic Syndrome." *Journal of Emergency Medical Services* 27, no. 4 (2002): 74–87.

McFarlane, K. "An Overview of Diabetic Ketoacidosis in Children." *Emergency Nursing* 23, no. 1 (2011): 14–19.

National Eye Institute. U.S. National Institutes of Health, 2012. Accessed January 2, 2012. http://www.nei.nih.gov/.

National Institutes of Health. National Diabetes Education Program, 2012. Accessed January 2, 2012. http://ndep.nih.gov.

Nattrass, M. "Diabetic Ketoacidosis." *Medicine* 38, no. 12 (2010): 667–70.

Plotnick, L. P., L. M. Clark, F. L. Brancati, and T. Erlinger. "Safety and Effectiveness of Insulin Pump Therapy in Children and Adolescents with Type 1 Diabetes." *Diabetes Care* 26, no. 4 (2003): 1142–47.

Quinn, L. "Diabetes Emergencies in the Patient with Type 2 Diabetes." *The Nursing Clinics of North America* 36, no. 2 (2001): 341–60.

Research, Science and Therapy Committee of the American Academy of Periodontology. "Diabetes and Periodontal Diseases." *American Academy of Periodontology* 71, no. 4 (2000): 664–78.

Vanelli, M., and F. Chiarelli. "Treatment of Diabetic Ketoacidosis in Children and Adolescents." *Acta BioMedica* 74, no. 3 (2003): 59–68.

WebMD Health. Diabetes Health Center, 2005. Accessed August 2, 2005. http://my.webmd.com/content/article/46/1667_50935?z=1667_50936_6504_00_08.

White, J. R., and R. K. Campbell. "Inhaled Insulin: An Overview." *Clinical Diabetes* 19, no. 1 (2001): 13–16.

Wilson, M. H., J. J. Fitzpatrick, N. S. McArdle, L. F. A. Stassen. "Diabetes Mellitus and Its Relevance to the Practice of Dentistry." *Journal of the American Dental Association* 56, no. 3 (2010): 128–33.

Wipf, J. E., and D. S. Paauw. "Ophthalmologic Emergencies in the Patient with Diabetes." *Endocrinology and Metabolism Clinics of North America* 29, no. 4 (2000): 813–29.

Woodrum, J. L. "Diabetes Quiz. How Much Do You Know about Diabetes?" *Diabetes Self-Management* 16, no. 2 (1999): 29–30.

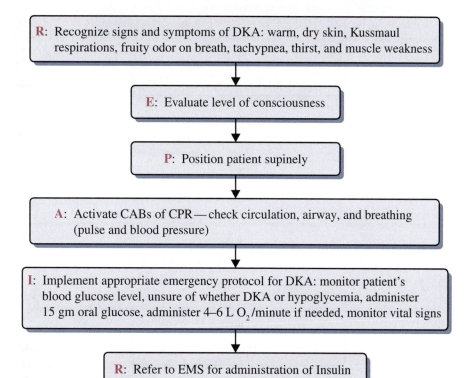

**TREATMENT OF
DIABETIC KETOACIDOSIS
R.E.P.A.I.R.**

R: Recognize signs and symptoms of DKA: warm, dry skin, Kussmaul respirations, fruity odor on breath, tachypnea, thirst, and muscle weakness

E: Evaluate level of consciousness

P: Position patient supinely

A: Activate CABs of CPR—check circulation, airway, and breathing (pulse and blood pressure)

I: Implement appropriate emergency protocol for DKA: monitor patient's blood glucose level, unsure of whether DKA or hypoglycemia, administer 15 gm oral glucose, administer 4–6 L O_2/minute if needed, monitor vital signs

R: Refer to EMS for administration of Insulin

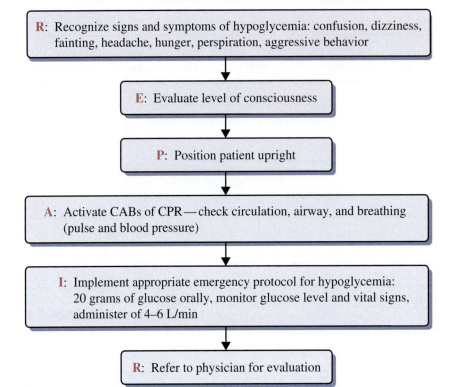

TREATMENT OF HYPOGLYCEMIA
R.E.P.A.I.R.

R: Recognize signs and symptoms of hypoglycemia: confusion, dizziness, fainting, headache, hunger, perspiration, aggressive behavior

E: Evaluate level of consciousness

P: Position patient upright

A: Activate CABs of CPR—check circulation, airway, and breathing (pulse and blood pressure)

I: Implement appropriate emergency protocol for hypoglycemia: 20 grams of glucose orally, monitor glucose level and vital signs, administer of 4–6 L/min

R: Refer to physician for evaluation

17

Adrenal Insufficiency and Crisis

LEARNING OBJECTIVES

Upon reading the material in this chapter, the reader will be able to:

- ☑ State the function of the adrenal glands.
- ☑ List several etiologies causing adrenal insufficiency.
- ☑ Discuss the pathophysiology of adrenal crisis.
- ☑ Recognize specific signs and symptoms associated with adrenal crisis.
- ☑ Determine suggested treatment modalities for patients experiencing adrenal crisis.
- ☑ Explain strategies for preventing adrenal crisis.

Case Study ....➤

Scenario

Your mid-afternoon patient, Nancy Van Riper, arrives for her dental hygiene appointment. She is a 56-year-old woman who explains that she is a severe dental phobic and other than her initial examination a week ago has not had dental hygiene care for 16 years. She is scheduled for one quadrant of periodontal debridement with local anesthetics. While reviewing her medical history, you notice that she reports that she has Addison's disease and takes 30 mg of hydrocortisone daily. As you are preparing for treatment, your patient states that she is nauseous and not feeling well. You take her pulse, and she is tachypneic, with a pulse rate of 118 beats/minute and it is thready. Her respiration rate is 24 breaths/minute, and she is quite hypotensive, with a blood pressure of 78/54 mmHg. From what medical emergency is your patient suffering?

Introduction

The adrenal glands are endocrine glands located on the top of both kidneys. They are triangular shaped and measure about one-half inch in height and 3 inches in length. (See Figure 17.1 ■) Each gland consists of a **medulla** (the center of the gland) surrounded by the **cortex**. The medulla is responsible for producing epinephrine and norepinephrine. The adrenal cortex produces other hormones, such as **cortisol** and **aldosterone**. Cortisol mobilizes nutrients, modifies the body's response to inflammation, stimulates the liver to raise the blood sugar level, and helps control the amount of water in the body. Aldosterone regulates salt and water levels, which affect blood volume and blood pressure.

Adrenal insufficiency can be divided into two major categories: primary and secondary. Primary adrenal insufficiency or **Addison's disease** is a result of the destruction of the adrenal cortex of the adrenal gland. Common causes of this form of adrenal insufficiency are autoimmune disease, tuberculosis, adrenal hemorrhage, adrenal metastases, and AIDS. The prevalence of primary adrenal insufficiency is 93–140 per 1 million individuals. It usually occurs in the fourth decade of life, and women are more frequently affected. Clinical symptoms do not usually occur until at least 90% of both adrenal cortices have been destroyed.

Secondary adrenal insufficiency occurs when there is an insufficient amount of **adrenocorticotropic hormone (ACTH)** to stimulate the adrenal cortex. This condition is often found in individuals on glucocorticoid therapy (oral or topical medications). It can also be found in individuals with diseases of the pituitary or hypothalamus glands, where the adrenal-stimulating hormones are produced. The prevalence of secondary adrenal insufficiency is estimated at 150–280 per 1 million individuals. It usually affects women in their sixth decade of life.

Patients with adrenal insufficiency will exhibit symptoms such as weakness, weight loss, anorexia, fatigue, nausea and vomiting, orthostatic hypotension, and abdominal pain. These symptoms will become more acute when severe insufficiency occurs.

Treatment of both types of adrenal insufficiency is replacement of **glucocorticoids** and **mineralocorticoids** as necessary. The most common form of replacement is hydrocortisone. New evidence suggests that the addition of (DHEA) dehydroepiandrosterone, a hormone naturally made by the body that can be synthetically produced, may improve the well-being of patients with adrenal insufficiency; however, long-term trials still need to be completed.

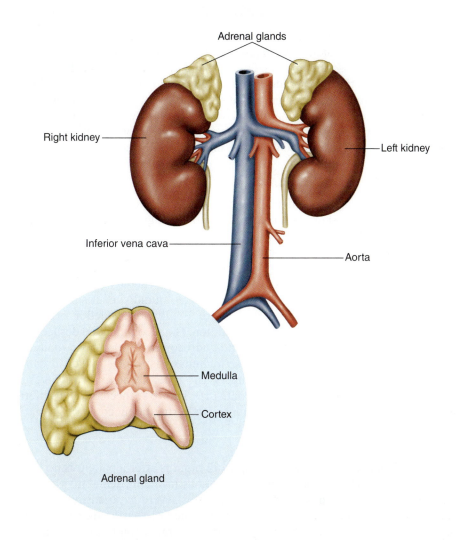

Adrenal glands

Right kidney

Left kidney

Inferior vena cava

Aorta

Medulla

Cortex

Adrenal gland

FIGURE 17.1 The adrenal glands.

Adrenal Crisis

Adrenal crisis is a life-threatening condition that occurs when the body is severely lacking cortisol. This condition can happen in one of two ways. One possible scenario is that the individual has not yet been diagnosed with adrenal insufficiency and is now at a point where the body is in severe need of cortisol to maintain normal carbohydrate and protein metabolism, as well as to help control the immune system. This is a common occurrence because adrenal insufficiency is often unrecognized in its early stages and can mimic other disorders, such as gastrointestinal illness or psychiatric disease. The second scenario is that a patient with adrenal insufficiency is placed in a stressful situation where the body requires additional cortisol, but is unable to produce the necessary amount. In many instances, individuals who are on corticosteroid therapy (use of exogenous corticosteroids) for long periods of time for conditions such as lupus erythematosus or asthma will experience a reduction in ACTH production, and eventually atrophy of the adrenal cortex will occur, necessitating an increase in glucocorticoid dosage. This scenario can lead to an increased likelihood of adrenal crisis if the individual encounters a stressful situation. In addition, vomiting and diarrhea, as occurs when a patient is experiencing the flu, have been known to commonly trigger an adrenal crisis. Major infections are also risk factors, and there has been at least one report of an adrenal crisis experienced by an undiagnosed Addison pediatric patient due to a severe dental infection.

Table 17.1 Signs and Symptoms of Adrenal Crisis

- Fatigue
- Lethargy
- Muscular weakness
- Headache
- Confusion
- Fever
- Nausea
- Vomiting
- Abdominal pain
- Hypotension
- Tachycardia
- Diaphoresis
- Dehydration
- Cyanosis
- Sunken eyes
- Dyspnea
- Dizziness
- Somnolence

Signs and Symptoms of Adrenal Crisis

Signs and symptoms of adrenal crisis include fatigue, lethargy, muscular weakness, headache, cyanosis, confusion, fever, nausea, vomiting, abdominal pain, hypotension, tachycardia, diaphoresis, sunken eyes, dyspnea, and dehydration. (See Table 17.1 ■) Hypotension without the appropriate amount of glucocorticoids during times of stress can lead to shock and cardiovascular collapse. If the hypotension is left untreated, death can result. The symptoms of adrenal crisis evolve slowly over a period of a few hours, and ultimately a severe exacerbation of these symptoms is manifested. An ACTH stimulation test aids in the definitive diagnosis of the condition.

Treatment of Adrenal Crisis

Management of an individual suffering from adrenal crisis requires stabilization until EMS arrives. The airway should be maintained, and vital signs should be continuously monitored. If the patient is experiencing dyspnea, oxygen should be administered at a rate of 2–5 L/minute via a nasal cannula. EMS will likely begin intravenous sodium chloride fluid therapy to replace fluid volume and correct sodium deficiency. Essentially this patient requires the administration of glucocorticoids as quickly as possible. Mineralocorticoids will need to be administered in individuals suffering from primary adrenal insufficiency; however, they are usually not needed in individuals suffering from the secondary form of the condition. The recommended dosage is 100 mg bolus of hydrocortisone intravenously and fludrocortisone 0.1 mg once daily. This therapy should help alleviate any cardiac arrhythmias, gastrointestinal disturbances, hypotension, and blood electrolyte imbalances. The generally accepted rule is that it is better to overtreat than to undertreat patients who are suspected to be suffering from adrenal crisis because the ramifications of undertreatment could be grave.

Prevention of Adrenal Crisis

The risk of adrenal crisis can occur for up to 12 months after a patient is no longer taking exogenous corticosteroids. Stressful situations, including dental treatment, can trigger an adrenal crisis whose primary symptom is severe hypotension; therefore, patients who have been on corticosteroids during the last year or are currently suffering from adrenal insufficiency may need to temporarily reintroduce or increase their corticosteroid therapy when stress is anticipated. Consultation with the patient's physician is essential to determine the appropriate course of treatment.

Most patients taking corticosteroids do not require additional corticosteroids referred to as "stress coverage" for dental treatment unless they are severe dental phobics or are undertaking a major surgical procedure. The risk of adrenal crisis is determined by the drugs administered, health of the patient, and degree of pain control. Some patients take a small additional dose of 5–10 mg of hydrocortisone if they find dental work stressful. Profound anesthesia during dental treatment and provision of postoperative analgesics will help reduce the stress of these patients and reduce the likelihood of adrenal crisis. These patients should wear a medical alert bracelet or necklace and carry an emergency medical information card that indicates the diagnosis, medications, and doses, as well as the physician to call in the event of an emergency. By doing so, the patient is more likely to obtain the necessary treatment for his or her condition in a timely manner.

Case Resolution and Conclusion

Adrenal crisis is an emergency that can occur in the dental office because of the increased stress level that some patients experience. In Nancy's case, the stress caused her body to require additional cortisol to maintain adequate body functions, and she, like all individuals suffering from adrenal insufficiency, was unable to produce that added hormone. Nancy, therefore, began to exhibit shock-like symptoms, such as fatigue, lethargy, muscular weakness, headache, confusion, fever, nausea, vomiting, abdominal pain, hypotension, tachycardia, diaphoresis, and dehydration. Nancy was positioned supinely, and EMS was contacted immediately. While waiting for EMS to arrive, Nancy was administered supportive care in the form of 4 L O_2/minute and the continual monitoring of her vital signs. Once in the hospital, Nancy received 100 mg of hydrocortisone intravenously. Timely treatment of this emergency prevented Nancy from experiencing cardiovascular collapse and death.

Review Questions

1. All of the following are causes of primary adrenal insufficiency *except* one. Which one is the *exception*?

   A. AIDS
   B. autoimmune disease
   C. tuberculosis
   D. diabetes

2. Which of the following is a sign of adrenal crisis?

   A. hypotension
   B. bradycardia
   C. dry skin
   D. chest pain

3. A patient suffering from adrenal crisis is in need of

   A. thyroxine
   B. glucocorticoids
   C. glucose
   D. none of the above

4. Which is the most important vital sign to monitor in a patient suspected of adrenal crisis?

   A. pulse
   B. respiration
   C. blood pressure
   D. temperature

5. The dental office is a very stressful experience for your midafternoon patient who is taking corticosteroids. The likelihood of adrenal crisis is increased because stress increases the need for cortisol, and patients who suffer from adrenal insufficiency are unable to produce additional cortisol.

   A. The first sentence is true and the second sentence is false.
   B. The first sentence is false and the second sentence true.
   C. Both sentences are true.
   D. Both sentences are false.

6. Your dental-phobic patient with a history of lupus erythematosus who takes corticosteroids daily is scheduled for a dental extraction. What treatment modifications should be made?

   A. No modifications are necessary.
   B. Have the patient double his dosage of corticosteroid an hour before the appointment.
   C. Contact his physician for appropriate treatment modification.
   D. None of the above.

7. What is the most common medication prescribed for patients with adrenal insufficiency?

   A. hydrocortisone
   B. thyroxine
   C. epinephrine
   D. cephalexin

8. All of the following are likely to trigger an adrenal crisis in patients who suffer from adrenal insufficiency *except* one. Which one is the *exception*?

   A. infection
   B. stress
   C. flu
   D. weight loss

Bibliography

Anderson, D. M., J. Keith, P. D. Novak, and M. A. Elliot, eds. *Mosby's Medical, Nursing & Allied Health Dictionary*. 6th ed. St. Louis, MO: Mosby-Year Book, Inc., 2008.

Arlt, W., and B. Allolio. "Adrenal Insufficiency." *The Lancet* 361 (2003): 1881–93.

Bablenis-Haveles, E. *Applied Pharmacology for the Dental Hygienist*. 6th ed. St. Louis, MO: Mosby-Elsevier, Inc., 2011.

Bain, S., and V. S. Igar. "Physical Signs for the General Dental Practitioner. Case 87. Adrenal Insufficiency." *Dental Update* 38, no. 7 (2011): 501.

Bennett, J. D., and M. B. Rosenberg. *Medical Emergencies in Dentistry*. 1st ed. Philadelphia, PA: W. B. Saunders, 2002.

Bsoul, S. A., G. T. Terezhalmy, and W. S. Moore. "Addison Disease." *Quintessence International* 34, no. 10 (2003): 784–85.

Chang, S. S., S. J. Liaw, M. J. Bullard, T. F. Chiu, J. C. Chen, and H. C. Liao. "Adrenal Insufficiency in Critically Ill Emergency Department Patients: A Taiwan Preliminary Study." *Academic Emergency Medicine* 8, no. 7 (2001): 761–64.

Don-Wauchope, A. C., and A. D. Toft. "Diagnosis and Management of Addison's Disease." *The Practitioner* 24, no. 4 (2000): 794–99.

Dorin, R. I., C. R. Qualls, and L. M. Crapo. "Diagnosis of Adrenal Insufficiency." *Annals of Internal Medicine* 139, no. 3 (2003): 194–204.

Gibson, N., and J. W. Ferguson. "Steroid Cover for Dental Patients on Long-Term Steroid Medication: Proposed Clinical Guidelines Based Upon a Critical Review of the Literature." *British Dental Journal* 197, no. 11 (2004): 681–85.

Hahner, S., and B. Allolia. "Therapeutic Management of Adrenal Insufficiency." *Best Practice & Research Clinic Endocrinology & Metabolism* 23, no. 2 (2009): 167–79.

Handerhan, B. "Recognizing Adrenal Crisis." *Nursing* 22, no. 4 (1992): 33.

Jones, A., and A. Catling. "The Patient with Endocrine Disease." *Surgery* 28, no. 9 (2010): 446–51.

Kearney, K. "Adrenal Crisis." *American Journal of Nursing* 100, no. 7 (2000): 49–50.

Mah, P. M., R. C. Jenkins, A. Rostami-Hodjegan, J. Newell-Price, A. Doane, V. Ibbotson, G. T. Tucker, and R. J. Ross. "Weight-Related Dosing, Timing and Monitoring Hydrocortisone Replacement Therapy in Patients with Adrenal Insufficiency." *Clinical Endocrinology* 61 (2004): 367–75.

Malamed, S. F. *Medical Emergencies in the Dental Office*. 6th ed. St. Louis, MO: Mosby Publishing Company, 2007.

Marzotti, S., and A. Falorni. "Addison's Disease." *Autoimmunity* 37, no. 4 (2004): 333–36.

Milenkovic, A., D. Markovic, D. Zdravkovic, T. Peric, T. Milenkovic, and R. Vukovic. "Adrenal Crisis Provoked by Dental Infection: Case Report and Review of the Literature." *Oral Surgery, Oral Medicine, Oral Pathology, Oral Radiology, and Endodontics* 110, no. 3 (2010): 325–29.

Miller, C. S., J. W. Little, and D. A. Falace. "Supplemental Corticosteroids for Dental Patients with Adrenal Insufficiency." *Journal of the American Dental Association* 132, no. 11 (2001): 1570–79.

Nieman, L. K. "Dynamic Evaluation of Adrenal Hypofunction." *Journal of Endocrinological Investigation* 26, no. 7 (2003): 74–82.

Oelkers, W., S. Diederich, and V. Bahr. "Therapeutic Strategies in Adrenal Insufficiency." *Annales d'Endocrinologie* 62, no. 2 (2001): 212–16.

Perry, R. J., E. A. McLaughlin, and P. J. Rice. "Steroid Cover in Dentistry: Recommendations Following a Review of Current Policy in UK Dental Teaching Hospitals." *Dental Update* 30, no. 1 (2003): 45–47.

Raisbeck, E. "Recognising Adrenal Insufficiency." *Emergency Nurse* 10, no. 4 (2002): 24–26.

Salvatori, R. "Adrenal Insufficiency." *Journal of the American Medical Association* 294, no. 19 (2005): 2481–88.

Shenker, Y., and J. B. Skatrud. "Adrenal Insufficiency in Critically Ill Patients." *American Journal of Respiratory Critical Care Medicine* 163, no. 7 (2001): 1520–23.

Stanhope, R. "Management of Adrenal Crisis—How Should Glucocorticoids Be Administered?" *Journal of Pediatric Endocrinology & Metabolism* 16, no. 8 (2003): 1099–100.

Ten, S., M. New, and N. Maclaren. "Addison's Disease." *The Journal of Clinical Endocrinology & Metabolism* 86, no. 7 (2001): 2909–22.

White, K., and W. Arlt. "Adrenal Crisis in Treated Addison's Disease: A Predictable But Under-Managed Event." *European Journal of Endocrinology* 162, no. 1 (2010): 115–20.

Willenberg, H. S., S. R. Bornstein, and G. P. Chrousos. "Adrenal Insufficiency." In: G. Fink, ed., *Encyclopedia of Stress*, pp. 47–52, 2010. Waltham, MA: Academic Press.

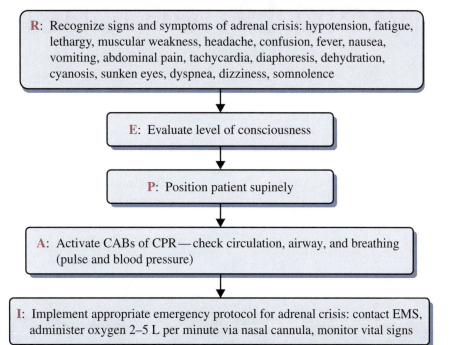

TREATMENT OF ADRENAL CRISIS
R.E.P.A.I.R.

R: Recognize signs and symptoms of adrenal crisis: hypotension, fatigue, lethargy, muscular weakness, headache, confusion, fever, nausea, vomiting, abdominal pain, tachycardia, diaphoresis, dehydration, cyanosis, sunken eyes, dyspnea, dizziness, somnolence

E: Evaluate level of consciousness

P: Position patient supinely

A: Activate CABs of CPR—check circulation, airway, and breathing (pulse and blood pressure)

I: Implement appropriate emergency protocol for adrenal crisis: contact EMS, administer oxygen 2–5 L per minute via nasal cannula, monitor vital signs

R: Refer to emergency department immediately

18

Thyroid Emergencies

LEARNING OBJECTIVES

Upon reading the material in this chapter, the reader will be able to:

- ✓ State the function of the thyroid gland.
- ✓ Differentiate between hyperthyroidism and hypothyroidism.
- ✓ Discuss the pathophysiology of thyroid storm and myxedema coma.
- ✓ Compare and contrast specific signs and symptoms associated with thyroid storm and myxedema coma.
- ✓ Determine suggested treatment modalities for patients experiencing thyroid storm and myxedema coma.

Case Study ·····················➤

Scenario

Your second patient on this January day in your Vermont dental office is Bryan Thomas, a 78-year-old male in fair health. His medical history reveals that he has hypothyroidism and is supposed to take Synthroid daily before breakfast. He informs you that he is on a fixed income and could not afford the medication for the past two months. He also informs you that he has just recovered from a bout of pneumonia. His voice seems rather hoarse, and you notice that his skin is dry, scaly, and cool to the touch. His hair is coarse and sparse. He seems much more confused and apathetic than he was at his previous appointments, but you assume that it is because of his age. You take his pulse and find that he is bradycardic, with a pulse rate of 50 beats/minute. His blood pressure is 122/98 mmHg. His respiration rate is 12 breaths/minute, and his breaths are weak. You decide to take his temperature as he is complaining of being cold, and you find he is hypothermic, with a body temperature of 95°F. When you begin the intraoral examination, you notice that his tongue is quite enlarged. In light of his vital signs, you decide to postpone dental hygiene treatment as you suspect the patient is suffering a medical emergency that requires immediate attention by a physician. Which medical emergency do you suspect?

Introduction

The **thyroid gland** is a butterfly-shaped organ that is located anterior to the trachea. The normal size of the thyroid gland is 2 to 2.5 cm in width and 3 to 5 cm in length. The action of thyroid hormones produced by the thyroid gland is threefold; they determine metabolic rate, growth rate, and other specific body mechanisms. **Euthyroid** is the term used to describe an individual with a normally functioning thyroid gland. If not enough or too much thyroid hormone is produced, there can be significant effects on the body. (See Figures 18.1 and 18.2 ■)

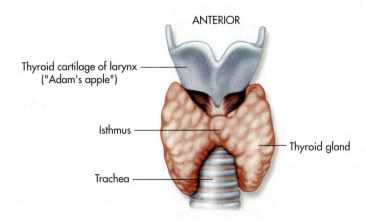

FIGURE 18.1 The thyroid gland.

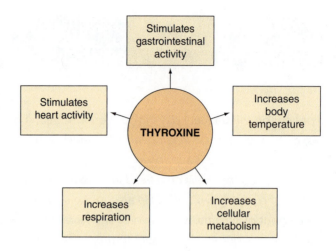

FIGURE 18.2 Effects of thyroxine.

In **hypothyroidism** or **myxedema**, insufficient thyroid hormone is produced by the thyroid gland. Causes of hypothyroidism include autoimmune disorders, such as **Hashimoto's thyroiditis**, pituitary tumors, surgery, or irradiation. Certain medication can also cause thyroid dysfunction. Individuals with hypothyroidism are continually medicated with a synthetic thyroid hormone. This medication is some form of levothyroxine. Patients with documented hypothyroidism should be asked the following questions: (1) Are they taking their medications? (2) Is their dosage stabilized? (3) Do they have routine blood work performed to insure adequate medication levels?

In young individuals myxedema manifests as cold intolerance, weight gain, dry skin, constipation, and mental and physical slowing. In elderly patients the same symptoms may apply; however, the symptoms may be more difficult to decipher because elderly individuals may have additional chronic diseases that can mimic the symptoms of hypothyroidism. In addition, musculoskeletal and mobility disorders are common in the elderly with hypothyroidism. Carpal tunnel syndrome, depression, high cholesterol levels, anemia, decreased memory, and slowed speech and thinking are also associated with hypothyroidism in the geriatric population. (See Figure 18.3 ■)

In **hyperthyroidism**, too much thyroid hormone is produced by the thyroid gland. The condition is also known as **thyrotoxicosis** and is often the result of a condition called Graves' disease. **Graves' disease** is a disorder associated with an enlarged thyroid gland, which will feel soft on palpation. The origin is unknown, but the disease is hereditary in nature and is suspected to be an autoimmune disorder. Another cause of hyperthyroidism is **nodular goiter**, which is an enlarged thyroid gland with multiple nodules. The goiter may become toxic and produce thyroid hormone on its own, causing hyperthyroidism. (See Figure 18.4 ■) Additionally, hyperthyroidism can be caused by inflammation of the thyroid gland or thyroiditis. It occurs in about 2% of women and 0.2% of men. Hyperthyroidism displays signs such as weight loss, nervousness, insomnia, bulging eyes (exophthalmos) (see Figure 18.5 ■), tremors, increased sweating, rapid heart rate, and diarrhea. These symptoms are the opposite of the symptoms of hypothyroidism.

Hyperthyroid patients are treated in one of three ways: surgery, **ablation therapy**, or antithyroid drugs. Surgery is now the last resort as several complications can arise, such as hemorrhage, hypoparathyroidism, and vocal cord paralysis. It is recommended only when the other two treatment options are unsuccessful. Ablation therapy involves using radioactive iodine to disable the thyroid gland. This will cause the patient to be hypothyroid, and he or she will need to be medicated with a synthetic hormone replacement. There are several antithyroid medications that can be used to control hyperthyroidism, including methimazole and propylthiouracil. Unfortunately, relapses usually occur so this is often a temporary treatment option. Moreover, side effects of these drugs include **agranulocytosis** and **hepatitis**.

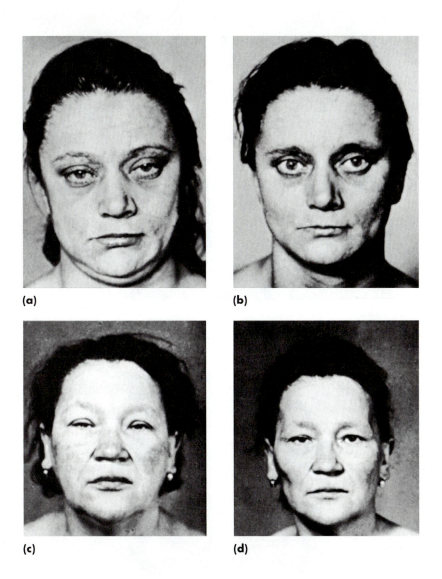

(a) (b)

(c) (d)

FIGURE 18.3 (a) A 29-year-old myxedema patient showing facial puffiness, muscle weakness, and drooping eyelids, which give a sleepy appearance. (b) The same patient after two months of thyroxine replacement. (c) A 62-year-old patient with myxedema exhibiting marked edema of the face and a somnolent look. The hair is stiff and without luster. (d) The same patient after three months of treatment with thyroxine.

Thyroid Emergencies

When thyroid hormone levels become too low, the patient may experience a potentially life-threatening condition called **myxedema coma**. If thyroid hormone levels become too high, the patient will most likely experience a serious condition called **thyroid storm**. These two conditions are fairly rare, but the dental healthcare provider should be knowledgeable of their signs, symptoms, and appropriate treatment.

Myxedema Coma

Myxedema coma occurs when the body is unable to compensate for the severe deficiency of the thyroid hormones often because of some precipitating event. The term *coma* is somewhat of a misnomer as the patient may or may not be in a comatose state. Myxedema coma can result from undiagnosed hypothyroidism; incorrect treatment; or a precipitating factor such as a trauma, infection or sepsis, hemorrhage, hypoglycemia, or surgery. Certain medications can also trigger the condition. Barbiturates,

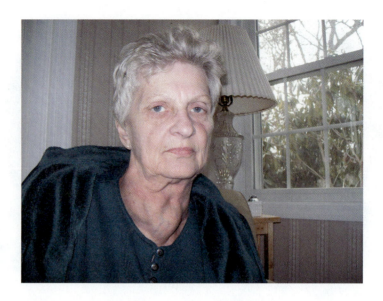

FIGURE 18.4 A 72-year-old woman with nodular goiter.

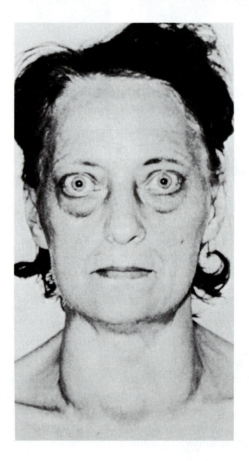

FIGURE 18.5 A Graves' disease patient with marked exophthalmos. The eyes have a fixed, staring expression. Note marked swelling of neck because of an enlarged thyroid.

beta-blockers, diuretics, lithium, narcotics, phenothiazines, phenytoin, and tranquilizers have been known to precipitate myxedema coma.

Myxedema coma is more common in women. It is more commonly found in individuals over 70 years of age and is rarely seen in individuals younger than 60. This

Table 18.1   **Signs and Symptoms of Myxedema Coma**

- Deterioration of the patient's mental state: confusion, apathy, depression, or psychosis
- Hypothermia (temperature <95°F)
- Hair loss
- Certain facial conditions: puffiness, macroglossia, ptosis, periorbital edema
- Cool, dry skin with nonpitting edema
- Bradycardia
- Changes in blood pressure with elevation in the early stages and lowered blood pressure in later stages
- Constipation
- Seizures
- Impaired mobility
- Hypoventilation
- Coma, which is rare

emergency is seen more frequently in the winter months, because the patient could be suffering from hypothermia.

SIGNS AND SYMPTOMS   The cardinal feature of myxedema coma is deterioration of the patient's mental state, with the patient possibly exhibiting confusion, apathy, depression, or psychosis. Other features may include hypothermia (temperature < 95°F), lethargy, hair loss, certain facial conditions (puffiness, macroglossia, **ptosis**, periorbital edema), cool, dry skin with nonpitting edema, bradycardia, changes in blood pressure with elevation in the early stages and lowered blood pressure in later stages, constipation, seizures, impaired mobility, delayed deep tendon reflexes, hypoglycemia, and **hypoventilation**. Airway compromise caused by the condition can lead to death. Coma is possible, but it is rare. (See Table 18.1 ■)

TREATMENT   The major goal when treating myxedema coma is to normalize the patient's temperature and maintain respirations. The patient must be admitted to the hospital as soon as possible as myxedema coma can be fatal if left untreated. The patient will most likely be treated in the intensive care unit as he or she may need ventilatory support with possible mechanical ventilation. Sedatives and tranquilizers should not be used as they will increase the risk of respiratory arrest. Intravenous administration of thyroid hormone replacement is required, and corticosteroids are also often administered until adrenal insufficiency is ruled out. The patient will need to be rewarmed using regular blankets as rapid rewarming can lead to hypotension and vascular collapse. Prophylactic antibiotics are often administered as this condition is commonly caused by infections. The cardiac status of the patient should be closely monitored, and the patient's blood pressure requires stabilization. The mortality rate for a patient with myxedema coma has been reported as 30% to 60%; therefore, this condition requires rapid, definitive treatment.

Thyroid Storm

Thyroid storm is a life-threatening emergency characterized by an exacerbation of a hyperthyroid state. It is often the result of undiagnosed thyroid disease; overzealous treatment of hypothyroidism; discontinuance of antithyroid medication; or a precipitating factor such as trauma, infection, diabetic ketoacidosis, cerebrovascular accident, stress, toxemia of pregnancy, fright, or surgery. Statistics indicate that 10% to 50% of thyroid storm cases are fatal.

SIGNS AND SYMPTOMS   The clinical features of thyroid storm can be described as an exaggeration of an uncomplicated hyperthyroid state. The classic symptom of thyroid storm is fever (possibly as high as 108°F) accompanied by diaphoresis. (See Figure 18.6 ■) The central nervous system is often affected, leading to restlessness, confusion, anxiety, or even psychosis. The patient may also suffer from gastrointestinal

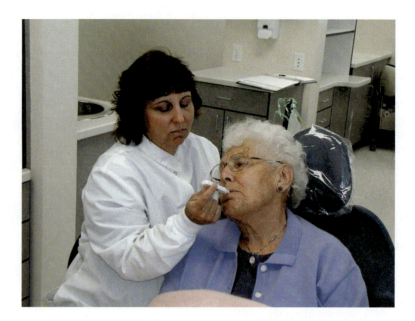

FIGURE 18.6 Using blanket and taking temperature of a patient suspected of myxedema coma.

Table 18.2 Signs and Symptoms of Thyroid Storm

- Fever (possibly as high as 108°F)
- Diaphoreses
- Restlessness
- Confusion
- Anxiety
- Psychosis
- Gastrointestinal symptoms: nausea, vomiting, diarrhea, jaundice
- Increased systolic blood pressure
- Tachycardia
- Widened pulse pressure
- Arrhythmias

symptoms, such as nausea, vomiting, diarrhea, or even jaundice. Increased systolic blood pressure, tachycardia, widened pulse pressure, and arrhythmias are also common in individuals suffering from thyroid storm. (See Table 18.2 ■)

TREATMENT   Thyroid storm treatment is directed at stabilization until the patient is transported to the emergency department. In the dental office the clinician should ensure that the patient is in a comfortable position, administer oxygen 4–6 L/minute, and monitor vital signs. Once EMS arrives, the patient will likely be placed on IV fluids. Propylthiouracil and methimazole are the drugs of choice to treat this condition. In addition, a beta-blocker may be administered to help control the heart rate and reduce cardiac output and workload. Corticosteroids are also often administered as thyroid storm can lead to adrenal insufficiency. To lower the patient's body temperature, a regulating blanket may be used and acetaminophen administered. Aspirin is contraindicated as it increases serum levels of T_3 and T_4. Care should be taken to ensure that shivering does not occur as this can increase cardiac demands and temperature. Once the patient is stabilized, the determination will be made as to which of the three courses of treatment will be followed to remedy the condition: antithyroid drugs, ablation therapy, or surgery.

Case Resolution and Conclusion ·····························➤

The thyroid gland is an important structure that helps maintain and support many of the body's metabolic processes by its production of thyroid hormones. These hormones are essential in determining the metabolic rate and body temperature; regulating protein, fat, and carbohydrate catabolism; maintaining appropriate growth rate; promoting central nervous system development; and synthesizing various enzymes. The overproduction or underproduction of these hormones has a negative impact on the body and can lead to debilitating conditions. If the rate of production of these hormones becomes extreme, two conditions can occur: myxedema coma and thyroid storm. In the case scenario presented at the beginning of this chapter, the patient states that he has a history of hypothyroidism; however, he could not afford his medication for some time. In addition, he just recently recovered from pneumonia. The clinician notices symptoms of severe hypothyroidism, such as hoarse voice; dry, scaly, cool skin; coarse hair; confusion; apathy; complaining of cold; large tongue; bradycardia; and weak respirations. These signs and symptoms alert the clinician to take the patient's temperature, and it is determined that Bryan is hypothermic. The clinician deduces that the patient is suffering from severe hypothyroidism (myxedema coma) and takes the appropriate steps. The patient is positioned supinely, and EMS is contacted immediately. Blankets are applied to the patient in an attempt to increase the patient's body temperature. Six liters per minute of oxygen is administered to improve respiration. Vital signs of the patient are continuously monitored until EMS arrives. Once hospitalized, Bryan was administered levothyroxine intravenously and rewarmed with blankets. He was informed about the importance of taking his medication on a regular basis as this condition can be fatal, and he was released from the hospital after a few days of close observation.

Review Questions

1. The most accepted method for treating hyperthyroidism is

    A. surgery
    B. ablation therapy
    C. antithyroid medication
    D. beta-blockers

2. Which of the following is a sign of thyroid storm?

    A. fever
    B. macroglossia
    C. bradycardia
    D. hypoventilation

3. All of the following are strategies for managing thyroid storm *except* one. Which one is the *exception*?

    A. wrapping in blankets to increase body temperature
    B. administering oxygen 4–6 L/minute
    C. administering acetaminophen
    D. administering beta-blockers

4. Hypothyroidism is characterized by

    A. weight loss
    B. cold intolerance
    C. diarrhea
    D. low cholesterol

5. The emergent condition arising from severe hypothyroidism is

   A. thyroid storm
   B. thyrotoxicosis
   C. myxedema coma
   D. diabetic ketoacidosis

6. The most common medication a patient would take for hypothyroidism is

   A. levothyroxine
   B. beta-blocker such as vasotec
   C. acetaminophen
   D. none of the above

7. All of the following are treatment management strategies for myxedema coma *except*

   A. slowly rewarming the patient
   B. administering IV levothyroxine
   C. administering IV corticosteroids
   D. administering sedatives and tranquilizers

8. The hereditary autoimmune disorder whereby the individual has an increased level of thyroid hormone production is known as

   A. myxedema coma
   B. Grave's disease
   C. Hashimoto's disease
   D. euthyroid

Bibliography

Anderson, D. M., J. Keith, P. D. Novak, and M. A. Elliot, eds. *Mosby's Medical, Nursing & Allied Health Dictionary*. 6th ed. St. Louis, MO: Mosby-Year Book, Inc., 2008.

Bennett, J. D., and M. B. Rosenberg. *Medical Emergencies in Dentistry*. 1st ed. Philadelphia, PA: W. B. Saunders, 2002.

Birrell, G., and T. Cheetham. "Juvenile Thyrotoxicosis: Can We Do Better?" *Archives of Disease in Childhood* 89, no. 8 (2004): 745–50.

Charles, R. A., and S. Goh. "Not Just Gastroenteritis: Thyroid Storm Unmasked." *Emergency Medicine Australasia* 16, no. 3 (2004): 247–49.

Franklyn, J. "Thyrotoxicosis." *Clinical Medicine* 3, no. 1 (2003): 11–15.

Ghobrial, M. W. "Coma and Thyroid Storm in Apathetic Thyrotoxicosis." *Southern Medical Journal* 95, no. 5 (2002): 552–54.

Greco, L. K. "Hypothyroid Emergencies." *Topics in Emergency Medicine* 23, no. 4 (2001): 44–51.

Grimes, C. M., C. H. Muniz, and W. H. Montgomery. "Intraoperative Thyroid Storm: A Case Report." *American Association of Nurse Anesthetists Journal* 72, no. 1 (2004): 53–55.

Jao, Y. T. F. N., Y. Chen, W. Lee, and F. Tai. "Thyroid Storm and Ventricular Tachycardia." *Southern Medical Journal* 97, no. 6 (2004): 604–607.

Jones, A., and S. Catling. "The Patient with Endocrine Disease." *Surgery* 28, no. 9 (2010): 446–51.

Lee, C. H., and C. R. Wira. "Severe Angioedema in Myxedema Coma: A Difficult Airway in a Rare Endocrine Emergency." *American Journal of Emergency Medicine* 27, no. 8 (2009): 1021e1–2021e2.

Lien Munson, B. "Myths and Facts about Thyroid Storm." *Nursing 2004* 34, no. 5 (2004): 24.

Malamed, S. F. *Medical Emergencies in the Dental Office*. 6th ed. St. Louis, MO: Mosby Publishing Company, 2007.

Martindale, J. L., E. L. Senecal, Z. Obermeyer, E. S. Nadel, and D. F. M. Brown. "Case Presentations of the Harvard Affiliated Emergency Medicine Residencies." *Journal of Emergency Medicine* 39, no. 4 (2010): 491–96.

Migneco, A., V. Ojette, A. Testa, A. DeLorenzo, and N. Gentloni Silveri. "Management of Thyrotoxic Crisis." *European Review for Medical and Pharmacological Sciences* 9, no. 1 (2005): 69–74.

Pickett, F. A., and J. R. Gurenlian. *Preventing Medical Emergencies: Use of the Medical History*. 2nd ed. Philadelphia, PA: Lippincott Williams & Wilkins, 2010.

Rehman, S. U., D. W. Cope, A. D. Senseney, and W. Brzezinski. "Thyroid Disorders in Elderly Patients." *Southern Medical Journal* 98, no. 5 (2005): 543–49.

Rodriquez, I., E. Fluiters, L. F. Perez-Mendez, R. Luna, C. Paramo, and R. V. Garcia-Mayor. "Factors Associated with Mortality of Patients with Myxoedema Coma: Prospective Study in 11 Cases Treated in a Single Institution." *Journal of Endocrinology* 180, no. 2 (2004): 347–50.

Savage, M. W., P. M. Mah, A. P. Weetman, and J. Newell-Price. "Endocrine Emergencies." *Postgraduate Medical Journal* 80, no. 947 (2004): 506–15.

Shagham, J. Y. "Thyroid Disease: An Overview." *Radiologic Technology* 73, no. 1 (2001): 25–44.

Simmons Holcomb, S. "Thyroid Diseases." *Dimensions of Critical Care Nursing* 21, no. 4 (2002): 127–33.

Simmons Holcomb, S. "Detecting Thyroid Disease, Part 2." *Nursing 2003* 33, no. 9 (2003), 32cc1–32cc4.

Simmons Holcomb, S. "Detecting Thyroid Disease." *Nursing 2005* 35, no. 10 (2005): 4–9.

Simmons Holcomb, S. "Thyroid Storm." *Nursing* 39, no. 11 (2009): 72.

Simmons Holcomb, S. "A Delicate Balance: Detecting Thyroid Disease." *Nursing* 40, no. 7 (2010): 22–30.

Vora, N. M., F. Fedok, and B. C. Stack. "Report of a Rare Case of Trauma-Induced Thyroid Storm." *Ear, Nose & Throat Journal* 81, no. 8 (2002, August): 570–74.

Wall, C. R. "Myxedema Coma: Diagnosis and Treatment." *American Family Physician* 62, no. 11 (2000): 2485–90.

Young, J. "Myxedema Coma." *Nursing 99* 29, no. 1 (1999a, January): 64.

Young, J. "Thyroid Storm." *Nursing 99* 29, no. 8 (1999b, August): 33.

TREATMENT OF MYXEDEMA COMA
R.E.P.A.I.R.

R: Recognize signs and symptoms of myxedema coma: deterioration of the patient's mental state, confusion, apathy, depression or psychosis, hypothermia (temperature <95°F), hair loss, facial puffiness, macroglossia, cool, dry skin with nonpitting edema, bradycardia, elevated BP, seizures, impaired mobility, and hypoventilation, hypoglycemia

E: Evaluate level of consciousness—coma is rare

P: Position patient supinely

A: Activate CABs of CPR—check circulation, airway, and breathing (pulse and blood pressure)

I: Implement appropriate emergency protocol for myxedema coma: contact EMS normalize temperature with blankets, maintain respirations, administer O₂ 4–6 liters per minute, monitor vital signs

R: Refer to emergency department immediately

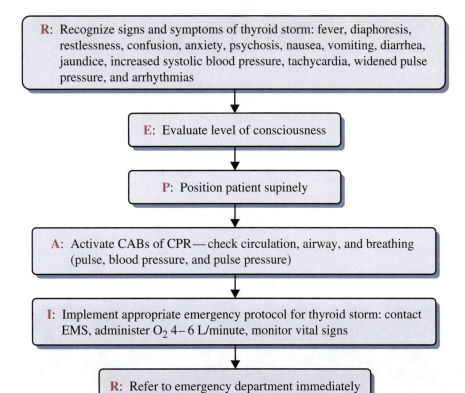

TREATMENT OF THYROID STORM
R.E.P.A.I.R.

R: Recognize signs and symptoms of thyroid storm: fever, diaphoresis, restlessness, confusion, anxiety, psychosis, nausea, vomiting, diarrhea, jaundice, increased systolic blood pressure, tachycardia, widened pulse pressure, and arrhythmias

E: Evaluate level of consciousness

P: Position patient supinely

A: Activate CABs of CPR—check circulation, airway, and breathing (pulse, blood pressure, and pulse pressure)

I: Implement appropriate emergency protocol for thyroid storm: contact EMS, administer O_2 4–6 L/minute, monitor vital signs

R: Refer to emergency department immediately

Epistaxis

LEARNING OBJECTIVES

Upon reading the material in this chapter, the reader will be able to:

- ✓ Discuss potential causes of epistaxis in the dental office.

- ✓ Recognize specific signs and symptoms associated with epistaxis.

- ✓ Determine suggested treatment modalities for patients experiencing epistaxis.

- ✓ Explain strategies for preventing epistaxis.

Case Study ·······································➤

Scenario

Your patient, Lee Wong, a 68-year-old man, is waiting for his 10:00 A.M. dental hygiene appointment in your Phoenix, Arizona, office. Suddenly he sneezes and realizes that his nose is bleeding and informs your office receptionist. The receptionist becomes alarmed at the amount of bright red blood present and seeks your assistance. What should you do?

Introduction

Nosebleeds or epistaxis is a common occurrence in the general population and therefore may occur in the dental office. Sixty percent of individuals will experience epistaxis in their lifetime. Six percent of individuals with epistaxis will require medical attention for the condition. Nosebleeds can range from a minor condition to a life-threatening condition.

For the most part nosebleeds are caused by digital manipulation (nose picking) and are therefore common in children; however, they are more serious if they occur in adults. Nosebleeds occur more frequently in men. Eighty percent of nosebleeds are idiopathic. They are more common in the fall and winter months because of the dry, cold weather; however, there is some evidence that weather is not an indicator of the incidence of epistaxis.

Most nosebleeds (85%) are referred to as anterior bleeds and are usually easy to manage. Anterior nosebleeds usually occur at **Kiesselbach's plexus** or **Little's area**, which is a group of blood vessels located anterior to the septal wall and close to the mucosal surface, and due to their location, they can be easily broken. Kiesselbach's plexus is the area where several arteries meet: the sphenopalatine, greater palatine, superior labial, and anterior ethmoidal arteries. Posterior nosebleeds, which occur more often in the geriatric population, tend to be more difficult to manage. This type of nosebleed usually occurs at **Woodruff's plexus**, where the following arteries coalesce: posterior nasal, sphenopalatine, and ascending pharyngeal. These arteries are also located superficially and can be readily damaged. (See Figure 19.1 ■)

There are multiple etiologies of epistaxis, and these are often divided into either local or systemic factors. Local factors include, but are not limited to, allergies, cocaine, environmental irritants, foreign bodies, nasal sprays, digital manipulation, septal deviation or perforation, sinusitis, trauma, upper respiratory infections, sneezing, and neoplasm. Systemic factors tend to be significantly more serious and include, but are not limited to, anemia, anticoagulant therapy, **arteriosclerosis**, blood dyscrasia (i.e., **hemophilia**, **thrombocytopenia**, **von Willebrand's disease**), chronic obstructive pulmonary disease (COPD), **Osler-Weber-Rendu syndrome (hereditary hemorrhagic telangiectasia [HHT])**, and hypertension. Hypertension as an etiology of epistaxis is a controversial issue. Some evidence indicates that individuals with hypertension are three times more likely to experience epistaxis than those who are normotensive; however, this blood pressure elevation may be due to the stress of experiencing a nosebleed. It has been determined that epistaxis incidence in patients with hypertension is not related to hypertension severity. Several medications and herbal supplements, including aspirin, warfarin, clopidogrel, ginseng, garlic, ginkgo biloba, heparin, NSAIDs, ticlopidine, and dipyridamole, have anticoagulant properties and can lead to epistaxis. In addition, there is a relationship between alcohol consumption and epistaxis.

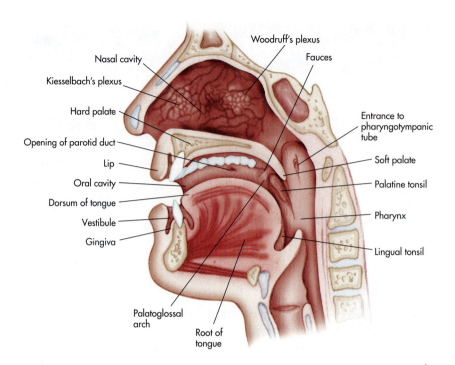

FIGURE 19.1 Nasal anatomy.

Table 19.1 Signs and Symptoms of Epistaxis

Anterior Epistaxis	Posterior Epistaxis
• Oozing blood • Bright red blood	• Profuse bleeding • Dark red blood • Gagging • Coughing • Vomiting

Signs and Symptoms of Epistaxis

The signs and symptoms of this emergency are readily apparent—blood exuding from the nasal cavity. If the nosebleed is from the anterior region of the nasal cavity, the blood will usually ooze and be bright red. If, however, the nosebleed is from the posterior portion of the nasal cavity, the bleeding will be profuse, dark red, and often bilateral. One major problem with posterior nosebleeds is that they tend to drain into the mouth and cause gagging and coughing, which can lead to vomiting or pneumonitis. (See Table 19.1 ■)

Treatment of Epistaxis

The first step when treating epistaxis is to identify the mechanism of injury and define the severity. This will determine the course of action. The clinician should wear personal protection attire. The CABs should be performed to ensure that the patient has appropriate circulation, has an open airway, and is breathing. Suction may be needed to remove blood from the mouth to maintain an airway. Position the patient upright and have his or her head tilted slightly forward to prevent blood from entering the throat. Have the patient apply direct pressure by pinching the lower part of the nose for at least 15 minutes and up to 20 minutes. Be sure to have the patient breathe through the mouth. Have a basin of some type available so the patient can spit out all blood and saliva. Place an ice pack over the bridge of the nose (doing so may help with vasoconstriction). The patient should not blow his or her nose, although doing so may aid in **hemostasis**. Most nosebleeds will stop with direct pressure; however, if the bleeding does not stop, it could be a more serious condition and the patient should be referred to the emergency department for evaluation and treatment. Treatments that may need to be performed in the emergency department include **cauterizing** the area using silver nitrate or packing the nostrils. If sufficient blood loss occurs, the patient may require a blood transfusion. Laboratory tests may be performed to help determine the etiology of the epistaxis. Additionally, the patient may need to be examined by an ear, nose, and throat (ENT) specialist, and in some cases surgery is needed.

Prevention of Epistaxis

To prevent the recurrence of a nosebleed, the patient should be instructed to keep his or her head elevated for four hours and not to blow the nose for several hours. Heavy lifting and bending at the waist should be avoided for 24 hours. Patients should use a humidifier at home to prevent dryness. In addition, they should apply a pea-sized amount of a lubricating cream to each nostril one to three times per day. Water intake should be increased, and patients should avoid taking any medications containing aspirin, which could cause bleeding.

Case Resolution and Conclusion ·······························➤

Although epistaxis is usually a benign condition, it can be an etiology of a more severe health problem. Nosebleeds can be alarming for both clinician and patient, so it is important to understand the possible cause(s) and appropriate treatment. In the case presented, Lee Wong was having excessive bright red blood exiting his nasal cavity. Lee lives in a dry, warm climate, so the clinician assumed that the condition was caused by damage to the blood vessels in the anterior portion of the nose as they lie close to the mucosal surface. The clinician donned her personal protective equipment and ensured that Lee had a patent airway. He was then asked to tilt his head forward and apply pressure to his nostrils for 20 minutes. The clinician then placed an ice pack on the bridge of Lee's nose. The bleeding dissipated within a few minutes, so referral to the emergency department for additional procedures and testing was deemed unnecessary.

Review Questions

1. For what amount of time should pressure be applied for a nosebleed?

   A. 5 minutes.
   B. 20 minutes.
   C. 45 minutes.
   D. Pressure should not be applied for a nosebleed.

2. All of the following are useful recommendations to prevent a recurrence of epistaxis *except* one. Which one is the *exception*?

   A. avoiding medications with anticoagulant properties
   B. avoiding bending at the waist for 24 hours
   C. keeping the head elevated for four hours
   D. using a dehumidifier in the home

3. Profuse bleeding of dark red blood out of both nostrils is indicative of which type of nosebleed?

A. anterior
B. posterior
C. mucosal
D. septal

4. The most common site for epistaxis is

A. the nares
B. Woodruff's plexus
C. Kiesselbach's plexus
D. none of the above

5. The most common cause of epistaxis is

A. digital manipulation
B. hypertension
C. blood dyscrasia
D. foreign body

6. All of the following are systemic conditions that are often associated with epistaxis *except* one. Which one is the *exception*?

A. neoplasm
B. thrombocytopenia purpura
C. anemia
D. arteriosclerosis

7. Applying ice to the nose during epistaxis is helpful as it provides

A. cauterization
B. angioedema
C. vasoconstriction
D. vasodilation

8. All of the following are agents that have anticoagulant properties *except* one. Which one is the *exception*?

A. acetaminophen
B. aspirin
C. ginkgo biloba
D. clopidogrel

Bibliography

Anderson, D. M., J. Keith, P. D. Novak, and M. A. Elliot, eds. *Mosby's Medical, Nursing & Allied Health Dictionary.* 6th ed. St. Louis, MO: Mosby-Year Book, Inc., 2008.

Barbarito, C. "Hypertension Induced Epistaxis." *American Journal of Nursing* 98, no. 2 (1998): 48.

Bennett, J. D., and M. B. Rosenberg. *Medical Emergencies in Dentistry.* 1st ed. Philadelphia, PA: W. B. Saunders, 2002.

Bishow, R. M. "Current Approaches to the Management of Epistaxis." *Journal of the Academy of Physician Assistants* 16, no. 5 (2003): 52–69.

Bond, F., and A. Sizeland. "Epistaxis—Strategies for Management." *Australian Family Physician* 20, no. 10 (2000): 933–38.

Bray, D., C. E. B. Giddings, P. Monnery, N. Eze, S. Lo, and A. G. Toma. "Epistaxis: Are Temperature and Seasonal Variations True Factors of Incidence?" *The Journal of Laryngology & Otology* 119, no. 9 (2005): 724–26.

Crown, L. A., and R. D. Criner. "Epistaxis: A Practical Approach to Treatment." *Patient Care for the Nurse Practitioner, Thomson Gale* (2004). Accessed Infotrac, June 5, 2006. http://globalrph.medwire.com/main/Default.aspxzp=conte/6articleID=110037.

Fletcher, L. M. "Epistaxis." *Surgery* 27, no. 12 (2009): 512–17.

Frazee, T. A., and M. S. Hauser. "Nonsurgical Management of Epistaxis." *Journal of Oral and Maxillofacial Surgery* 58, no. 4 (2000): 419–24.

Friese, G., and R. F. Wojciehoski. "The Nose: Bleeds, Breaks, and Obstructions." *Emergency Medical Services* 34, no. 8 (2005): 129–37.

Herkner, H., C. Havel, M. Mullner, G. Gamper, A. Bur, A. F. Temmel, A. N. Laggner, and M. M. Hirschl. "Active Epistaxis at ED Presentation Is Associated with Arterial Hypertension." *American Journal of Emergency Medicine* 20, no. 2 (2002): 92–95.

Knopfholz, J., E. Lima-Junior, D. Precoma-Neto, and J. R. Faria-Neto. "Association Between Epistaxis and Hypertension: A One Year Follow-Up after an Index Episode of Nose Bleeding in Hypertensive Patients." *International Journal of Cardiology* 134, no. 3 (2009): e106–e109.

Leong, S. C. L., R. J. Roe, and A. Karkanevatos. "No Frills Management of Epistaxis." *Emergency Medicine Journal* 22, no. 7 (2005): 470–72.

Manes, R. P. "Evaluating and Managing the Patient with Nosebleeds." *Medical Clinics of North America* 94, no. 5 (2010): 903–12.

McErlane, K., and C. Pence. "Epistaxis." *Nursing 2004* 34, no. 8 (2004): 88.

Pallin, D. J., Y. Chng, M. P. McKay, J. A. Emond, A. J. Pelletier, and C. A. Camargo. "Epidemiology of Epistaxis in US Emergency Departments." *Annals of Emergency Medicine* 46, no. 1 (2005): 77–81.

Pope, L. E. R., and C. G. L. Hobbs. "Epistaxis: An Update on Current Management." *Postgraduate Medicine Journal* 81 (2004): 309–14.

Shellenbarger, T. "Nosebleeds: Not Just Kid's Stuff." *RN* 63, no. 2 (2000): 50–56.

Sparacino, L. L. "Epistaxis Management: What's New and What's Noteworthy." *Lippincott's Primary Care Practice* 4, no. 5 (2000): 498–507.

Vaghela, H. "Using a Swimmer's Nose Clip in the Treatment of Epistaxis in the A & E department." *Accident and Emergency Nursing* 13, no. 4 (2005): 261–63.

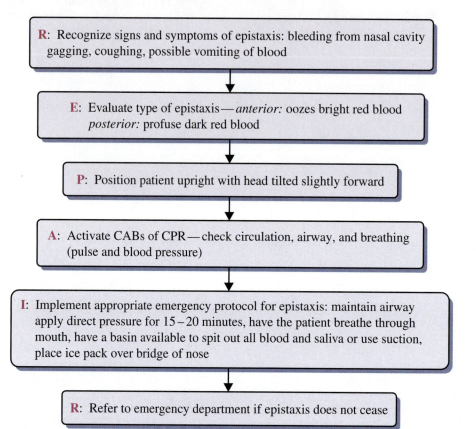

TREATMENT OF EPISTAXIS
R.E.P.A.I.R.

R: Recognize signs and symptoms of epistaxis: bleeding from nasal cavity gagging, coughing, possible vomiting of blood

E: Evaluate type of epistaxis—*anterior:* oozes bright red blood *posterior:* profuse dark red blood

P: Position patient upright with head tilted slightly forward

A: Activate CABs of CPR—check circulation, airway, and breathing (pulse and blood pressure)

I: Implement appropriate emergency protocol for epistaxis: maintain airway apply direct pressure for 15–20 minutes, have the patient breathe through mouth, have a basin available to spit out all blood and saliva or use suction, place ice pack over bridge of nose

R: Refer to emergency department if epistaxis does not cease

20

Excessive Bleeding Following an Extraction

LEARNING OBJECTIVES

Upon reading the material in this chapter, the reader will be able to:

- ✓ Identify the signs and symptoms of excessive bleeding levels following oral surgery.

- ✓ List the possible causes and contributing factors associated with excessive bleeding after extraction.

- ✓ Establish proper treatment modalities for excessive bleeding both during and after oral surgery.

- ✓ Determine precautions for preventing excessive bleeding during and after oral surgery.

- ✓ Discuss the international normalized ratio as it relates to patient treatment.

Case Study

Scenario

Your patient, Margaret Barclay, arrives for her scheduled recall dental hygiene appointment. Ms. Barclay is a 62-year-old woman in fair health, who is on a regular four-month recall schedule. Her history consists of high cholesterol and a past episode of angina pectoris in 2004. Daily medications for Margaret are listed as Lipitor (20 mg), aspirin (0.81 gm), and a multivitamin. She confirms that her medical history and her medications have not altered since her last recall visit. Ms. Barclay complains of pain in the area of tooth #32, and after completing blood pressure, pulse, respiration (all within normal limits), and her intra- and extraoral examinations, you conclude that further examination of that area is warranted. After taking both a panograph and a periapical film of #32, you determine that #32 is abscessed and consult with the dentist with whom you work, who confirms your diagnosis. Upon completion of your hygiene appointment, a referral to an oral surgeon for extraction of #32 is given to Ms. Barclay.

Several days later, Ms. Barclay returns to your office. She complains of excessive bleeding at the site of extraction and says the problem has been ongoing for several hours and began shortly after her surgery was completed that morning. She has been unable to contact the oral surgeon and has come to your office for help. What do you do?

Introduction

As in any surgery, possible complications during or after extraction can include excessive bleeding, infection, or a reaction to the anesthetic agent used during the procedure. The majority of patients who undergo routine dental extractions are unaffected with excessive bleeding, and most surgery is completed without problem; however, there are exceptions to this rule, and at-risk patients can often be identified and managed pretreatment to minimize their bleeding potential. Some of the causes of bleeding problems during or after extractions will be discussed in this chapter, as will possible prevention methods.

One group that is at risk for excess bleeding postsurgery is hemophiliacs. Hemophilia is "a group of hereditary bleeding disorders characterized by a deficiency of one of the factors necessary for coagulation of the blood."[1] Dental extraction in this group is associated with a high risk of bleeding. Of the three types of hemophilia, type A is the most common, and patients who have any type of this disease can have a form that is rated from mild to severe.

Although bleeding disorders are relatively rare, 1% of the population is affected by von Willebrand's disease (VWD). VWD is a genetic disease; patients who present with this disease have insufficient levels of von Willebrand factor (VWF), a blood protein that is necessary for normal blood clotting. This deficiency indicates the patient may be prone to excessive and long-lasting bleeding after a dental extraction

---

[1]Anderson, K. N. and L. E. Anderson. *Mosby's Dictionary of Medicine, Nursing & Allied Health* (5th ed.), 1998. St. Louis, MO: Mosby-Year Book, Inc.

or surgery, and precautions must be taken by the health professional prior to initiation of treatment.

Another sector of the population that is prone to excessive bleeding is those taking **anticoagulants**. These medications include warfarin, heparin, clopidogrel, dabigatran etexilate, prasugrel, and aspirin, and are often prescribed for health management post myocardial infarction, angina pectoris, cerebrovascular accident, **coronary arterial bypass graft surgery**, deep vein **thrombosis**, atrial fibrillation, and **embolism**. Although all of the previously listed medications are considered anticoagulants, they vary in potency. The risk of excessive bleeding can depend greatly on the type and dosage of drug the patient is receiving.

All patients should always be questioned through a thorough medical history review prior to any type of dental treatment. In the case of extraction or scaling and root planing, a review of all medications is extremely important. Not only may prescribed medications such as those listed in the preceding paragraph increase the risk of bleeding during any dental procedure, but the clinician should also be informed if a patient is taking any supplements or herbal medications. Several of these (e.g., St. John's wort and ginkgo biloba) may increase bleeding during or after invasive dental procedures, and patients may be advised to discontinue their use for a period of time.

Hematoma caused by a local anesthetic injection has also been indicated as a culprit in profuse bleeding post extraction. A hematoma is a collection of blood trapped beneath the skin and is usually caused by trauma. If an artery or one of its branches is severely traumatized during injection, hemorrhage can occur, and this may result in potential complications. Hemorrhage is the second most common problem in dental surgery, and, once initiated, a hematoma can continue to expand, causing decreased oxygen saturation and altered mental capacity.

Signs and Symptoms of Excessive Bleeding

The symptoms of excessive bleeding post extraction are easily recognized. In a normal case scenario, and assuming the patient has followed the instructions given to him or her by the dental professional, there should be no bleeding at an excessive rate or heavy flow. If bleeding from the extraction site is heavy, unaffected by compression, and lasts up to two hours, the patient needs to be aware that this reaction is not within normal limits and further steps must be taken to resolve this potentially dangerous situation. In addition to excessive bleeding, other signs of an abnormal reaction post extraction are fever, hypotension, altered mental capacity, and hematoma.

Treatment and Prevention of Excessive Bleeding

The treatment and prevention of excessive bleeding in both the medically compromised and uncompromised patient will be presented as this chapter proceeds. As noted in the Introduction, there are several identifiable groups at risk for heavy uncontrolled bleeding during or after oral surgery. There are also individuals who may have an undiagnosed systemic illness that can be a precursor to complications once surgery is complete. These illnesses can lie dormant until induced by trauma, such as oral surgery. Finally, the treatment and prevention of hematoma will be addressed.

Medically Uncompromised Patients

After a routine dental extraction, patients should be given instructions on how to manage bleeding and other side effects. These instructions include no exercise for 12 to 24 hours after surgery, lying down with the head elevated for several hours, and placing gauze over the tooth socket and applying pressure for at least two hours. Application of pressure is considered the most effective way to control bleeding, and another option in place of plain gauze is to moisten a tea bag with water, wrap it in

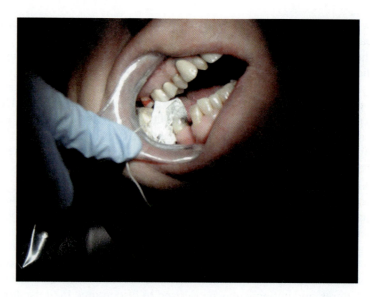

FIGURE 20.1 Use of tea bag following extraction.

gauze, place it over the socket, and apply pressure by biting on it. (See Figure 20.1 ■) Tea contains tannic acid, which may help to reduce bleeding for some patients. There are also a variety of materials, such as hemostatic collagen products, cellulose products, or hemostatic bandages, that can be placed into the tooth socket by the oral surgeon postsurgery. Although it is normal for some blood to ooze from the site for 12 hours, it is not normal for the bleeding to be a steady flow.

If the patient follows these instructions and bleeding is still occurring at a steady or heavy rate, follow-up treatment is indicated. Patients who note excessive bleeding or other unusual side effects such as a fever, hypotension, or hematoma should call their dentist or oral surgeon immediately. If the dental professional cannot be reached, patients should proceed to a hospital emergency department for care.

Patients with Hemophilia

Dental extraction in hemophiliacs requires a multidisciplinary approach and rigid protocol that should be decided by the physician, oral surgeon, and patient before surgery. At this time, no consensus exists as to the oversight of hemophiliacs who need dental extractions, but there are several options that may be employed. Management using a systemic treatment and/or local hemostasis has two of these options. Systemically, replacement therapy given through recombinant factor injections or IV can be utilized one hour before surgery. The type of recombinant factor used is dependent on the severity of hemophilia in the particular patient. After replacement therapy and immediately before extraction, hemostasis assessment should be carried out. Locally, hemostasis can be achieved through local anesthesia before extraction and through glues, gelatin packing, and compressive splints postsurgery. In all cases, local anesthesia with a vasoconstrictor is the anesthetic of choice as it reduces bleeding during surgery.

Postsurgery, the **alveolus** should be thoroughly cleaned and biological glue inserted. This is followed by insertion of a gelatin packing that is then covered by a layer of glue. The alveolus is then sutured with absorbable sutures that are covered with biological glue. Intermittent compression is required of the patient for the next three days, with directions given for time and type of compression. Following these protocols for treatment and prevention, the hemophiliac can safely withstand routine extraction work, and delayed bleeding several days after the procedure is usually limited.

Patients with Von Willebrand Disease

Von Willebrand's disease is the most common inherited bleeding disorder. VWD manifests itself through defects in the VWF, an important protein for hemostasis. Treatment prior to extraction for patients with VWD is dependent upon the category of VWD (type 1, 2, or 3) with which the patient presents. For most type 1 and some type 2 patients, drug treatment may consist of desmopressin acetate, which promotes the release of VWF. Patients who have a more severe deficiency of the protein complex and do not respond to desmopressin therapy may require treatment with pooled human plasma. As with hemophiliacs, the key to successful surgery with minimal postoperative bleeding is a multidisciplinary approach that includes the physician, oral surgeon, and patient, and often involves a combination of drug therapy and conservative surgical practices.

Patients Taking Anticoagulants

The effect of anticoagulants on the amount of bleeding during and after oral surgery varies and is dependent on the potency and dosage of the drug, as well as the host's response to a particular drug. The medications discussed in this chapter are warfarin, heparin, clopidogrel, dabigatran etexilate, prasugrel, and aspirin. As previously mentioned, these drugs are used to manage post myocardial infarction, angina pectoris, cerebrovascular accident, coronary arterial bypass graft surgery, deep vein thrombosis, atrial fibrillation, and embolism. It is important that the dental professional consult with the patient's medical provider when indicated prior to invasive procedures such as extraction. Recent research has argued that inappropriate adjustments in anticoagulation therapy place the patient at far greater risk of stroke than hemorrhage during most dental procedures.

Warfarin (coumadin) drugs are used for prevention and treatment of thrombosis disorders. Patients who are taking warfarin and need to undergo dental extraction are usually placed into one of three risk categories: low, moderate, and high. Low risk indicates no change in medication. Moderate risk indicates medication withdrawal 48 hours before the procedure. High risk indicates further consultation with the patient's physician, who will base his or her decision on the type of surgery to be performed, patient risk factor, and clinical judgment. Completely eliminating the drug will not necessarily reduce bleeding and may lead to **hypercoagulability**. One method of determining category placement is by using the **international normalized ratio** (INR) test. The INR was developed to determine clotting time for individual patients and is used during routine monitoring of warfarin therapy. By determining the INR, the physician can identify clotting time and establish the best course of treatment related to medication dosage prior to oral surgery. A target range of 2.0 to 3.0 is indicated for best clotting results, but the most current research indicates that patients with an INR of between 2 and 4 may be treated safely. All patients taking warfarin should have testing completed before any type of surgery is attempted.

Heparin may be used for treatment of thrombogenic episodes or for hospitalized patients who are undergoing complicated surgery. Heparin reduces blood clotting immediately, but it is short acting and there is usually no need to discontinue therapy for simple procedures, such as dental hygiene treatment or an oral extraction.

Clopidogrel (Plavix), prescribed for a multitude of thrombosis disorders, blocks platelet aggregation and therefore may prolong bleeding time. If a patient is taking this medication, the patient and the dental professional should consult with the patient's physician; for elective general dental surgery, it may be recommended that clopidogrel use be temporarily discontinued (usually for 5–10 days) in order to restore platelet function prior to any extraction.

Dabigatran etexilate (Pradaxa) is a medication used for prevention of stroke and systemic embolism in patients with nonvalvular atrial fibrillation. Pradaxa causes bleeding by inhibiting thrombin-induced platelet aggregation. At this time, there is no scientific evidence to warrant discontinuation of dabigatran etexilate prior to dental surgery. Although patients may have a higher risk of bleeding if they are over 75 years of age and taking aspirin, long-term NSAIDs (nonsteroidal anti-inflammatory drugs), clopidogrel, or prasugrel (to be discussed in the next paragraph) in combination with dabigatran etexilate, the recommendation remains that dabigatran etexilate continue to be administered as discontinuation places the patient at an increased risk of stroke.

Prasugrel (Effient) is prescribed to reduce the likelihood of thrombotic cardiovascular events. Like other medications previously discussed, prasugrel acts by blocking platelet aggregation and, therefore, may prolong bleeding time. At this time, however, there is no scientific evidence to warrant discontinuing prasugrel prior to dental surgery.

Aspirin is commonly used to treat angina, **ischemic heart disease**, post myocardial infarction, post bypass surgery, post angioplasty, and post stroke, and transient ischemic attacks. Often the risk of excessive bleeding will prompt a physician to discontinue the use of aspirin in patients who are on a low-dose regimen; however, recent studies have determined that minor oral surgery such as extraction can be performed at little or no risk to the patient receiving low-dose aspirin on a regular basis, and it has been concluded that when surgery is performed using a local anesthetic and the patient is compliant with follow-up procedures, the incidence of postextraction bleeding is minor.

Patients with Hematoma

A hematoma is a collection of blood trapped beneath the skin and is caused by trauma that can include local anesthetic injection technique. Because local anesthetic is commonly used during extraction, there is always some risk of hematoma complication. The best way to prevent hematoma is a careful and knowledgeable approach to injection; however, in cases where hematoma cannot be avoided, treatment includes applying firm pressure with gauze until the hematoma is no longer expanding and placing a cold pack on the area. If pressure does not quell the expansion, the patient should be transported by ambulance to the hospital for further treatment and investigation into underlying systemic causes.

Case Resolution and Conclusion

Some of the causes of and treatment for excessive bleeding following a routine dental extraction have been examined in this chapter. In our original case scenario, it would appear Ms. Barclay was having difficulty with bleeding because of her long-term regimen of aspirin as follow-up treatment for a past episode with angina pectoris; however, a low dose of aspirin is no longer implicated in excessive bleeding postsurgery, so the dental professional should refer Margaret to the hospital and to her physician for further investigation of a possible systemic cause for the bleeding. The dental professional should attempt to quell Margaret's bleeding through applying pressure or using a tea bag, but if these methods fail, she should be transported to the hospital immediately.

Dental professionals need to be aware of oral manifestations of systemic health and understand that traumatic dental treatment may aggravate a

(continued)

subclinical form of a disease. The dental professional must always obtain and maintain an updated and accurate medical history for each patient. This may help in determining the underlying cause of postsurgical complications and, more important, should help to prevent these complications.

Review Questions

1. A low dosage of aspirin over a long period of time

   A. has been implicated in excessive postsurgical bleeding
   B. has minimal or no effect on excessive bleeding
   C. should be avoided entirely if surgery is to be performed
   D. should be minimized before surgery

2. The medical consensus involving treatment of hemophiliacs before dental surgery is

   A. to stop all medication 48 hours before surgery
   B. that all dental extractions be performed in a hospital setting
   C. that local hemostasis and systemic treatment *must* be combined

3. After a dental extraction, the patient should *not*

   A. exercise for 12–24 hours
   B. lie down with head elevated
   C. be concerned if blood continues to flow heavily from the extraction site
   D. apply pressure to extraction site for more than 20 minutes

4. The second most common problem in dental surgery is

   A. fear and anxiety
   B. hemorrhage
   C. infection
   D. lack of patient compliance with postsurgical instructions

5. A hematoma is

   A. an unavoidable side effect of dental extraction
   B. often caused by an incorrect choice of local anesthetic
   C. a collection of bacteria trapped beneath the skin
   D. most often caused by trauma

6. Which of the following anticoagulation medications is most likely to be discontinued prior to dental surgery?

   A. aspirin
   B. heparin
   C. Plavix
   D. Pradaxa

Bibliography

Ardekian, L. "Does Low-Dose Aspirin Therapy Complicate Oral Surgical Procedures?" *Journal of the American Dental Association* 131, no. 3 (2000): 331–88.

Frachon, X. "Management Options for Dental Extraction in Hemophiliacs: A Study of 55 Extractions." *Oral Surgery, Oral Medicine, Oral Pathology, Oral Radiology, and Endodontics* 99, no. 3 (2000–2002): 270–75.

Jeske, A. H., G. D. Suchko, ADA Council on Scientific Affairs and Division of Science, and Journal of the American Dental Association. "Lack of a Scientific Basis for Routine Discontinuation of Oral Anticoagulation Therapy before Dental Treatment." *Journal of the American Dental Association* 134, no. 11 (2003): 1492–97.

Knies, Robert C. *Research Applied to Clinical Practice: International Normalized Ratio (INR).* Accessed July 28, 2006. http://ENW.org/Research-INR.htm.

Maden, G. A. "Minor Oral Surgery Without Stopping Daily Low-Dose Aspirin Therapy: A Study of 51 Patients." *Journal of Oral and Maxillofacial Surgery* 63, no. 9 (2005): 1262–65.

Malamed, S. F. *Medical Emergencies in the Dental Office.* 5th ed. St. Louis, MO: Mosby Publishing Company, 2000.

Malmquist, J. P. "Complications in Oral and Maxillofacial Surgery: Management of Hemostasis and Bleeding Disorders in Surgical Procedures." *Oral and Maxillofacial Surgery Clinics of North America* 23, no. 3 (2011): 387–94.

Moghadam, H. G., and Caminiti, M. F. "Life-Threatening Hemorrhage after Extraction of Third Molars: Case Report and Management Protocol." *Journal of the Canadian Dental Association* 68, no. 11 (2002): 670–74.

Peters, K. A. "Disseminated Intravascular Coagulopathy: Manifestations after a Routine Dental Extraction." *Oral Surgery, Oral Medicine, Oral Pathology, Oral Radiology, and Endodontics* 99, no. 4 (2005): 419–23.

Piot, B. "Management of Dental Extractions in Patients with Bleeding Disorders." *Oral Surgery, Oral Medicine, Oral Pathology, Oral Radiology, and Endodontics* 93, no. 3 (2002): 247–56.

Sabar, R., A. D. Kaye, and E. A. Frost. "Perioperative Considerations for the Patient on Herbal Medicines." *Middle East Journal of Anesthesiology* 16, no. 3 (2001): 287–314.

Scully, C. "Oral Surgery in Patients on Anticoagulant Therapy." *Oral Surgery, Oral Medicine, Oral Pathology, Oral Radiology, and Endodontics* 94, no. 1 (2002): 57–64.

Wynn, R. L., T. M. Meiller, and H. L. Crossley, eds. *Drug Information Handbook for Dentistry*. Hudson, OH: Lexicomp, 2010.

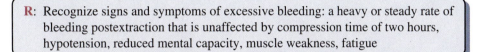

TREATMENT OF EXCESSIVE BLEEDING FOLLOWING AN EXTRACTION
R.E.P.A.I.R.

R: Recognize signs and symptoms of excessive bleeding: a heavy or steady rate of bleeding postextraction that is unaffected by compression time of two hours, hypotension, reduced mental capacity, muscle weakness, fatigue

E: Evaluate type of bleeding flow, reassess medical history and interview patient for overlooked conditions that may be the cause of heavy bleeding

P: Position patient with head elevated

A: Activate CABs of CPR—check circulation, airway, and breathing (pulse and blood pressure)

I: Implement appropriate emergency protocol for excessive bleeding: Place gauze on extraction site and apply pressure, if needed use tea bag and hold with firm pressure for 20 minutes

R: Refer to oral surgeon for follow-up treatment and refer to physician for investigation into underlying systemic cause, if necessary, or refer to emergency department if heavy bleeding persists

21

Intraocular Foreign Body

LEARNING OBJECTIVES

Upon reading the material in this chapter, the reader will be able to:

- ☑ Discuss potential causes of intraocular foreign bodies in the dental office.

- ☑ Recognize specific signs and symptoms associated with intraocular foreign body.

- ☑ Determine suggested treatment modalities for patients experiencing intraocular foreign body.

- ☑ Explain strategies for preventing intraocular foreign body.

Case Study

Scenario

Your first patient of the day, Shirley Goldman, arrives for her recare dental hygiene appointment. She is a 62-year-old female who brushes only once per day, does not floss, and tends to have a great deal of supragingival calculus at each visit. You have completed Shirley's medical history, vital signs recording, and intra/extra oral examination, and all were within normal limits. While reviewing her personal oral hygiene technique, you determine that she is noncompliant with your previous recommendations regarding brushing and flossing, and you find moderate calculus deposits. You begin debriding the mandibular anterior teeth using your H6/7 scaler, and a piece of calculus enters Shirley's eye. You realize that you had forgotten to place the protective eyewear on your patient before treatment. Shirley says, "There is something in my eye" and begins to rub her eye vigorously. What should you do?

Introduction

The advent of standard precautions (mask, gloves, protective eyewear for both the operator and the patient) makes the case scenario fairly unlikely, although accidents do occur. An intraocular foreign body may not just occur to patients, it can also affect dental professionals' coworkers, family members, or even themselves. In the United States in 2004, there were over 36,000 cases of work-related eye injuries. Men represent the majority of individuals suffering from this emergency. The home is gradually replacing the workplace as the most common site of injury. Hammering is the most common source; however, bungee cords also cause a significant proportion of eye injuries as they tend to snap back into the eye with great force. Figure 21.1a and b, ■

(a)

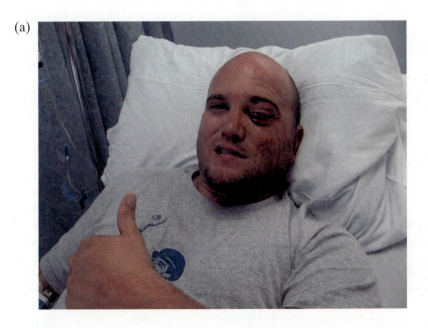

(b)

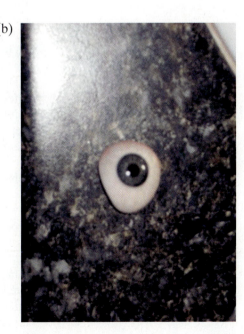

FIGURE 21.1 (a) Eye injury from bungee cord. (b) prosthetic eye for patient on left

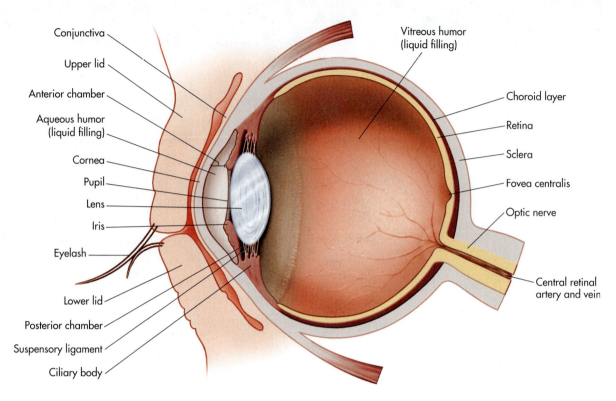

FIGURE 21.2 Internal structures of the eye.

respectively, depicts a young male who lost most of his right eye due to a bungee cord accident and the prosthetic appliance he now wears.

The eyes are approximately 2.5 cm in diameter, and the direct and open location of the eye makes it vulnerable to blunt or penetrating objects. Two common areas of the eye affected by foreign objects are the **cornea** and the **sclera**. The cornea is a nonvascular, transparent coat that covers the colored iris. The sclera is the white of the eye and consists of a coat of a dense connective tissue. It covers the entire eyeball except the cornea and protects the inner parts. The **conjunctiva** is the thin layer that covers the sclera of the eyes and the inside of the eyelids and can also be affected by an intraocular foreign body. (See Figure 21.2■)

Consequences of a foreign body in the cornea or sclera can range from discomfort to impaired vision and even blindness. Other complications include local infection, meningitis, and hemorrhage. Superficial foreign bodies and chemical splash injuries primarily affect the cornea, and the severity of the injury depends on the depth of the injury within the corneal layers. Prompt assessment and appropriate treatment will help reduce the damage.

The form and composition of the foreign body is extremely important in determining the best modality for diagnosis, treatment, and management. A foreign body is essentially classified as either organic or inorganic. Organic foreign bodies include a wide variety of substances, such as dirt, wood, or other vegetable matter. These types of foreign bodies are associated with a higher incidence of complications, such as bacterial or fungal infections. Inorganic foreign bodies are subdivided into metallic and nonmetallic substances. Metallic foreign bodies include steel, iron, lead, aluminum, and other metal alloys. Interestingly, metal compounds are well tolerated by the eye, with the exception of copper and iron, which have been noted to cause severe infections. Inorganic nonmetallic foreign bodies include stone, plastic, glass, or other minerals. These are also usually well tolerated by the eye unless they are sharp or large in size.

Signs and Symptoms of Intraocular Foreign Body

Intraocular foreign bodies are usually detected by the individual feeling some sensation in the eye, ranging from burning or itching to severe pain. Other symptoms include tear production, double vision, and/or light sensitivity. Appropriate treatment requires that several factors regarding the foreign body need to be determined: pain level, velocity of the foreign body entering the eye, composition of the foreign body—organic or inorganic (metallic or nonmetallic), and alteration to patient's vision or sensitivity to light.

Superficial bodies that do not involve the cornea usually cause discomfort rather than severe pain. If the cornea is involved, commonly the pain will be more intense, and uncontrolled muscle contraction of the eyelids (known as **blepharospasm**) is often observed.

Low-velocity foreign bodies will normally be found on the conjunctiva or the cornea, whereas high-velocity objects can enter the **globe** or the orbit of the eye. Very small, high-velocity objects can penetrate the eye and show little or no obvious external damage. Either of these types of foreign bodies can cause globe rupture and can threaten vision.

Determination of the material composing the foreign body is very important. Metallic objects can rust and be extremely difficult to remove. In addition, they can result in a severe inflammatory reaction. If the individual was wearing contact lenses or spectacles, they may have been damaged and their fragments may also be involved in the injury.

Reduction in visual acuity is unlikely to occur if the foreign body is superficial and on structures, such as the eyelid or conjunctiva. Moreover, low-velocity objects usually do not cause severe visual impairment, whereas high-velocity foreign objects will be more likely to cause vision loss and particularly sensitivity to light.

Treatment of Intraocular Foreign Body

Removal of superficial intraocular foreign bodies can be performed in one of two ways. In both methods, instruct the patient not to rub his or her eyes as doing so can cause corneal abrasions. Wash your hands and reglove for infection control purposes. To locate the object, gently pull down the lower lid and have the patient look upward. If the foreign body is obvious, it can be removed with a cotton swab using the following method. Any force used can create a corneal abrasion, so this method should be used only for superficial objects. Moisten a cotton-tipped applicator with saline and mop the subtarsal plate, which is a fibrous layer that gives the eyelids shape, strength, and a place for muscles to attach. Always direct the object away from the pupil. Usually the patient will experience immediate relief. (See Figure 21.3■)

The second method of removal is to irrigate the eye with either saline solution or water. The emergency eyewash station or an eye cup can be used. Before having the

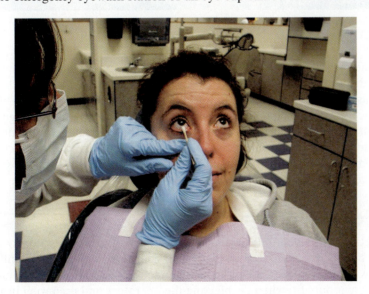

FIGURE 21.3 Use of cotton-tipped applicator for intraocular foreign body removal.

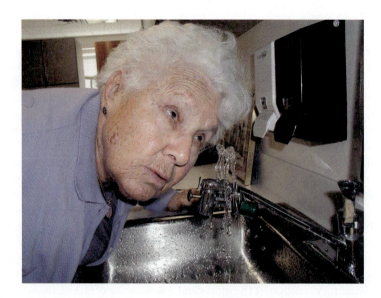

FIGURE 21.4 Removal of intraocular foreign body using eyewash station.

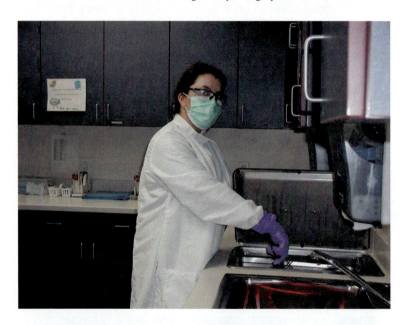

FIGURE 21.5 Use of protective eyewear in sanitization area.

fluid enter the eye, allow it to run on the cheek for a moment. Irrigation should occur from the medial to the lateral portion of the eye. Do not pour the fluid directly onto the cornea as this will be extremely uncomfortable for the patient. The irrigation method should also be used for any liquid or chemical that has entered the eye. (See Figure 21.4 ■)

Avoid attempting to remove embedded objects. These types of intraocular foreign bodies should be treated by eye specialists. Cover both eyes lightly with a clean cloth to limit eye movement, and seek immediate emergency medical care. This procedure should also be followed for any foreign body that cannot be removed easily.

Prevention of Intraocular Foreign Body

The best method to prevent intraocular foreign body is for the operator to wear eye protection. The use of proper safety eyewear with sideshields should significantly reduce the risk of eye injury. In the dental office, eye protection should be worn not just during patient treatment but also when disinfecting the operatory and preparing instruments for sterilization. (See Figure 21.5■) Chemicals used in ultrasonic baths, radiographic developing, and surface disinfection can also cause eye injury if splash occurs, so it is essential that eyewear be worn when performing procedures using these substances. Moreover, patients should always wear eye protection during treatment. These preventive methods are essential to reduce the risk of ocular trauma, thereby eliminating the potential of visual impairment and loss.

Case Resolution and Conclusion

Eye injuries from foreign bodies remain prevalent in the workplace and at home. Protective eyewear should be used anytime there is a risk for eye injury; however, accidents do occur, and dental healthcare professionals may be required to remove an intraocular foreign body. In the case scenario, Shirley had a piece of calculus enter her eye and was rubbing it vigorously. The clinician instructed Shirley to stop rubbing her eye. The foreign body was a low-velocity, organic object, so the clinician decided to attempt to remove it using the emergency eyewash station. She escorted Shirley to the sink, turned on the water, pulled the knob for the eyewash, and asked Shirley to place her eye in the water stream. After a few seconds, Shirley blinked a few times and determined that the object was removed. If the object had not been removed, referral to the emergency department would have been necessary.

Review Questions

1. Which of the following intraocular foreign bodies will be more likely to cause an infection?

   A. glass
   B. calculus
   C. instrument tip
   D. study model stone

2. All of the following are symptoms of a foreign body in the eye *except* one. Which one is the *exception*?

   A. burning in the eye
   B. tear production
   C. double vision
   D. epistaxis

3. The cotton-tipped applicator method of intraocular foreign body removal is best used for removal of which type of foreign body?

   A. embedded
   B. superficial
   C. chemical
   D. none of the above

4. When using the irrigation method of intraocular foreign body removal, the solution should be

   A. applied directly onto the cornea
   B. applied from the lateral portion of the eye to the medial portion of the eye
   C. applied from the medial portion of the eye to the lateral portion of the eye
   D. heated before application

5. Which method of intraocular foreign body removal is best to use for a chemical splash?

   A. cotton-tipped applicator
   B. irrigation method
   C. rub the eye vigorously until the object is removed

6. The nonvascular transparent coat that covers the colored iris is the

   A. cornea
   B. globe
   C. sclera
   D. pupil

Bibliography

Al-Thowaibi, A., M. Kumar, and I. Al-Matani. "An Overview of Penetrating Ocular Trauma with Retained Intraocular Foreign Body." *Saudi Journal of Ophthalmology* 25 (2011): 203–205.

Anderson, D. M., J. Keith, P. D. Novak, and M. A. Elliot, eds. *Mosby's Medical, Nursing & Allied Health Dictionary*. 6th ed. St. Louis, MO: Mosby-Year Book, Inc., 2008.

Bennett, J. D., and M. B. Rosenberg. *Medical Emergencies in Dentistry*. 1st ed. Philadelphia, PA: W. B. Saunders, 2002.

Hollander, D. A., and A. J. Aldave. "Ocular Bungee Cord Injuries." *Current Opinion in Ophthalmology* 13, no. 3 (2002): 167–70.

Jone, G. "Foreign Bodies in the Eye." *Accident & Emergency Nursing* 6, no. 2 (1998): 66–69.

Kanoff, J. M., A. V. Turalba, A. T. Andreoli, and C. M. Andreoli. "Characteristics and Outcomes of Work-Related Open Globe Injuries." *American Journal of Ophthalmology* 150, no. 2 (2010): 265–69.

Kuhn, F., T. Halda, C. D. Witherspoon, R. Morris, and V. Mester. "Intraocular Foreign Bodies: Myths and Truths." *Journal of Ophthalmology* 6, no. 4 (1996): 464–71.

Lee, C. H., L. Lee, L. Y. Kao, K. K. Lin, and M. L. Yang. "Prognostic Indicators of Open Globe Injuries in Children." *American Journal of Emergency Medicine* 27, no. 5 (2009): 530–35.

Lustrin, E. S., J. H. Brown, R. Novelline, and A. L. Weber. "Radiologic Assessment of Trauma and Foreign Bodies of the Eye and Orbit." *Neuroimaging Clinics of North America* 6, no. 1 (1996): 219–33.

Malamed, S. F. *Medical Emergencies in the Dental Office*. 6th ed. St. Louis, MO: Mosby Publishing Company, 2007.

Marieb, E. N., and K. Hoehn. *Human Anatomy & Physiology*. 8th ed. San Francisco, CA: Pearson Education, Inc., 2010.

Mayo Foundation for Medical Education and Research. "Removing a Foreign Body from Your Eye." *Mayo Clinic Health Letter* 20, no. 3 (2002): 3.

Mester, V., and F. Kuhn. "Intraocular Foreign Bodies." *Ophthalmology Clinics of North America* 15, no. 2 (2002): 235–42.

Owens, J. K., J. Scibilia, and N. Hezoucky. "Corneal Foreign Bodies—First Aid, Treatment and Outcomes." *American Association of Health Nurses Journal* 49, no. 5 (2001): 226–30.

Reich, J. "Investigating a Foreign Body." *Australian Family Physician* 29, no. 11 (2000): 1086–87.

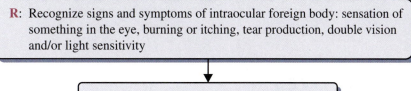

R: Recognize signs and symptoms of intraocular foreign body: sensation of something in the eye, burning or itching, tear production, double vision and/or light sensitivity

E: Evaluate type of foreign body

P: Position patient supinely if using cotton-tip applicator or over sink for either irrigation method

A: Activate CABs of CPR—check circulation, airway, and breathing (pulse and blood pressure) if necessary

I: Implement appropriate emergency protocol for intraocular foreign body:
Method 1: locate foreign body, lower eyelid, and have patient look up, saturate cotton-tip applicator with saline, and gently rub the tarsal or sclera area;
Method 2: irrigate with saline, lateral to medial surface of eye with eye up or use eyewash station

R: Refer to emergency department or eye specialist if object cannot be removed or if embedded

22

Broken Instrument Tip

LEARNING OBJECTIVES

Upon reading the material in this chapter, the reader will be able to:

☑ Discuss potential causes of broken periodontal instrument tips in the dental office.

☑ Recognize specific signs and symptoms associated with broken periodontal instrument tips.

☑ Determine suggested treatment modalities for patients experiencing broken periodontal instrument tip.

☑ Explain strategies for preventing broken periodontal instrument tips.

Case Study ·····································➤

Scenario

Your first patient after lunch is Lu Chen, a 35-year-old new patient who is scheduled for his first periodontal debridement with anesthesia appointment. Lu just recently relocated to the United States and has never had dental hygiene care. You review his medical history and find that he takes Effexor daily for anxiety and smokes one pack of cigarettes per day. His vital signs are pulse 82 beats/minute, respirations 16 breaths/minute, blood pressure 140/86 mmHg. He presents with moderate periodontitis with heavy tenacious accretions throughout the dentition. You have completed ultrasonic scaling the mandibular right quadrant and begin your hand scaling procedures. You find it necessary to use a great deal of pressure to remove the remaining deposits. You are using the Nevi 2 scaler interproximally on teeth #29 and #30, and when you remove your instrument from the sulcus, you realize that the instrument tip is missing. What should you do?

Introduction

Breaking a periodontal instrument tip can be a fairly common occurrence and can happen for various reasons. The most common cause of curette or scaler breakage is the continued use of an instrument that has been excessively thinned by sharpening. Each time an instrument is sharpened, a small amount of metal is removed from the instrument. Repeated sharpening can cause areas of the instrument to become thin and weak and can result in breakage during instrumentation. The application of excessive force, particularly when the dental hygienist is treating a patient with tenacious deposits, is another common variable for breakage. In addition, improper instrument selection for the area treated or faulty instrumentation technique are factors that can lead to instrument breakage. The production of defective instruments occurs infrequently as the manufacturing process is rigidly controlled; however, on occasion defective instruments can be produced if the company uses inferior materials, if there is a change in the manufacturing technique, or if there is ineffective quality control. Lastly, the clinician needs to be cognizant of instrument insertion, adaptation, and activation at all times to help prevent instrument breakage. (See Figure 22.1 ■)

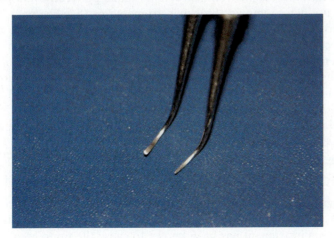

FIGURE 22.1 Thin instrument on right needing replacement due to high risk of breakage.

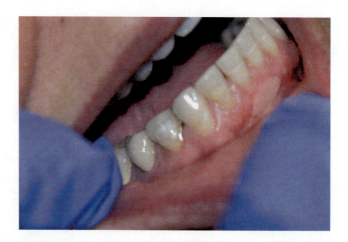

FIGURE 22.2 Broken instrument tip interproximally between teeth #27 and 28.

Signs and Symptoms of a Broken Periodontal Instrument Tip

The sign of a broken instrument tip is obvious in that the tip will be missing from the end of the instrument upon removal from the patient's oral cavity. In addition, patients may state that they feel something lodged between their teeth or in their gingival tissues. (See Figure 22.2 ■)

Treatment of a Broken Periodontal Instrument Tip

Once it has been determined that the instrument tip is broken, the debridement procedure should be immediately terminated and the area where you were working should be isolated with either gauze or cotton rolls. Cheek/lip retraction should be maintained. The clinician should try not to alarm the patient, but the patient should be asked not to swallow if possible and not to move his or her head. Suctioning, rinsing, or using compressed air is not recommended as these procedures might cause the removal of the tip unknowingly. Next, the immediate area (floor of the mouth, vestibule, tongue) should be examined in an effort to locate the tip. If the tip is not visible, adequate illumination should be used and gingival area where instrumentation was last performed should be blotted dry and examined closely. The gingival sulcus can then be carefully probed with a curette or explorer using a horizontal stroke. Care should be taken to avoid pushing the tip further into the gingiva or into the base of the sulcus. If the tip is located, it should be carefully removed with the curette. Autoclavable, magnetized instruments called **perioretrievers** are also available and are useful for removing broken instrument tips. (See Figure 22.3 ■) If the tip is not located, a periapical radiograph can be taken to help locate the tip, and then it should be carefully removed. After the tip has been removed, the patient should be informed regarding what has occurred and shown the removed tip. If the tip cannot be located with visual or radiographic inspection, then the situation should be treated as an aspirated or ingested foreign object (Refer to Chapter 14). Thorough documentation of the removal of the tip should be noted in the patient's chart. If the tip is located on the radiograph but cannot be removed, referral to an oral surgeon for removal is appropriate.

Prevention of a Broken Periodontal Instrument Tip

Maintaining instrument integrity through proper sharpening and replacement of thin instruments are two methods to help prevent tip breakage. Strong lateral pressure applied to a thin instrument has been known to cause the tip to break; therefore, it is essential to discard a curette that has reached the end of its useful life. Using the

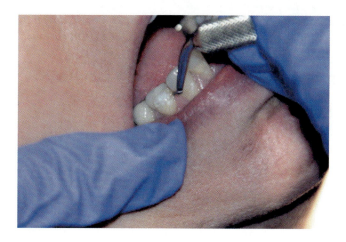

FIGURE 22.3 Removal of broken instrument tip with perioretriever.

proper instrument for the area being treated, as well as using the instrument correctly are two other mechanisms for reducing the risk of a broken instrument tip. In addition, using the ultrasonic scaler on patients with heavy accretions will reduce the amount of hand instrumentation required and reduce the risk of breaking an instrument tip.

Case Resolution and Conclusion

Broken periodontal instrument tips are likely to occur at some point in your dental hygiene career. Being prepared to treat the condition is essential to providing high-quality care for your patients. In the case scenario, the tip of the scaler was broken while the clinician was providing dental hygiene treatment to Lu Chen, who had heavy, tenacious calculus deposits. Lu was asked not to swallow while the clinician isolated the area with the gauze squares from her bracket table. The area was probed until the tip was located, and then the clinician dislodged the tip from the sulcus. A perioretriever was used to remove the tip from the oral cavity. The clinician showed the tip to Lu, explained what had happened, and thoroughly documented the incident in his chart. The hygienist then decided that it was best to use the ultrasonic scaler to remove the heavier deposits before attempting further hand instrumentation.

Review Questions

1. What is the first step to be performed once you have determined that you have broken your instrument tip?

   A. Isolate the area.
   B. Ask the patient to swallow.
   C. Sit the patient upright to prevent aspiration.
   D. Rinse the area with chlorhexidine.

2. All of the following are measures to help prevent broken instrument tips *except* one. Which one is the *exception*?

   A. use of the ultrasonic scaler on patients with heavy deposits
   B. proper instrument maintenance
   C. instrument retipping
   D. replacing worn instruments

3. What procedure is performed if the tip is located but cannot be removed?

 A. Refer to oral surgeon for removal.
 B. Anesthetize area and attempt to remove tip again.
 C. Take a radiograph to better locate tip.
 D. No treatment is necessary.

4. If the tip is not located by visual or radiographic inspection, the clinician should do which of the following?

 A. assume the tip was expectorated
 B. treat the situation as an ingested/aspirated foreign object
 C. rinse the area carefully and continue treatment
 D. none of the above

Bibliography

Carroll, D. P. "Take Extreme Care When Retrieving Broken Tips." *RDH* 13, no. 3 (1993): 8.

Gorokhovsky, V., B. Heckerman, P. Watson, and N. Bekesch. "The Effect of Multilayer Filtered Arc Coatings on Mechanical Properties, Corrosion, Resistance and Performance of Periodontal Dental Instruments." *Surface Coatings & Technology* 200, no. 18–19 (2006): 5614–30.

Johansson, B., and L. Krekmanov. "Fragment of Broken Instrument Removed from Field of Operation by an Electromagnet." *British Journal of Oral & Maxillofacial Surgery* 25, no. 3 (1987): 265–66.

Ruprecht, A., and A. Ross. "Location of Broken Instrument Fragments." *Journal of the Canadian Dental Association* 47, no. 4 (1981): 245.

Schwartz, M. "The Prevention and Management of the Broken Curet." *Compendium of Continuing Education in Dentistry* 19, no. 4 (1998): 418–25.

Wilkins, E. *Clinical Practice of the Dental Hygienist.* 9th ed. Philadelphia, PA: Lippincott Williams & Wilkins, 2009.

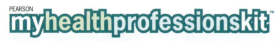

TREATMENT OF BROKEN INSTRUMENT TIP
R.E.P.A.I.R.

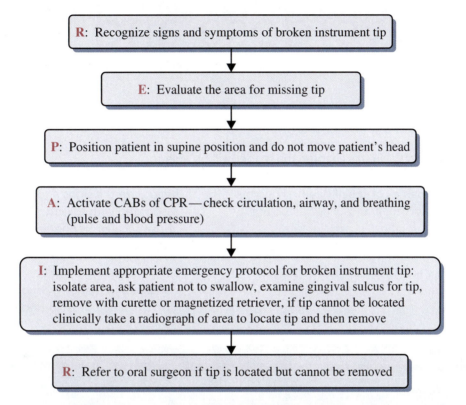

R: Recognize signs and symptoms of broken instrument tip

E: Evaluate the area for missing tip

P: Position patient in supine position and do not move patient's head

A: Activate CABs of CPR—check circulation, airway, and breathing (pulse and blood pressure)

I: Implement appropriate emergency protocol for broken instrument tip: isolate area, ask patient not to swallow, examine gingival sulcus for tip, remove with curette or magnetized retriever, if tip cannot be located clinically take a radiograph of area to locate tip and then remove

R: Refer to oral surgeon if tip is located but cannot be removed

23

Drug Overdose and Toxicity

LEARNING OBJECTIVES

Upon reading the material in this chapter, the reader will be able to:

✓ Recognize the names of specific central nervous system (CNS)–stimulant and CNS-depressant agents.

✓ Explain the mechanism of action of specific CNS-stimulant and CNS-depressant drugs in biological tissues.

✓ Recognize the signs and symptoms (toxidrome) associated with toxicity of common drugs of abuse such as amphetamines, cocaine, opioids, barbiturates, and benzodiazepine agents.

✓ Determine suggested treatment modalities for patients experiencing drug toxicity from specific CNS-stimulant or CNS-depressant drugs.

Case Studies ·······························➤

Scenario 1

Your new patient, Dorothy Wootton, a 25-year-old white woman, has just completed the medical and dental history form and is seated in your operatory for a new patient examination and prophylaxis. You notice that your patient appears anxious, is quite talkative, is sweating profusely, and seems agitated. You move closer to observe your patient's face and notice that her pupils are abnormally dilated. As you begin to review the patient's medical history, your patient reveals that she has abused amphetamines in the past, particularly methamphetamine, and has not obtained treatment for her addiction. Vital signs reveal a blood pressure of 200/110 mmHg, a pulse of 120 beats/minute, and respirations of 24 breaths/minute. Because of her vital signs, you decide to postpone dental hygiene treatment. From what medical emergency do you suspect your patient is suffering?

Scenario 2

Your 3:00 pm patient, Anna Kate Hoppe, is scheduled for a four-month periodontal maintenance appointment, and you notice that she arrives 15 minutes late. Once the patient is seated, you review her medical history and notice that she is lethargic and is slurring her speech as she responds to your questions. Upon closer observation, you notice that her pupils are abnormally small, almost pinpoint in size. Your patient tells you that she has been taking Roxicodone, an opioid analgesic, to alleviate severe back pain from a recent surgery. She tells you that her back pain is worse than usual today, so she took twice the normal dose of the prescribed medication. Your patient's vital signs reveal a blood pressure of 70/40 mmHg, pulse of 46, and respirations of 4. Because of her vital signs, you decide to postpone dental hygiene treatment. From what medical emergency do you suspect your patient is suffering?

Central Nervous System Stimulants

Amphetamines

Amphetamine agents are CNS stimulants and include drugs such as dextroamphetamine (Dexedrine), methylphenidate (Ritalin), amphetamine aspartate (Adderall), phentermine, and methamphetamine. Dextroamphetamine, methylphenidate, and amphetamine aspartate are used for the treatment of **narcolepsy** and attention-deficit hyperactivity disorder (ADHD). Phentermine is an **anorexiant** agent that is prescribed for weight loss. Methamphetamine is a common drug of abuse that can be taken orally, smoked, or injected intravenously, and is often referred to as "meth," "uppers," "crank," "speed," "chalk," "ice," "glass," "crystal," or "tina."

Amphetamine agents stimulate the CNS by activating a sympathetic autonomic nervous system (SANS) response. Stimulation of the SANS results in an increased heart rate, **mydriasis**, decreased digestion, dilation of bronchioles within the lungs, and increased flow of blood to the brain and skeletal muscles. This response is

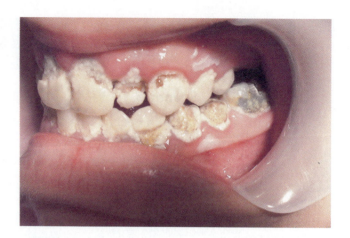

FIGURE 23.1 Patient with Meth mouth.

typically known as the fight-or-flight response of the SANS. Amphetamines prevent the neuronal reuptake of the excitatory neurotransmitters norepinephrine and dopamine within the SANS. Prevention of the reuptake of the neurotransmitters results in these **endogenous** chemicals constantly being released by **presynaptic neurons** originating within the CNS. The chemicals are then readily available to be transmitted through **postsynaptic neurons** to the target organ or tissue to exert their excitatory effects, instead of being "taken back up" and stored by neurons in an inactive state for future use.

Chronic methamphetamine users are likely to exhibit signs of bruxism and tooth wear due to an overall increase in energy and neuromuscular function experienced by the individual. Additionally, chronic methamphetamine abuse results in an oral condition termed "Meth mouth," referring to rampant caries that develop as a result of dehydration and **xerostomia**. (See Figure 23.1 ■) Methamphetamine users typically have poor oral hygiene and an increased intake of refined carbohydrates and high-calorie carbonated beverages, resulting in a reduction in the pH of the oral environment and subsequent caries formation.

Individuals currently using methamphetamine should not receive a local anesthetic agent with a **vasoconstrictor** for dental procedures. Methamphetamine use enhances the normal response of the SANS, which can result in myocardial ischemia and cardiac dysrhythmias. Methamphetamine combined with a local anesthetic vasoconstrictor agent such as epinephrine or levonordephrin will potentiate this **sympathomimetic** effect, which may result in **hypertensive urgency or emergency**, myocardial infarction, or stroke.

SIGNS AND SYMPTOMS OF AMPHETAMINE TOXICITY   Signs and symptoms of acute amphetamine (toxidrome) toxicity include **euphoria**, restlessness, talkativeness, anxiety, agitation, confusion, flushing, diaphoresis, anorexia, seizures, tachycardia, dysrhythmias, tachypnea, hypertension, chest pain, heart palpitations, and **hyperpyrexia**. Coma can occur as a result of the toxic effects of amphetamines within the CNS. Myocardial infarction can occur as a result of myocardial ischemia. The dental professional should use vasoconstrictors in as low a dose as possible as they may enhance the effects of the stimulant or vasoconstrictor.

TREATMENT OF AMPHETAMINE TOXICITY   If the patient exhibits signs and symptoms of amphetamine toxicity, EMS should be contacted immediately, and basic life support (BLS) measures must be provided as necessary. Vital signs should be monitored frequently until the patient can be transported to the emergency department. A benzodiazepine agent (CNS depressant) such as diazepam (Valium) can be administered to help control agitation and seizure activity. External cooling of the skin is recommended to aid in reduction of **hyperthermia**. External cooling can be achieved by placing the patient in a cool environment and spraying exposed skin with lukewarm water or using a tepid sponge to bathe the skin in combination with the use of air fans. If available, cooling blankets are advantageous in reducing hyperthermia. An **emetic drug** should not be given since vomiting can induce seizures in a patient with amphetamine toxicity.

Once the patient is in a hospital setting, systemic absorption can be prevented by the administration of activated charcoal. Activated charcoal will adsorb or attract and hold a substance to it when ingested. **Adsorption** of the toxic agent by the activated charcoal will prevent the absorption of the amphetamine agent from the gastrointestinal tract into the systemic circulation. Activated charcoal is a black powder that is combined with water to form a slurry. The usual dose of activated charcoal that is administered is one 50-gm bottle.

Cocaine

Cocaine is a drug that acts as a CNS stimulant and local anesthetic agent. Because of its potent vasoconstrictor effects, cocaine is used medically as a local anesthetic agent for mucous membranes, such as in nasal surgical procedures. Routes of administration for the street drug include snorting (intranasal administration), smoking, intravenous injection, and oral administration. The free base form of the drug, commonly known as "crack," is preferred for smoking because this pure form is more rapidly acting and powerful than the cocaine salt. The free base form of the drug can be created by dissolving the cocaine salt in an aqueous solution (often with sodium bicarbonate), evaporating the water through heating, and cooling and drying the free base until hard. Street names for cocaine include "crack," "rock," "snow," "coke," "toot," and "blow."

Within the SANS, cocaine prevents the reuptake of dopamine, norepinephrine, and serotonin, all excitatory neurotransmitters. Cocaine's mechanism of action is primarily as a dopamine reuptake inhibitor. As a result, dopamine-containing neurons within the brain constantly release dopamine for postsynaptic receptor attachment. This increase in dopamine levels produces feelings of euphoria and well-being for the cocaine user. Cocaine administration also stimulates the release of glutamate and aspartate, both proteinogenic amino acids. These substances have the effect of excitation on the CNS. With intranasal administration, effects of the drug are perceived in three to five minutes; thus it is rapidly acting with a peak effect in 10 to 30 minutes. The peak effect refers to the maximum response or effect of the drug within biological tissues. The drug's effects rarely last more than one hour. In addition to feelings of euphoria, the cocaine user will experience an increase in cardiac rate, blood pressure, and body temperature. Cocaine's rapid onset and short duration of action encourages the user to administer the drug frequently to maintain its effects.

The oral and intranasal use of cocaine can result in several orofacial complications. Cocaine is a potent vasoconstrictor; continued use can lead to ischemia and **necrosis** of the nasal septum, resulting in perforation of the nasal septum and palate. Palatal necrosis and perforation is more evident in women who are cocaine users than in men. Research suggests that the palatal connective tissue in women may be more susceptible than palatal connective tissue in men. Individuals who snort cocaine often have chronic sinusitis and a reduced sense of smell. An increase in dopamine levels produced by cocaine use may be associated with **bruxism** and tooth wear that is often evident with cocaine users. The incidence of dental caries increases among individuals using cocaine and is most likely due to increased carbohydrate intake. Gingival lesions can result at the site of application after repeated oral use of cocaine. Due to hyperactivity created by the drug, individuals using cocaine may exhibit signs of cervical abrasion and gingival laceration due to vigorous tooth brushing. Gingival recession and delayed healing may occur due to the vasoconstrictor effects of oral application of the drug.

With regard to dental or dental hygiene procedures, the use of local anesthetics with epinephrine is contraindicated for individuals using cocaine due to potential fatal effects. Cocaine's potent vasoconstrictor properties combined with a vasoconstrictor in a dental local anesthetic agent can produce an acute increase in blood pressure, leading to myocardial infarction or stroke.

SIGNS AND SYMPTOMS OF COCAINE TOXICITY   The toxic effects of cocaine depend on several factors, including patient tolerance and route of administration. Intravenous injection and smoking produce the highest levels of the drug within the brain and heart; thus these routes of administration are likely to produce rapid toxic effects, whereas snorting or oral ingestion may produce toxicity after a delayed period of time. The dental professional should avoid the use of vasoconstrictors with patients who have used cocaine within 24 hours of their appointment as it can lead to potentially fatal myocardial conditions. In addition, the chance of local anesthetic overdose is increased when it is administered to cocaine abusers.

Because of cocaine's rapid stimulation of the CNS and cardiovascular system, an individual with cocaine toxicity may exhibit signs and symptoms of anxiety, agitation, hyperthermia, chest pain, tachycardia, hypertension, cardiac arrhythmias, dyspnea, seizures, hallucinations, cerebral hemorrhage, ventricular fibrillation, myocardial infarction, and stroke. Additionally, the patient's pupils will be dilated, which is referred to as mydriasis.

TREATMENT OF COCAINE TOXICITY   An individual with cocaine overdose or toxicity must be transported to a hospital emergency room as quickly as possible. EMS should be called immediately, and BLS measures must be administered. Provide a calm, quiet environment for the patient, and monitor vital signs every 15 minutes until EMS arrives to transport the patient to the hospital. Hyperthermia may be treated with external cooling measures similar to those used in treatment of amphetamine toxicity. Vomiting should not be induced because it may produce seizures in a patient with cocaine toxicity.

Diazepam (Valium) can be administered to help control hyperactivity, tachycardia, anxiety, and seizures. Propranolol, a **beta-adrenergic blocker**, combined with a vasodilator, such as phentolamine, can be administered by trained hospital staff to treat hypertension induced by cocaine toxicity. The administration of an adsorbing agent such as activated charcoal is indicated only if the drug was orally ingested. If this is the case, a 50-gm bottle of activated charcoal is given to prevent further absorption of the drug.

Central Nervous System Depressants

Opioids

Opiates are derived from the juice of the naturally occurring poppy plant (*Papaver somniferum*). Opiates produced from this natural source are morphine and codeine. The drug class of opioids includes these agents, as well as semisynthetic and synthetically produced drugs, such as heroin, oxycodone, hydrocodone, meperidine, propoxyphene, fentanyl, buprenorphine, pentazocine, methadone, dextromethorphan, and tramadol. Some opioid drugs, such as oxycodone and hydrocodone are combined with ibuprofen or acetaminophen for pain relief. Common routes of administration are oral ingestion, smoking, and intravenous injection. All opioid agents produce depression within the CNS in the form of sedation, euphoria, and a reduction in pain perception.

The mechanism of action of opioid drugs involves the binding of the **exogenous** agent with specific opioid receptors in the CNS and spinal cord. The discovery of endogenous opioid-like agents (enkephalins, endorphins, dynorphins) helped to determine the presence of opioid receptors (mu, kappa, delta) within the body. The stimulation of these receptors produces the drug's effects within biological tissues. In addition to **analgesia**, sedation, and euphoria, opioids also depress the cough reflex mechanism in the medulla within the brain stem, producing an **antitussive** effect, and inhibit gastrointestinal motility, which can result in constipation.

SIGNS AND SYMPTOMS OF OPIOID TOXICITY   An individual suffering from opioid toxicity will exhibit signs and symptoms of **lethargy**, **miosis**, shallow respirations, hypotension, hypothermia, bradycardia, flaccid muscles, lack of response to external stimulation, and decreased bowel motility. Heroin is implicated in the production of pulmonary edema, whereas propoxyphene and meperidine are more likely to produce seizures. Severe overdose of any opioid agent will lead to coma, respiratory depression, and death. The dental professional should use local anesthetics in as low a dose as possible for individuals taking opioids as their use can increase the chance of local anesthetic overdose.

TREATMENT OF OPIOID TOXICITY   After calling EMS, BLS measures must be provided. Administration of oxygen 4–6 L/minute will aid in breathing for patients with shallow respirations. Vomiting should not be induced because of the possibility of increased lethargy and coma and because vomiting can increase the risk of an obstructed airway or aspiration in patients with poor muscle control. Vital signs should be monitored frequently until the patient is transported to the emergency room. External warming measures, such as wrapping the patient in a blanket, can help reduce hypothermia.

Once the patient is transported to the hospital emergency room, an **antidote** can be administered by qualified medical professionals to counteract the effects of the drug. An effective antidote is naloxone (Narcan), a competitive **opioid antagonist**. An antagonist drug counteracts the effects of an administered drug by displacing the drug from its receptor sites on the cell surface or from within the cell. In this case, the naloxone displaces the opioid agent from its cellular receptor sites (mu, kappa, delta) within the CNS, thus preventing the pharmacologic effects of the drug. As a result of the administration of naloxone, sedation will be decreased and respiration and blood pressure will return to a normal range. The usual dose of naloxone given as an antidote for opioid toxicity is 0.4–2 mg administered IV (intervals of 2–3 minutes, then 20–60 minutes up to 10 mg). If the opioid was orally ingested, administration of a 50-gm bottle of activated charcoal will adsorb the remaining drug within the gastrointestinal tract.

Barbiturates

Barbiturates are sedative-hypnotic agents that became popular in the 1950s and 1960s as short-acting prescription medications (secobarbital, pentobarbital) for the treatment of **insomnia**. Barbiturate use has mostly been replaced by a safer class of drugs known as benzodiazepines to alleviate anxiety and produce sedation. Ultrashort-acting barbiturates such as thiopental sodium (Pentothal) are effective for inducing general anesthesia. Phenobarbital (Luminal) is a commonly prescribed long-acting barbiturate with **anticonvulsant** properties that is effective in the prevention of epileptic seizures. Butalbital is a barbiturate that is sometimes combined with caffeine and an analgesic, such as acetaminophen (Fioricet) or aspirin (Fiorinal). Both medications are used in the treatment of headaches. All barbiturate agents produce depression of the CNS.

Barbiturates produce their effects within biological tissues by enhancing the effects of an inhibitory neurotransmitter within the CNS known as gamma-aminobutyric acid (GABA). Barbiturates are **GABA agonists**; the barbiturate agent "encourages" GABA to bind to its receptor sites to enhance its inhibitory effects. When GABA binds to cellular receptor sites, neuronal cell membranes open, allowing an influx of chloride ion into the cell. An influx of chloride ion inhibits excitation of the neuron. As a result of CNS depression by barbiturate agents, sedation or **hypnosis** is produced and anxiety is alleviated. The most common route of administration for barbiturates is orally; however, they can be delivered through intramuscular or intravenous injection or rectally via a suppository.

SIGNS AND SYMPTOMS OF BARBITURATE TOXICITY   The clinical presentation of barbiturate toxicity is dose dependent. An individual with mild to moderate toxicity will exhibit signs and symptoms of lethargy, slurred speech, ataxia, and **nystagmus**. Severe toxicity may result in hypothermia, miosis, hypotension, bradycardia, pulmonary edema, coma, and respiratory arrest.

TREATMENT OF BARBITURATE TOXICITY   For dental healthcare providers, treatment of patients with barbiturate toxicity is similar to the treatment of opioid toxicity. The first step is to call EMS and provide BLS measures as necessary. Monitor vital signs frequently until EMS arrives to transport the patient to the hospital emergency room. Provide external warming measures to prevent or treat hypothermia. Activated charcoal (50-gm bottle) will likely be administered once the patient has been transported to the emergency department; the charcoal promotes adsorption of the drug within the gastrointestinal tract.

Benzodiazepines

Benzodiazepine agents are now used in place of barbiturates for their sedative-hypnotic effects, including reduction of anxiety, and for their anticonvulsant and muscle relaxant properties. The majority of benzodiazepine agents are orally administered, but some can be delivered through intramuscular or intravenous injection, such as diazepam (Valium) or midazolam (Versed), a benzodiazepine used for preoperative sedation or induction of general anesthesia. Other examples of benzodiazepine agents include alprazolam (Xanax), clonazepam (Klonopin), lorazepam (Ativan), and triazolam (Halcion).

The mechanism of action of benzodiazepine agents is the same as that for barbiturate agents. It involves enhancement or potentiation of the inhibitory neurotransmitter GABA within the CNS. Enhancing the effects of GABA produces sedation, hypnosis, and **anxiolytic** effects. The dental professional should consider lowering the maximum dose of local anesthetics for patients taking depressants as they may enhance the effects of the depressant drug, possibly leading to respiratory arrest.

SIGNS AND SYMPTOMS OF BENZODIAZEPINE TOXICITY   Signs and symptoms associated with benzodiazepine toxicity include lethargy, slurred speech, ataxia, and mental confusion. Coma and respiratory arrest may occur, but because benzodiazepine agents have a wide therapeutic index (wide range of safe dosage), these serious complications are usually associated with the shorter-acting agents, such as triazolam (Halcion), and midazolam (Versed), or when combined with other CNS depressants. Patients in a benzodiazepine-induced coma exhibit miosis and hypothermia.

TREATMENT OF BENZODIAZEPINE TOXICITY   After calling EMS, breathing and circulation must be assessed and BLS measures must be provided as necessary. Placing the patient in a supine position is helpful for the treatment of hypotension. The patient's vital signs should be monitored until EMS arrives to transport the patient to the hospital emergency room. External warming measures should be provided to prevent or treat hypothermia.

Once the patient has been transported to the hospital emergency room, administration of a 50-gm bottle of activated charcoal will provide adsorption of the drug within the gastrointestinal tract. Flumazenil (Romazicon) can be administered as an antidote to counteract the effects of any benzodiazepine agent. Flumazenil acts within biological tissues as a benzodiazepine-receptor antagonist, binding to benzodiazepine cellular receptor sites and reversing the sedative effect of the drug.

The recommended initial dose of flumazenil is 0.2 mg administered IV, and may be repeated at one-minute intervals up to a total dose of 1 mg. The administration of flumazenil has been linked to the induction of seizures in patients taking benzodiazepines for seizure disorders and for conscious sedation, and in those suffering from flumazenil-induced withdrawal associated with benzodiazepine addiction. As a result, this antidote may not be appropriate for all patients exhibiting effects of benzodiazepine toxicity.

Case Resolution and Conclusion

After reviewing the medical history and noting the signs and symptoms of the patient in Scenario 1, Dorothy Wootton, it is evident that this patient was suffering from amphetamine toxicity. Signs and symptoms of dilated pupils; abnormally high blood pressure, pulse, and respirations; and diaphoresis, anxiousness, and talkativeness indicate possible toxicity from a CNS-stimulant drug. The signs and symptoms of amphetamine toxicity are very similar to those of cocaine toxicity. The patient's history of amphetamine abuse was the key to determining the specific drug involved in the production of the toxic effects. The dental operator placed Dorothy in a semisupine position (a supine position may have increased her blood pressure), placed a cool cloth on her forehead, and provided a cool mist spray to exposed skin. The operator also monitored Dorothy's vital signs until EMS arrived to transport the patient to the hospital. Once Dorothy arrived at the hospital's emergency room, diazepam (Valium) was administered to control agitation and prevent seizure activity, and activated charcoal was administered to prevent further absorption of the amphetamine into the systemic circulation. Dorothy made a complete recovery and upon advice from her physician and family members sought drug rehabilitation for methamphetamine abuse. She rescheduled her dental hygiene care appointment for after her drug rehabilitation was completed.

The patient in Scenario 2, Anna Kate Hoppe, exhibited the opposite clinical signs and symptoms of those of Dorothy Wootton. She displayed lethargy and was slurring her speech. Anna Kate's pupils were constricted, and her blood pressure, pulse, and respirations were well below normal. All of these conditions are consistent with the toxic effects of a CNS-depressant drug. Barbiturate and benzodiazepine drugs produce similar signs and symptoms as opioid drugs. The fact that Anna Kate was taking Roxicodone, an opioid analgesic, for her back pain, indicated to the operator the source of the toxic effects. After observing the clinical signs and symptoms, the dental operator placed Anna Kate in a supine position, monitored her vital signs frequently, and administered oxygen at 4–6 L/minute until EMS personnel arrived to transport her to the emergency room. The operator provided a blanket to warm the patient and help reduce the chances of hypothermia. Anna Kate lost

(continued)

consciousness on the way to the hospital. Despite the best efforts of the EMS and emergency room personnel, Anna Kate did not regain consciousness. Narcan was administered as an antidote to counteract the effects of the opioid drug, but without success. Blood levels of the Roxidone were much greater than expected, which indicated that Anna Kate had ingested a far greater amount of the drug than she described to the dental operator. As a result, she went into respiratory depression, suffered cardiac arrest, and died.

Drug overdose and toxicity from CNS-stimulant and CNS-depressant agents can result in serious, life-threatening outcomes for any individual self-administering these drugs. (See Table 23.1 ■) CNS stimulants, such as amphetamines and cocaine can produce myocardial infarction and stroke, whereas administration of CNS depressants such as opioids, barbiturates, or benzodiazepines can result in respiratory depression, coma, and death for the unsuspecting individual. Dental healthcare providers must be able to recognize signs and symptoms associated with drug toxicity and be proficient at providing basic life support measures while waiting for EMS to arrive. By doing so, dental practitioners significantly increase an individual's chance of survival.

Table 23.1 Signs and Symptoms of Drug Toxicity

Amphetamine Toxicity	Cocaine Toxicity	Opioid Toxicity	Barbiturate Toxicity	Benzodiazepine Toxicity
Euphoria	Anxiety	Lethargy	Lethargy	Lethargy
Restlessness	Agitation	Miosis	Slurred speech	Slurred speech
Talkativeness	Hyperthermia	Shallow respirations	Ataxia	Ataxia
Anxiety	Chest pain	Hypotension	Nystagmus	Mental confusion
Agitation	Tachycardia	Hypothermia	Hypothermia	Coma
Confusion	Hypertension	Bradycardia	Miosis	Respiratory arrest
Flushing	Cardiac arrhythmias	Flaccid muscles	Hypotension	
Diaphoresis	Dyspnea	Lack of response to external stimulation	Bradycardia	
Anorexia	Seizures		Pulmonary edema	
Seizures	Hallucinations		Coma	
Tachycardia	Cerebral hemorrhage		Respiratory arrest	
Hypertension	Ventricular fibrillation			
	Myocardial infarction			
Chest pains	CVA			
Heart palpitations				
Hyperpyrexia				
Mydriasis				

Review Questions

1. Which of the following drugs mimics the natural effects of the sympathetic autonomic nervous system (SANS)?

   A. benzodiazepines
   B. cocaine
   C. opioid drugs
   D. barbiturates

2. Which of the following is a sign of cocaine toxicity?

   A. bradycardia
   B. slurred speech
   C. hypertension
   D. respiratory depression

3. The purpose of activated charcoal in the treatment of drug toxicity is to

   A. act as an adsorbing agent
   B. induce vomiting
   C. provide an antidote
   D. achieve internal cooling

4. Which of the following oral effects may be evident in the cocaine user?

   A. dental caries
   B. gingival inflammation
   C. cervical abrasion
   D. all of the above

5. All of the following are strategies for managing opioid toxicity *except* one. Which one is the *exception*?

   A. wrap in blankets to increase body temperature
   B. administer oxygen 4–6 L/minute
   C. administer naloxone (Narcan)
   D. administer diazepam (Valium)

6. Which of the following is a sign of barbiturate toxicity?

   A. tachycardia
   B. unresponsiveness to external stimuli
   C. diaphoresis
   D. agitation

7. Benzodiazepines and barbiturates produce their effect within biological tissues by

   A. stimulating opioid receptors
   B. preventing the reuptake of dopamine
   C. enhancing the effect of GABA
   D. stimulating the SANS

8. Which of the following routes of administration produces the highest blood levels of a drug?

   A. oral ingestion
   B. intramuscular injection
   C. smoking
   D. intravenous injection

Bibliography

Abrams, A. C., and S. S. Pennington. *Foundations of Clinical Drug Therapy*. Philadelphia, PA: Lippincott Williams & Wilkins, 2005.

Bennett, J. D., and M. B. Rosenberg. *Medical Emergencies in Dentistry*. Philadelphia, PA: W. B. Saunders, 2002.

Brand, H. S., S. Gonggrijp, and C. J. Blanksma. "Cocaine and Oral Health." *British Dental Journal* 204, no. 7 (2008): 365–69. doi:10.1038/sj.bdj.2008.244.

Cooper, G. M., D. G. Le Couteur, D. Richardson, and N. A. Buckley. "A Randomized Clinical Trial of Activated Charcoal for the Routine Management of Oral Drug Overdose." *Journal of Toxicology: Clinical Toxicology* 40, no. 3 (2002): 313.

Hamamoto, D. T., and N. L. Rhodus. "Methamphetamine Abuse and Dentistry." *Oral Diseases* 15, no. 1 (2009): 27–37.

Haveles, E. B. *Applied Pharmacology for the Dental Hygienist*. 6th ed. Maryland Heights, MO: Mosby, Inc., Elsevier, Inc., 2011.

Kapila, Y. L., and K. Hoshang. "Cocaine-Associated Rapid Gingival Recession and Dental Erosion. A Case Report." *Journal of Periodontology* 68, no. 5 (1997): 485–88.

Kasper, D. L., and T. R. Harrison, eds. *Harrison's Principles of Internal Medicine*. 16th ed. New York: McGraw-Hill, 2005.

Malamed, S. F. *Handbook of Local Anesthesia*. 6th ed. St. Louis, MO: Mosby Publishing Company, 2011.

Maloney, W. J. "The Significance of Cocaine Use to Dental Practice." *The New York State Dental Journal*, 76, no. 6 (2010): 36–39.

Morton, P. G., D. Fontaine, C. M. Hudak, and B. M. Gallo. *Critical Care Nursing: A Holistic Approach*. 8th ed. Philadelphia, PA: Lippincott Williams & Wilkins, 2005.

Pallasch, T. J., and C. E. Joseph. "Oral Manifestations of Drug Abuse." *Journal of Psychoactive Drugs* 19, no. 4 (1987): 375–77.

Porth, C. M. *Essentials of Pathophysiology*. 3rd ed. Philadelphia, PA: Lippincott Williams, & Wilkins, 2011.

Queen, J. R., and J. Glauser. "A Young Man with Hyperthermia and New-Onset Seizures." *Cleveland Clinic Journal of Medicine* 69, no. 6 (2002): 453–62.

Shannon, M. W., S. W. Borron, and M. J. Burns. *Haddad and Winchester's Clinical Management of Poisoning and Drug Overdose.* 4th ed. Philadelphia, PA: Saunders, Elsevier, Inc., 2007.

Weinberg, M. A., C. Westphal, and J. B. Fine. *Oral Pharmacology for the Dental Hygienist.* Upper Saddle River, NJ: Pearson Education, Inc., 2008.

Wynn, R. L., T. F. Meiller, and H. L. Crossley, eds. *Drug Information Handbook for Dentistry.* 17th ed. Hudson, OH: Lexi-Comp, Inc., 2011.

Yagiela, J. A., F. J. Dowd, and E. A. Neidle. *Pharmacology and Therapeutics for Dentistry.* 5th ed. St. Louis, MO: Mosby, Inc., 2004.

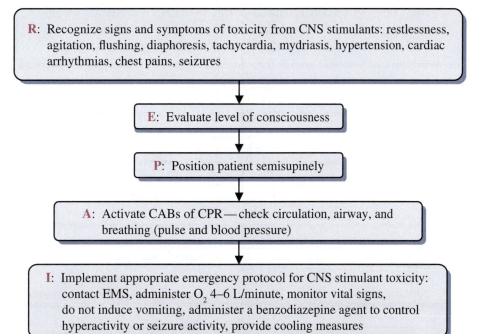

TREATMENT OF THE PATIENT WITH AMPHETAMINE OR COCAINE TOXICITY
R.E.P.A.I.R.

R: Recognize signs and symptoms of toxicity from CNS stimulants: restlessness, agitation, flushing, diaphoresis, tachycardia, mydriasis, hypertension, cardiac arrhythmias, chest pains, seizures

E: Evaluate level of consciousness

P: Position patient semisupinely

A: Activate CABs of CPR—check circulation, airway, and breathing (pulse and blood pressure)

I: Implement appropriate emergency protocol for CNS stimulant toxicity: contact EMS, administer O_2 4–6 L/minute, monitor vital signs, do not induce vomiting, administer a benzodiazepine agent to control hyperactivity or seizure activity, provide cooling measures

R: Refer to emergency department immediately

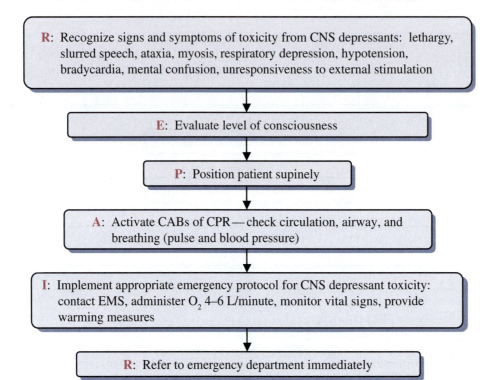

TREATMENT OF THE PATIENT WITH
OPIOID, BARBITURATE, OR
BENZODIAZEPINE TOXICITY
R.E.P.A.I.R.

R: Recognize signs and symptoms of toxicity from CNS depressants: lethargy, slurred speech, ataxia, myosis, respiratory depression, hypotension, bradycardia, mental confusion, unresponsiveness to external stimulation

E: Evaluate level of consciousness

P: Position patient supinely

A: Activate CABs of CPR—check circulation, airway, and breathing (pulse and blood pressure)

I: Implement appropriate emergency protocol for CNS depressant toxicity: contact EMS, administer O_2 4–6 L/minute, monitor vital signs, provide warming measures

R: Refer to emergency department immediately

Appendix

Medical Emergencies at a Glance

Emergency	Overview	Signs and Symptoms	Treatment
Adrenal Crisis	Severe reduction in cortisol production	Fatigue Lethargy Muscular weakness Headache Confusion Fever Nausea Vomiting Abdominal pain Hypotension Tachycardia Diaphoresis Dehydration	Contact EMS Administer O_2 4–6 L/minute Monitor vital signs
Allergic Reaction—Mild	Hypersensitive reaction to an allergen IgE response followed by the release of histamine and other chemical mediators	Localized redness, pruritus, edema, urticaria Conjunctivitis Pale or flushed skin Rhinitis	Administer chlorpheniramine 10 mg orally for three days
Allergic Reaction—Moderate	Hypersensitive reaction to an allergen IgE response followed by the release of histamine and other chemical mediators	Systemic redness, pruritus, edema, urticaria Rhinitis Abdominal pain Cramping Diarrhea Bronchospasm/mild dyspnea	Administer diphenhydramine 50 mg IM Administer chlorpheniramine 10 mg orally for three days Administer O_2 as needed Monitor vital signs
Allergic Reaction—Severe Anaphylaxis	Type I allergic reaction with an immediate hypersensitivity Most severe allergic response	Systemic redness, pruritus, edema, urticaria Rhinitis Angioedema of the lips, eyes, and larynx Bronchospasm with severe dyspnea and wheezing Hypotension Tachycardia/arrhythmias Decreased consciousness	Contact EMS Position patient supinely with legs elevated Administer epinephrine 0.2 mL–0.5 mL IM Administer O_2 4–6 L/minute Administer 100–500 mg hydrocortisone IM Administer diphenhydramine 50 mg IM Monitor vital signs
Angina Pectoris	Chest pain because of inadequate blood supply to heart muscle	Chest discomfort: pressure, burning, heaviness, squeezing, choking; radiates from shoulder down arm to neck, lower jaw, tongue Diaphoresis Nausea Pallor Duration of 1–15 minutes	Terminate procedure Position patient upright or semisupine Perform CABs of CPR Administer O_2 4–6 L/minute Monitor vital signs Administer nitroglycerine if patient is not hypotensive—patient's preferably, or spray from kit (can administer three doses in 15-minute period) If episode ceases, can resume treatment if patient feels well enough If pain more severe than normal or if pain does not cease, contact EMS and treat as myocardial infarction (MI)

Emergency	Overview	Signs and Symptoms	Treatment
Asthma Attack	Chronic respiratory disorder with narrowing of the bronchial airways	Dyspnea Wheezing Coughing Chest tightness Pallor	Position patient upright with arms forward Have patient self-administer own bronchodilator If patient does not have bronchodilator use one from emergency kit—albuterol Administer O_2 4–6 L/minute Monitor vital signs
Broken Instrument Tip	Broken instrument tip in gingival tissue	Missing tip from end of instrument	Isolate area Ask patient not to swallow Examine sulcus for tip Remove with curette or magnetized retriever If tip cannot be located clinically, take radiograph to locate tip and remove
Cardiac Pacemaker Malfunction/ Implantable Cardioverter Defibrillator	Malfunction of cardiac pacemaker or ICD possibly because of electromagnetic interference	Lightheadedness Dizziness Dyspnea Moist, pale skin Weakness Bradycardia or tachycardia depending on reason for implantation Chest pain Swelling in extremities Prolonged hiccoughing Muscle twitching Possible altered mental status	Position patient comfortably, probably upright Turn off interference Check pulse rate If normal pulse rate does not resume or if consciousness is lost, contact EMS and prepare for CPR
Cerebrovascular Accident	Abnormal condition of the brain characterized by occlusion or hemorrhage of a blood vessel resulting in a lack of oxygen to brain tissues	Severe headache Increased BP Neck pain or stiffness Inability to stand or walk Unequal pupils Vision changes Difficulty swallowing Nausea and vomiting Facial paralysis Paresthesia on one side of body Speech impairment Altered level of consciousness	Position patient semiupright Contact EMS Administer O_2 if needed Monitor vital signs
Diabetic Ketoacidosis	Severe hyperglycemia because of insufficient blood glucose levels	Poor skin turgor Warm, dry skin Thirst Muscle weakness Fatigue Nausea/vomiting Blurred vision Tachypnea/Kussmaul breathing Fruity odor on breath Hypotension Tachycardia	Contact EMS Determine blood glucose level Monitor vital signs Administer O_2 4–6 L/minute

Emergency	Overview	Signs and Symptoms	Treatment
Drug Toxicity			
Amphetamine Toxicity	Overdose of amphetamines resulting in overstimulation of the CNS	Euphoria Restlessness Talkativeness Anxiety Agitation Confusion Flushing Diaphoresis Anorexia Seizures Tachycardia Hypertension Intracranial hemorrhage Chest pains Heart palpitations	Contact EMS Provide basic life support (BLS) Monitor vital signs frequently Provide external cooling measures Can administer a benzodiazepine to control agitation
Cocaine Toxicity	Overdose of cocaine resulting in overstimulation of the CNS	Anxiety Agitation Hyperthermia Chest pain Tachycardia Hypertension Arrhythmias Dyspnea Seizures Hallucinations Cerebral hemorrhage Ventricular fibrillation MI Cardiovascular accident	Contact EMS Provide BLS Monitor vital signs frequently Provide external cooling measures Can administer a benzodiazepine to control agitation
Opiate/Opioid Toxicity	Overdose of opiates or opioids resulting in CNS depression	Lethargy Myosis Shallow respirations Hypotension Hypothermia Bradycardia Flaccid muscles Severe overdose: coma, respiratory depression, death	Contact EMS Provide BLS Administer O_2 4–6 L/minute Monitor vital signs frequently Provide external warming measures
Barbiturate Toxicity	Overdose of barbiturates resulting in CNS depression	Dose dependent Moderate toxicity: Lethargy Slurred speech Ataxia Nystagmus Severe toxicity: Hypothermia Myosis Hypotension Bradycardia Pulmonary edema Coma Respiratory arrest	Contact EMS Provide BLS Monitor vital signs frequently Provide external warming measures

Emergency	Overview	Signs and Symptoms	Treatment
Benzodiazepine Toxicity	Overdose of benzodiazepines resulting in CNS depression	Lethargy Slurred speech Ataxia Mental confusion Hypotension Coma Respiratory arrest	Contact EMS Position patient supinely Provide BLS Administer O_2 4–6 L/minute Monitor vital signs frequently Provide external warming measures
Epistaxis	Blood exuding from nasal cavity	Nasal bleeding Bright red color—anterior nosebleed Dark red color—posterior nosebleed	Use personal protective equipment Position patient upright Maintain airway Suction blood from mouth if necessary Have patient tilt head slightly forward Apply direct pressure by pinching lower part of nose for 15–20 minutes Have patient breathe through mouth Place ice pack over bridge of nose
Excessive Bleeding Following an Extraction	Heavy or steady bleeding for more than two hours following an extraction	Heavy or steady bleeding for more than two hours Hematoma Fatigue	Compression with gauze Tea bag with firm pressure for 20 minutes If bleeding persists, contact physician for follow-up treatment
Heart Failure	Clinical syndrome that occurs when the heart muscle is impaired and no longer effectively pumps sufficient volumes of blood		
	Left heart failure—inadequate blood pumped to circulation; blood coming to left ventricle from lungs "backs up," causing fluid to leak into the lungs	Dyspnea Orthopnea Nocturnal dyspnea Cheyne-Stokes respirations Dry, nonproductive cough Pallor Diaphoresis Elevated BP Rapid, thready pulse	Position patient upright or semiupright Perform CABs of CPR Administer O_2 3–5 L/minute Monitor vital signs Contact EMS if symptoms not alleviated
	Right heart failure—inability of heart to pump blood from systemic venous circulation to lungs for oxygenation systemic congestion in venous system	Fatigue, weakness Peripheral edema Pitting edema Reduction in renal blood flow Nocturia Distended jugular vein	Position patient upright or semiupright Perform CABs of CPR Administer O_2 3–5 L/minute Monitor vital signs Contact EMS if symptoms not alleviated
Hypertensive Emergency	Extremely high blood pressure with target end organ damage	BP > 220/140 Shortness of breath Chest pain Nocturia Dysarthria Weakness Altered consciousness Vision loss Seizures Congestive heart failure Nausea Vomiting Eventually coma	Retake BP to ensure accuracy Position conscious patient upright/unconscious patient supine Treat whatever target end organ damage is occurring Monitor vital signs/take blood pressure every five minutes Administer oxygen if needed Contact EMS

Emergency	Overview	Signs and Symptoms	Treatment
Hypertensive Urgency	Extremely high blood pressure without target end organ damage	BP > 180/110 Moderate to severe headache Anxiety Shortness of breath Edema epistaxis	Retake BP to ensure accuracy Position conscious patient upright/unconscious patient supine Monitor vital signs/take blood pressure every five minutes Administer O_2 if needed Contact EMS
Hyperventilation	Increased respirations that are faster and/or deeper than the metabolic needs of the body while eliminating more CO_2 than is produced	Prolonged, rapid, and deep respirations 22–40 breaths/minute Heart palpitations Impaired problem solving, motor coordination, balance and perceptual tasks Lightheadedness Dizziness Impaired vision Muscle twitching or carpopedal spasms Diaphoresis Circumoral paresthesia	Position patient upright Loosen tight clothing Work with patient to control breathing
Hypoglycemia	Severe hypoglycemia with a blood glucose level lower than 40–50 mg/dL	Confusion Seizures Dizziness Weakness Headache Hunger Cold, clammy skin Diaphoresis Irritability or aggressive behavior	*Conscious patient* Provide 20 gm of some form of sugar Maintain airway Monitor vital signs *Unconscious patient* EMS Glucagon 1 mg SC or IM 20 ml of 50% IV dextrose Monitor vital signs Administer O_2 4–6 L/minute
Intraocular Foreign Object	Foreign object in eye	Sensation in eye ranging from itching to severe pain Tear production Double vision Light sensitivity	Locate foreign body Lower eyelid and have patient look up Saturate cotton tip with saline and gently rub tarsal or sclera area OR Irrigate with saline from lateral to medial surface or use eyewash station
Myocardial Infarction	Necrosis of the myocardium because of total or partial occlusion of a coronary artery	Chest pain or discomfort lasting 20 minutes or longer: pressure, tightness, heaviness, burning, squeezing, or crushing—may radiate down arms, shoulders, neck, jaw, or back Weakness Dyspnea Diaphoresis Irregular pulse Nausea Vomiting Sense of impending doom Levine sign Women may have atypical discomfort, upper abdominal pain, shortness of breath, fatigue	Terminate treatment If history of angina treat for angina If no history of angina: Position patient comfortably Perform CABs of CPR Contact EMS Administer O_2 4–6 L/minute Monitor vital signs Administer nitroglycerine from kit if patient not hypotensive If pain not relieved in two to four minutes, administer two more doses of nitroglycerine If pain not relieved, administer 162–325 mg chewable aspirin Monitor vital signs Prepare for CPR if necessary

Emergency	Overview	Signs and Symptoms	Treatment
Myxedema Coma	Inability of the body to compensate for a severe deficiency of thyroid hormones	Confusion Apathy Depression Possible psychosis Hypothermia < 95°F Hair loss Facial changes Cool, dry skin Bradycardia Seizures	Position patient supinely Normalize temperature with blankets Administer O_2 4–6 L/minute Monitor vital signs Contact EMS
Obstructed Airway	Blocking of the airway by some object	Coughing Stridor Cyanosis Placing hands in throat area Eventual loss of consciousness if complete blockage	Sit patient upright Encourage coughing Do not apply back blows If total blockage suspected in conscious patient, use Heimlich maneuver If total blockage suspected in unconscious patient, place patient in supine position and perform procedure for obstructed airway determined by the American Heart Association or American Red Cross
Pulmonary Edema	Result of swift, abrupt accumulation of fluid in the alveolar spaces of lungs often as a result of heart failure	Gasping for air Rapid pulse Cool, moist skin Cyanotic lips, nail beds Anxiety Cough with frothy, blood-tinged sputum Crackle sound in lungs	Position patient upright or semiupright Perform CABs of CPR Contact EMS Administer O_2 10 L/minute Monitor vital signs Perform bloodless phlebotomy Use a vasodilator (nitroglycerine) Perform CPR if necessary
Seizures			
Generalized Tonic-Clonic	Generalized electrical abnormality throughout the brain with a loss of consciousness	Four Phases: Prodromal—aura (sensation that preceded seizure) Preictal—loss of consciousness Ictal—muscle contraction and relaxation Postictal—cessation of seizure with generalized depression	Position patient supinely Maintain open airway Prevent injury to patient Gently restrain patient Monitor vital signs
Generalized Absence	Generalized electrical abnormality throughout the brain without a loss of consciousness	Brief change in level of consciousness Blinking or eye rolling Blank stare Duration of 5–30 seconds	Reassure patient Most resolve without incident
Shock			
Hypovolemic Shock	Failure of the cardiovascular-pulmonary system to deliver enough oxygenated blood to body tissues because of fluid loss	Rapid, thready pulse Cool skin Reduced urine output	Position the patient supinely Arrest cause of fluid loss Contact EMS Perform CABs of CPR Monitor vital signs Oxygenate 4–6 L/min Administer fluid therapy required

Emergency	Overview	Signs and Symptoms	Treatment
Cardiogenic Shock	Failure of the cardiovascular-pulmonary system to deliver enough oxygenated blood to body tissues because of decreased cardiac output	Decreased BP systolic < 90 mmHg Fast, weak pulse Cool, clammy skin Cyanosis Nonspecific chest pain Shortness of breath Reduced urine output Mental confusion	Position patient supinely Contact EMS Perform CABs of CPR Monitor vital signs Oxygenate 4–6 L/min Administer fluid and drug therapy required
Septic Shock	Failure of the cardiovascular-pulmonary system to deliver enough oxygenated blood to body tissues because of bacterial invasion	Fever Vasodilation Increased cardiac output Tissue edema Pink, warm skin	Position patient supinely Contact EMS Perform CABs of CPR Monitor vital signs Oxygenate 4–6 L/min Aggressive fluid therapy required Antimicrobial therapy required Possible surgical intervention
Neurogenic Shock	Failure of the cardiovascular-pulmonary system to deliver enough oxygenated blood to body tissues because of pathology of the brain stem or spinal cord	Hypotension Bradycardia Peripheral vasodilation	Position patient supinely Contact EMS Perform CABs of CPR Monitor vital signs Administer O_2 4–6 L/minute Drug therapy must be provided by trained professional
Obstructive Shock	Failure of the cardiovascular-pulmonary system to deliver enough oxygenated blood to body tissues because of indirect heart pump failure	Severe hypotension Dyspnea	Position patient supinely Contact EMS Perform CABs of CPR Monitor vital signs Administer O_2 4–6 L/minute Treatment of the source of obstruction must be provided by trained professional
Syncope	Transient loss of consciousness and postural tone most often caused by loss of cerebral oxygenation and perfusion	Presyncopal: Pupil dilation Diaphoresis Excitation of piloerector muscles Weakness Dizziness Vertigo Nausea Yawning Sighing Visual changes Increased BP and pulse Shortness of breath Heart palpitations Chest pain Syncope: Loss of consciousness Weak, slow pulse	Remove objects from oral cavity Position patient in supine position with feet elevated Open airway Assess circulation Loosen tight clothing Administer O_2 4–6 L/minute If unconsciousness persists, contact EMS

Emergency	Overview	Signs and Symptoms	Treatment
Thyroid Storm	Exacerbation of hyperthyroid state	Fever Diaphoresis Restlessness Confusion Anxiety Psychosis Nausea/vomiting Increased systolic BP Tachycardia Widened pulse pressure	Position patient supinely Contact EMS Administer O_2 4–6 L/minute Monitor vital signs

Glossary

ablation therapy: use of radioactive iodine to disable the thyroid gland

absence seizure: mild form of an epileptic seizure

acidosis: a condition of low blood pH

acute myocardial infarction or myocardial infarction: irreversible damage or death to the heart muscle as a result of an acute reduction in oxygenated blood flow to the myocardium; it is most commonly the result of blockage of a coronary vessel due to the formation of a thrombosis. It is commonly known as a heart attack.

acute pulmonary edema: sudden accumulation of excessive fluid in the lungs, usually the result of left ventricular heart failure

Addison's disease: condition of adrenal insufficiency that occurs as a result of the destruction of the adrenal cortex of the adrenal gland

adrenal crisis: life-threatening condition that occurs when the body is severely lacking cortisol

adrenal insufficiency: deficient output of mineralocorticoids and glucocorticoids

adrenocorticotropic hormone: hormone produced by the pituitary gland that stimulates the adrenal cortex

adsorption: attracting and holding a substance

agranulocytosis: a severe decrease in the number of white blood cells, resulting in neutropenia

air hunger: feeling of suffocation

aldosterone: hormone produced by the adrenal gland that regulates salt and water levels

alkalosis: a condition of high blood pH

allergen: substance that causes an allergic reaction

allergy: a hypersensitive reaction to a common, usually harmless substance

alveolus: socket that holds the tooth roots

ammonia inhalants: smelling salts: an active compound of ammonium carbonate used for arousing consciousness

analgesia: absence of feelings of pain without loss of consciousness

anaphylactic shock: a sudden, massive vasodilation and circulatory collapse caused by the individual being exposed to an allergen for which he or she is extremely sensitive.

anaphylaxis: a life-threatening hypersensitive reaction to a previously encountered antigen

angina pectoris: chest pain caused by a transient deficiency in blood delivery to the myocardium

angioedema: painless swelling seen in an allergic reaction

anorexia: inability to eat due to a loss of appetite

anorexiant: a substance such as a drug that causes suppression of appetite

antagonist: any agent that exerts an opposite action to that of another

antibody: immunoglobulin, protein secreted in response to an antigen

anticoagulant: any substance used to suppress blood clotting

anticonvulsant: a drug that prevents or controls seizures

antidote: an agent that counteracts the effects of another substance, such as a poison

antigen: a substance that has the ability to provoke an immune response

antitussive: an agent that suppresses or relieves cough

anxiolytic: a substance or drug that provides relief from feelings of anxiety

aortic dissection: a tear in the inner wall of the aorta causing blood to flow between the layers of the wall of the aorta, which forces the layers apart

apnea: absence of respirations

arrhythmia: irregular heart beat

arterial stenosis: narrowing of arterioles

arteriosclerosis: hardening and thickening or hardening of the inner walls of large and medium-sized elastic and muscular arteries

aspiration: inhaling or drawing something into the lungs or respiratory passages

asthma: chronic respiratory disorder in which there is increased responsiveness of the trachea, bronchi, and bronchioles to various triggers, resulting in the narrowing of the airways

asystole: absence of a heartbeat, cardiac arrest

ataxia: an impairment in the ability to control voluntary muscle movement often observed as an unsteady gait and muscular incoordination

atherosclerosis: hardening and thickening of the artery walls specifically due to an accumulation of fibrolipid plaques containing, among other things, cholesterol

atherosclerotic heart disease: coronary artery disease as a result of an accumulation of fibrolipid plaques on the walls of the coronary arteries. This can result in occlusion of the artery directly or by formation of a thrombus, causing angina, myocardial infarction, stroke, or death

atrial fibrillation: irregular and rapid heartbeat causing poor blood flow

aura: sensory hallucination experienced prior to a seizure

auscultatory gap: disappearance and reappearance of Korotkoff sounds that can occur during blood pressure measurements

automatism: repetitive, nonpurposeful activity

bag-mask device: a device composed of a manually compressible container with a plastic bag of oxygen at one end and at the other a one-way valve and mask used for resuscitation

basophils: rare white blood cells

beta-adrenergic blocker: a drug that blocks beta receptor stimulation within the sympathetic autonomic nervous system (SANS), producing a reduction in the rate and force of heart contractions, smooth muscle vasoconstriction, and bronchoconstriction

beta 2 receptor: an (adrenergic) cellular receptor within the sympathetic autonomic nervous system (SANS) that when stimulated causes smooth muscle relaxation in the bronchi and vasodilation

Biot's respirations: cyclic breathing patterns characterized by periods of shallow breathing alternating with periods of apnea

biphasic: having two stages

bronchodilation: increasing the diameter of the bronchial lumen allowing increased airflow to and from the lungs

blepharospasm: uncontrolled muscle contraction of the eyelids

blood pressure: force exerted by the blood against the blood vessel walls

bradyarrhythmia: slow, irregular heartbeat

bradycardia: heart rate less than 60 beats per minute

bradypnea: abnormally slow respiratory rate

bronchodilator: a substance that relaxes contractions of the smooth muscle of the bronchioles of the lungs to improve ventilation

bronchoscopy: use of a viewing tube through the nose or mouth to examine the internal surface of the main bronchi in the lung

bronchospasm: abnormal contraction of the smooth muscle of the bronchi, resulting in acute narrowing and obstruction of the airways

bruxism: clenching or grinding of the maxillary and mandibular teeth while in occlusion

cachexia: wasting syndrome characterized by muscle atrophy, fatigue, weakness, and significant loss of appetite

cardiac arrhythmia: see *arrhythmia*

cardiac output: amount of blood pumped out by each ventricle in one minute

cardiac pacemaker: device composed of a pulse generator and leads that provide pacing impulses to the heart as necessary

cardiac syncope: loss of consciousness resulting from an inadequate cardiac output and usually occurs as a result of serious underlying heart disease

cardiac tamponade: compression of the heart produced by blood accumulating in the pericardial sac

cardiogenic shock: type of shock caused by a reduction in tissue perfusion caused by a decrease in cardiac output

cardiovascular collapse: failure of the circulatory system

cardioversion: delivery of a synchronized electric shock to restore the heart's normal sinus rhythm

carpopedal spasms: sharp flexion of the wrist and ankle joints

catecholamines: a sympathomimetic compound many of which are produced naturally by the body and function as key neurologic chemicals to help regulate the biological clock and play a role in emotional behavior

cauterizing: to burn tissues by some form of heat

cerebral edema: brain swelling

cerebral infarction: necrosis of an area of brain tissue secondary to an interruption in the blood supply

cerebrovascular accident: a condition that occurs when blood circulation to the brain is interrupted and brain tissue dies

challenge dose: second exposure to an allergen that produces the allergic response

chemical mediators: a neurotransmitter chemical that is released during an allergic response

Cheyne-Stokes respirations: cyclic breathing patterns characterized by periods of respirations of increased rate and depth alternating with periods of apnea

cholesterol: a waxy fat produced by the liver and found in the outer layer of every cell in the human body. It has numerous roles that are crucial to normal body functioning. It is carried by lipoprotein molecules (HDL, LDL, and triglycerides) in the blood stream. High levels of cholesterol in the blood stream can result in coronary artery disease

chronic obstructive pulmonary disease: a progressive and irreversible condition characterized by diminished respiratory capacity

chronotropic: factors that increase the heart rate

Chvostek's sign: abnormal spasm of the facial muscles elicited by light taps on the facial nerve

circumoral paresthesia: numbness or tingling around the oral cavity

coma: total unresponsiveness to sensory stimuli for an extended period

computerized axial tomography (CT) scan: a computer device that translates radiographic images into a detailed, cross-sectional picture of each body region scanned

congestive heart failure: inability of the blood circulation by the heart to meet the needs of the body tissues

conjunctiva: thin layer that covers the sclera of the eyes and the inside of the eyelids

conjunctivitis: inflammation of the conjunctiva

contact dermatitis: condition of itching, redness, and swelling possibly with blister formation caused by exposure of the skin to an allergen

convulsions: torrent of electrical discharges in groups of the brain neurons that cause uncontrolled body movements

cornea: nonvascular, transparent coat that covers the colored iris

coronary arterial bypass graft surgery: procedure to bypass blocked coronary arteries to improve blood flow to the heart

coronary artery disease: narrowing of the small vessels that supply oxygenated blood to the heart, also called coronary heart disease and atherosclerotic heart disease

cortex: outer layer of adrenal gland that produces the hormones cortisol and aldosterone

cortisol: a hormone produced by the adrenal glands that mobilizes nutrients, modifies the body's response to inflammation, stimulates the liver to raise the blood sugar, and helps to control the amount of water in the body

cyanosis: blue or purplish appearance to the skin or mucous membranes due to lack of oxygenation of the tissues

cytolytic: the destruction of the living cell

defibrillation: electrically shocking the heart by interrupting the chaotic twitching by depolarizing the entire myocardium

degranulation: rupture of the cell surface allowing the cell contents to spill out

diastolic blood pressure: force of the blood against the blood vessel walls during ventricular relaxation

diabetes mellitus: autoimmune metabolic disorder characterized by hyperglycemia

diabetic ketoacidosis (DKA): diabetic coma—life-threatening complication of uncontrolled diabetes characterized by extremely high blood glucose levels

diabetic nephropathy: damage to the small blood vessels in the kidneys, impairing their ability to filter impurities from blood for excretion in the urine due to diabetes

diabetic retinopathy: a disorder of the blood vessels of the retina characterized by capillary microaneurysms, hemorrhage, exudates, and the formation of new vessels and connective tissues

diaphoresis: profuse sweating

distributive shock: type of shock caused by vasodilation and abnormal distribution of fluids within the circulatory system

dysarthria: difficulty speaking

dysphagia: inability to swallow

dyspnea: labored breathing

dysrhythmia: a disturbance in the normal rhythmic pattern of the heart

eczema: skin rash characterized by itching, blistering, oozing, and scaling of the skin

edema: swelling of a tissue due to inflammation

electroencephalogram: a device that records the electrical activity of the neurons of the brain

embolism: obstruction of a blood vessel usually caused by a blood clot

emetic drug: a drug that induces vomiting

encephalitis: inflammation of the brain

endogenous: originates or develops within a biological cell or tissue

endoscopy: visual examination of a body cavity with a flexible tubelike device called an endoscope

epilepsy: a group of neurological disorders characterized by recurrent seizures, sensory disturbances, abnormal behavior, loss of consciousness, or all of these

epileptogenic: seizure provoking

epistaxis: nosebleed

erythema: reddened skin

euphoria: a mental or emotional state of well-being, elation, and happiness

euthyroid: having a normal-functioning thyroid gland

exogenous: originates or is produced outside of the body

external respiration: occurs when oxygen is taken into the body and carbon dioxide is eliminated via the lungs

fetal macrosomia: newborn with excessive birth weight

fibrinolysis: the breaking down of fibrin that occurs as part of a process designed to dissolve a clot or prevent a clot from forming

flow meter: the dial that allows for the appropriate amount of oxygen to be delivered

GABA agonist: a drug that mimics or enhances the effect of gamma-aminobutyric acid (GABA), an inhibitory neurotransmitter in the central nervous system, by binding to GABA cellular receptor sites

gait: an individual's walking style including speed, stance, and rhythm

gangrene: necrosis of a tissue usually the result of ischemia, bacterial invasion with subsequent putrefaction

generalized tonic-clonic seizure: most severe form of epileptic seizures where the individual loses consciousness and convulses

gestational diabetes: glucose intolerance with initial onset during pregnancy

globe: hollow portion of the eye that is composed of a wall enclosing a cavity filled with fluid

glomerulonephritis: inflammation of the glomeruli of the kidney leading to permeability of the filtration membrane

glucocorticoid: a hormone released by the adrenal glands that influences energy metabolism of most body cells and helps the person to resist stressors

glucometer: a device that measures the approximate concentration of glucose in the blood

glycated hemoglobin test (HbA1c): test that reveals the average blood glucose level over a two- to three-month period

Graves' disease: disorder associated with an enlarged thyroid gland

Hashimoto thyroiditis: an autoimmune disease in which the thyroid gland is attacked by B and T lymphocytes and results in hypothyroidism

heart failure: a clinical syndrome that occurs when the heart muscle becomes impaired and no longer effectively pumps sufficient volumes of oxygenated blood to the body's tissues and organs

Heimlich maneuver: procedure in which air in the victim's lungs is used to expel an obstruction from the airway

hepatitis: inflammation of the liver often caused by a viral infection

hematoma: swelling of clotted blood in tissue

hemophilia: hereditary bleeding disorder caused by a deficiency of various clotting factors

hemostasis: the cessation of bleeding

hepatorenal: pertaining to the kidneys and the liver

hereditary hemorrhagic telangiectasia (HHT): genetic bleeding disorder that leads to abnormal blood vessel formation in the skin, mucous membranes, and often in some organs

high-density lipoprotein (HDL): known as the "good" cholesterol and is thought to prevent arterial disease; carries cholesterol away from the cells and back to the liver where it is broken down or expelled as waste

histamine: a chemical found in cells that has the ability to cause an allergic reaction when released

hyperbilirubinemia: an excess of bilirubin in the blood of the newborn

hypercoagulability: tendency to develop blood clots

hyperglycemia: elevated blood glucose levels

hyperpyrexia: excessively high fever

hyperosmolar hyperglycemic state: a diabetic coma in which the level of ketone bodies is normal

hypersensitive: an immune response to a perceived threat that is usually harmless to the body

hypertension: a disorder characterized by elevated blood pressure exceeding 140/90 mmHg

hypertensive emergency: extremely high blood pressure with target end organ damage

hypertensive urgency: extremely high blood pressure without target end organ damage

hyperthermia: abnormally high body temperature

hyperthyroidism: thyrotoxicosis, too much thyroid hormone is produced by the thyroid gland

hyperventilation: condition in which the patient breathes faster and/or deeper than the metabolic needs of the body, thus eliminating more carbon dioxide than is being produced

hypocalcemia: reduction in the calcium levels in the bloodstream

hypocapnia: lack of carbon dioxide in the arterial blood system

hypoglycemia: low blood glucose levels

hypnosis: a trance-like state of altered consciousness resembling sleep

hypotension: low blood pressure with a systolic pressure below 100 mmHg

hypothermia: state in which an individual's body temperature is reduced below his or her normal range

hypothyroidism: myxedema, insufficient thyroid hormone is produced by the thyroid gland

hypoventilation: insufficient ventilation to meet the body's metabolic needs

hypovolemic shock: type of shock caused by inadequate venous return to the heart

hypoxia: inadequate delivery of oxygen to body tissues

hypoxaemia: a state in which the oxygen level of arterial blood is below normal

ictus: see *ictal*

ictal: seizure

Immunoglobulin E (IgE): humoral antibody produced by the body in response to an antigen and is responsible for causing an allergic reaction

infective endocarditis: a bacterial infection of the innermost lining of the myocardium

initial stage of shock: first stage when cells are deprived of oxygen, which inhibits their ability to produce energy

insomnia: chronic inability to sleep

inotropic: pertaining to the force of muscular contraction

insulin: a protein that is responsible for lowering blood glucose levels by transporting glucose to body cells, inhibiting the breakdown of glycogen to glucose and inhibiting the conversion of amino acids or fats to glucose

internal cardioverter defibrillator: a device implanted within the body that is designed to recognize certain types of abnormal heart rhythms (arrhythmias) and correct them by electrically shocking the heart

internal respiration: the use of oxygen, the production of carbon dioxide, and their exchange between cells and blood

International normalized ratio (INR): standardized system used to report the results of blood clotting tests

ischemic heart disease: heart disease caused by inadequate flow of blood to the heart

Kiesselbach's plexus: a convergence of small arteries and veins located superficially on the anterosuperior part of the nasal septum

Kussmaul respirations: increased depth and rate of respirations

Korotkoff sounds: the sounds heard when taking a manual blood pressure measurement

laryngeal edema: swelling as a result of fluid accumulation in the soft tissues of the larynx

left ventricular heart failure: loss of the left ventricle's ability to contract normally, resulting in a fall in cardiac output; the force of the ventricular contraction is inadequate and not enough

lethargy: a state of lowered level of consciousness characterized by apathy, sluggishness, or sleepiness

Levine sign: clenched fist held over the chest indicating that the individual may be experiencing chest pain, including angina pectoris or myocardial infarction

Little's area: a convergence of small arteries and veins located superficially on the anterosuperior part of the nasal septum

local anesthetics: a substance used to prevent the transmission of nerve impulses to eliminate sensation

lumbar puncture: procedure used to remove cerebrospinal fluid for testing

macroangiopathy: characterized by accumulation of lipids and blood clots within large blood vessel walls, obstructing blood flow; complication of diabetes resulting in an increased risk for cardiovascular disease

magnetic resonance imaging: produces high-contrast images of soft tissues

malignancy: tendency of a medical condition to become progressively worse and to potentially result in death

mast cell: white blood cell that releases chemical mediators during an inflammatory response

medulla of adrenal gland: area in the center of the gland

meningitis: inflammation of the connective tissue membrane that covers the central nervous system structures

microangiopathic: a disease of the small blood vessels in which the basement membrane of the capillaries thickens

mineralocorticoid: a substance that regulates the electrolyte concentration in the extracellular fluids

myosis: abnormal, prolonged constriction of the pupil of the eye

mydriasis: abnormal, prolonged dilation of the pupil of the eye

myocardium: heart muscle

myxedema: hypothyroidism, insufficient thyroid hormone is produced by the thyroid gland

myxedema coma: condition that occurs when the body is unable to compensate for the severe deficiency of thyroid hormones

myocardial infarction: necrosis of the myocardial tissues caused by an interruption of blood flow

narcolepsy: a chronic sleep disorder characterized by uncontrollable attacks of deep sleep or excessive sleepiness

nasal cannula: a device for delivering oxygen by way of two small tubes that are inserted into the nostrils

necrosis: death of biological cells or tissue due to causes such as infection, inflammation, infarction, toxins, or trauma

neurally mediated syncope: disorder of the autonomic nervous system, which results in hypotension, bradycardia, and loss of consciousness

neurocardiac syncope: loss of consciousness due to a decrease in blood flow to the brain

neurocardiogenic syncope: vasovagal syncope—loss of consciousness due to a decrease in blood flow to the brain

neurogenic shock: results from the loss of sympathetic nerve activity from the brain's vasomotor center following an emotional trauma, a disease, a drug, or traumatic injury to the brain stem or spinal cord

nocturia: the need to urinate during the night

nodular goiter: enlarged thyroid gland with multiple nodules

noncardiac syncope: syncope associated with various conditions that do not affect the heart, such as seizures, orthostatic hypotension, situational occurrences, hyperventilation, and metabolic diseases

non-rebreathing face mask: an oxygen delivery device that is a plastic mask that has a reservoir bag attached

NSAID: nonsteroidal antiinflammatory drug—any of a group of drugs having analgesic, antipyretic, and antiinflammatory effects

nystagmus: rapid rhythmic involuntary movement of the eyeball. Movements can be rotary, horizontal, or vertical

obstructive shock: shock associated with obstruction of the vessels or the heart

oliguria: reduced urine output

opioid antagonist: a drug that prevents the normal effects or action of an opioid agent by blocking opioid cellular receptor sites in the central nervous system

orthostatic hypotension: a sudden drop in systolic blood pressure caused by a change in body position, usually moving from a supine to a sitting position

Osler-Weber-Rendu syndrome: an inherited condition characterized by hemorrhagic telangiectasia of the skin and mucosa

palpitation: racing or pounding of the heart

paresthesia: the sensation of tingling or numbness of the skin

paroxysmal: an episodic seizure, convulsion, fit, or spasm

paroxysmal nocturnal dyspnea: attacks of severe shortness of breath and coughing that generally occur at night, usually awakening the person from sleep

piloerector muscle: clusters of smooth muscle fibers that connect to the hair follicle to the upper regions of the dermis

pitting edema: term for type of edema where, after pressure is applied to the edematous area, the indentation persists for some time after the release of the pressure, usually seen in the legs and ankles, symptom of right ventricular heart failure

postsynaptic neuron: a neuron that receives an electrical impulse through chemical signaling from a presynaptic neuron and passes that signal to a muscle or gland to produce an effect

postural hypotension: a sudden drop in systolic blood pressure caused by a change in body position, usually moving from a supine to a sitting position

prehypertension: sustained elevated blood pressure with systolic reading between 120 and 139 mmHg and diastolic reading between 80 and 89 mmHg

presynaptic neuron: a neuron that transmits an electrical impulse (by releasing a chemical neurotransmitter) through a synaptic space to a postsynaptic neuron cell body or dendrite(s)

presyncopal: state consisting of muscular weakness, lightheadedness, and feeling faint

Prinzmetal's angina: also called *variant angina*; caused by a transient spasm of a coronary artery, causing a brief occlusion of the vessel. The majority of these anginal episodes occur while the person is at rest (neither emotional stress nor physical exertion triggers an attack) and at odd hours of the day or night. It is more common in women under 50 and those thought to be at low risk for CAD

prodromal: pertaining to early symptoms that may mark the onset of a disease or condition

proteinogenic: a substance capable of producing proteins

pruritus: itching

ptosis: upper eyelid drooping

pulmonary edema: a condition characterized by the accumulation of fluid in the air sacs of the lungs, creating breathing difficulty

pulmonary embolism: blockage of the pulmonary artery by some type of obstruction, such as fat, air, a tumor, or thrombus

pulse pressure: difference between the systolic pressure and the diastolic pressure

pulsus alternans: presence of an arterial pulse alternating between weak and strong beats; almost always indicative of left ventricular heart failure

pyrexia: abnormal elevation in body temperature

reducing valve: portion of the regulator allows for the safe release of the highly pressurized oxygen contained in the cylinder

regulator: a common unit of the oxygen tank in which the reducing valve and flow meter are joined together.

renal insufficiency: condition in which the kidneys fail to adequately filter toxins and waste products from the blood

respiration: the process by which oxygen and carbon dioxide are exchanged within the body

respiratory alkalosis: an increase in the pH of the circulating blood

respiratory arrest: continued absence of respirations, not compatible with life

rhinitis: inflammation of the mucous membranes of the nose because of the effect of histamine on the mucosa of the nasal passages

right ventricular heart failure: usually occurs shortly after left ventricular heart failure as a result of damage to the right side of the heart due to increased fluid pressure. It results in the inability of the heart to pump oxygen-poor blood from the systemic venous circulation into the lungs for oxygenation. The major clinical symptom is the development of peripheral edema

sclera: white of the eye consisting of a coat of a dense connective tissue

seizure: torrent of electrical discharges in groups of the brain neurons that cause uncontrolled body movements

sensitizing dose: first exposure to the antigen

septic shock: type of shock that occurs when certain bacteria invade the bloodstream

shock: condition produced when the cardiovascular-pulmonary system fails to deliver enough oxygenated blood to body tissues to support the metabolic needs of those tissues and leads to abnormal cellular and tissue function

sigh: breath of deep inspiration and prolonged expiration

somnolence: condition of being drowsy or sleepy

sphygmomanometer: device used to take a blood pressure reading

stable angina: the most common form of angina and is usually related to coronary artery disease

stage 1 hypertension: sustained elevated blood pressure with systolic reading between 140 and 159 mmHg and a diastolic reading between 90 and 99 mmHg

stage 2 hypertension: sustained elevated blood pressure with systolic reading 160 mmHg or higher or a diastolic reading 100 mmHg or higher

status asthmaticus: total airway obstruction and respiratory tract failure

status epilepticus: recurrence of any type of seizure without recovery between seizure episodes

stridor: harsh sound made during inspiration

stroke volume: the amount of blood pumped out by one ventricle with each heart beat

stupor: state of unresponsiveness in which the individual is unaware of the surroundings

subarachnoid hemorrhage: intracranial bleeding into the cerebrospinal fluid–filled space on the surface of the brain

sympathetic division of the autonomic nervous system: one of the three parts of the autonomic nervous system whose action is to mobilize the body's nervous system fight-or-flight response and maintain homeostasis

syncope: fainting, brief loss of consciousness

systolic blood pressure: force of the blood against the blood vessel walls during ventricular contraction

tachyarrhythmia: rapid, irregular heartbeat

tachycardia: A rapid pulse rate of more than 100 beats/minute

tachypnea: abnormally fast respiratory rate

target-organ damage: damage occurring in major organs fed by the circulatory system due to uncontrolled hypertension, hypotension, or hypovolemia

tetany: condition caused by hypocalcemia that results in loss of sensation, muscle twitches, cramps, and sharp flexion of the wrist and ankle joints

thrombocytopenia: deficiency in the number of circulating platelets

thrombosis: localized clotting of the blood

thrombus: blockage in a blood vessel that forms at its point of origin

thyroid gland: butterfly-shaped organ that is located anterior to the trachea

thyroid storm: life-threatening emergency characterized by an exacerbation of a hyperthyroid state

thyrotoxicosis: hyperthyroidism, too much thyroid hormone is produced by the thyroid gland.

tinnitus: ringing or clicking in the ears without auditory stimuli

transcutaneous electrical nerve stimulators (TENS): a method of pain control by use of electrical impulses to the nerve endings

triglyceride: main constituent of animal fat and vegetable oils; in association with cholesterol, they form the plasma lipids (blood fat). Triglycerides in plasma originate either from fats in our food, or are made in the body from other energy sources, such as carbohydrates. Unused calories are converted into triglycerides and are stored in fat cells to be used as energy when no food source is available. High levels of triglycerides are associated with atherosclerosis

unstable angina: a clinical syndrome that falls between stable angina and acute myocardial infarction and represents an imbalance between myocardial oxygen supply and demand. Angina pectoris is considered unstable if it presents with at least one of the following three features: (1) the angina occurs at rest or with minimal exertion and lasts more than 20 minutes without the interruption of nitroglycerin, (2) the onset is new and the pain is severe and definite, (3) the pain is more severe, more frequent, and more prolonged (can last up to 30 minutes) than angina experienced in the past.

uremia: the presence of urea and other nitrogen waste products in the blood often associated with renal failure

urticaria: a pruritic skin lesion characterized by transient wheals of varying shapes and sizes with well-defined erythematous margins and pail centers

Valsalva maneuver: any forced expiratory effort against a close airway

vasodepressor syncope: sudden loss of consciousness due to a decrease in blood flow to the brain

vasoconstrictor: an endogenous chemical or exogenous substance such as a drug that causes contraction of the muscular walls of blood vessels

vasovagal syncope: neurocardiogenic syncope, loss of consciousness due to a decrease in blood flow to the brain

venipuncture: the transcutaneous puncture of a vein by a sharp rigid stylet or cannula carrying a flexible plastic catheter or by a steel needle attached to a catheter or syringe

ventricular fibrillation: condition in which there is chaotic electrical activation of the ventricles

ventricular tachycardia: a rapid heartbeat that starts in the ventricles and is represented by a pulse rate of more than 100 beats/minute, with at least three irregular heartbeats in a row. There are numerous causes including presentation as an early or late complication of a heart attack

ventricular tachycardia: rapid contractions of the ventricles that are not coordinated with atrial activity

von Willebrand's disease: an inherited disorder characterized by abnormally slow clotting of the blood caused by a deficiency of a component of factor VIII

wheezing: a high-pitched sound that is usually heard on expiration

Woodruff's plexus: area in the nasal cavity where the posterior nasal, sphenopalatine and ascending pharyngeal arteries coalesce.

xerostomia: abnormal dryness of the oral cavity caused by a reduction in salivary flow

Index

Note: Numbers in *italics* refer to figures; those followed by *t* refer to tables.

Coronary artery disease (CAD) *(continued)*
  obesity and, 100
  overview, 96
  premature, 98
  risk factors, 96–100
  tobacco use and, 98
Cortex, 180
Corticosteroids
  for adrenal crisis, 181, 182
  emergency kit, dental office, 14
Cortisol, 180
CPR. *See* Current cardiopulmonary
    resuscitation (CPR)
CPSS. *See* Cincinnati Prehospital Stroke
    Scale (CPSS)
Crack, 231
Current cardiopulmonary resuscitation (CPR), 4
Cyanosis, 144
  heart failure and, 116
  seizures and, 78

D

Dabigatran etexilate, 209–210
Defibrillation, 126
Degranulation, 153
Dehydration, 172, 182, 230
  hypovolemic shock and, 59
Dental office
  emergencies
    management of, 5
    simulations, 4
    team structure, 4–5, 5*t*
    treatment record, 5, *6*
Diabetes mellitus (DM)
  atherosclerosis and, 99
  dental professional's role in, 171
  diagnosis of, 167
  gestational, 167
  hypertension and, 99
  medications/treatments for, 169–171
  mortality rate, 99
  obesity and, 100
  systemic complications, 167–169, 168*t*
  type 1, 166, 167
  type 2, 166, 167
  types of, 166, 166*t*
Diabetic ketoacidosis (DKA)
  cerebral edema and, 172

signs and symptoms of, 171–172, 172*t*
    treatment of, 172
Diabetic nephropathy, 168
Diabetic neuropathy, 167
Diabetic retinopathy, 167
Diaphoresis, 51, 67, 104, 182, 230
  hyperventilation and, 67
Diazepam, 232
  in hyperventilation, 68
Diphenhydramine, 156, *156*
  emergency kit, dental office, 10*t*, 12, *13*
Distributive shock, 59*t*–60*t*, 60–61
  anaphylactic, 60
  neurogenic, 61
  septic, 60–61
Drug-induced asthma, 135
Dysphagia, 145
Dyspnea, 25
  heart failure and, 115–116
  paroxysmal nocturnal, 116
  shock and, 61
Dysrhythmia, 104
Dysrhythmias, 79

E

Eczema, 153
Edema, pulmonary, 113, 118–119
Education courses, 5
Electroencephalogram (EEG), 73
Emetic drug, 231
Encephalitis, 75
Endogenous chemicals, 230
Epileptic cry, 78
Epileptogenic, 74
Epinephrine, 9, 230, 232
  administration of, 156, 157
  allergies, 156, 157
  angina pectoris and, 101
  asthma and, 135
  biphasic anaphylaxis and, 156, 157
  emergency kit, dental office, 10, 10*t*, 11, *11*
  heart failure and, 117
  syncope and, 48
  systolic blood pressure and, 61
Epistaxis
  etiologies of, 199
  local factors for, 199
  prevention of, 201

M

Macroangiopathy, 99

Magnetic resonance imaging (MRI), 75

Mast cells, 153

Medical history, accuracy of, 2

Medulla, 180

Meningitis, 75

Meperidine, 119, 233

Metallic foreign bodies, 216

Methamphetamine, 229, 230

Meth mouth, 230, *230*

Mineralocorticoids, 182

MRI. *See* Magnetic resonance imaging (MRI)

Myocardial infarction (MI)

    amphetamine use and, 230

    cardiogenic shock and, 60

Myocardial ischemia

    hyperventilation and, 68

    methamphetamine use and, 230

Myxedema coma

    overview, 189–191

    signs and symptoms of, 191, *191t*

    treatment of, 191

N

Naloxone, 233

Narcolepsy, 229

Nasal anatomy, *200*

Nasal cannula, 43, *43*

National Heart, Lung, and Blood Institute, 31

National Institutes of Health (NIH), 90

Nervous systems, parasympathetic and sympathetic, 48, *50*

Neurally mediated syncope. *See* Neurocardiac syncope

Neurocardiac syncope, 48

Neurocardiogenic syncope. *See* Neurocardiac syncope

Neurogenic shock, 61

    signs and symptoms, 61

    treatment, 61

NIH. *See* National Institutes of Health (NIH)

Nitroglycerin, *102*

    acute myocardial infarction and, 105

    acute pulmonary edema and, 119

    administration of, 101

    angina pectoris, 100, 101, 102, 103

    emergency kit, dental office, 10t, 11, *12*

    hypertensive emergency and, 36

Nodular goiter, 188, *190*

Noncardiac syncope, 48, 49, 51

Nonmetallic foreign bodies, 216

Nonsteroidal antiinflammatory drugs (NSAID), 135, 152, 190, 210

Norepinephrine, 48

Nosebleeds. *See* Epistaxis

Noxious stimuli, 48

NSAID. *See* Nonsteroidal antiinflammatory drugs (NSAID)

O

Obesity, 100

Obstructive/mechanical syncope, 51

Obstructive shock, 59t–60t, 61

    signs and symptoms, 61

    treatment, 61

OGTT. *See* Oral glucose tolerance test (OGTT)

Opiates, 232

Opioid antagonist, 233

Opioids, 232–233

    administration routes, 232

    mechanism of action, 232–233

Oral glucose tolerance test (OGTT), 167

Organic foreign bodies, 216

Orthopnea, 116

Orthostatic hypotension, 36–37

    symptoms, 36

    syncope and, 48, 49

Osler-Weber-Rendu syndrome, 199

Oxygen

    administration of, 42–44, *43, 44*

    emergency kit, dental office, 10

Oxygen delivery rate, 42

Oxygen tanks, 42, *42*

P

Pacemakers, *125,* 125–126, *126*

    for arrhythmias, 126

    defined, 125

    lead apron over, 127, *128*

    local anesthetics for, 128

Pacemakers, malfunction of, 126–129

    causes of, 127

    risk for, 126–127

    signs and symptoms of, 129, *129*

    treatment of, 129

Semisynthetic drugs, 232
Sensitization exposure, 153
Sensitizing dose, 153
Septal deviation, 199
Septic shock, 60–61
  signs and symptoms, 61
  treatment, 61
Serotonin, 231
Serum glucose test, 75
Shock
  defined, 58
  stages, 58–59
    compensatory, 58
    initial stage, 58
    progressive, 59
    refractory, 59
  treatment for, 60, 61
  types, 58, 59t–60t
    anaphylactic, 60
    cardiogenic, 60
    distributive, 60–61
    hypovolemic, 59
    neurogenic, 61
    obstructive, 61
    septic, 60–61
Sighs, 26
Simple partial seizures, 76–77
Sinusitis, 199, 231
Skin color, 4, 136, 136t, 144
Skin prick test, 158
Skin scratch test, 158–159
Sleep deprivation, 75
Smoking, 3
  angina pectoris, 103
  cocaine toxicity and, 231, 232
  coronary artery disease and, 98
Sodium, thiopental, 233
Sodium bicarbonate, 231
Sodium bisulfite, 135, 152
Sodium chloride, 60, 182
Sodium nitroprusside, 36
Somnolence, 49
Sphygmomanometer, 28
Status asthmaticus, 136
Status epilepticus, 79–80
  mortality, 79
Steroids, 14
Stethoscope, 29
Stress, respirations in, 26

Stridor, 25–26
Stroke, 2, 23, 86
  embolic, 89
  hemorrhagic, 87, 87t, 88, 89t, 90
  intracerebral hemorrhagic, 88
  ischemic, 87, 87t, 88, 89, 89t
  occlusive, 88
  thrombotic, 89
  See also Cerebrovascular accident (CVA)
Stroke scales, 90
Stroke volume (SV), 23
Stupor, 144
Subarachnoid hemorrhage, 88
  seizure and, 75
  symptoms of, 90
Substance abuse, 88
  amphetamines, 229–231
  barbiturates, 233–234
  benzodiazepines, 234–235
  cocaine, 231–232
  opioids, 232–233
Suffocation, 68, 118, 144
Supplemental drugs, 14
Surgery, conditions related to
  coma, myxedema, 189
  hemorrhagic stroke, 91
  hyperthyroidism, 188
  pulmonary embolism, 67
  thyroid storm, 191, 192
  tooth extraction, 206–210
Sympathetic autonomic nervous system (SANS), 229–230
Sympathomimetic drugs, 26, 157
Sympathomimetic effect, 230
Syncope, 2
  angina pectoris and, 103
  bradypnea and, 23
  cardiac, 51
  in children, 47
  conditions related to, 47
  defined, 47
  mortality rate, 48
  neurocardiac, 48
  noncardiac, 48, 49, 51
  obstructive/mechanical, 51
  overview, 47–48
  pacemaker, malfunction of, 126, 129
  seizures and, 74
  signs and symptoms of, 51–52, 51t
  tachyarrhythmias, 126

Syncope, 2 (*continued*)
    treatment of, 52–53
    types and etiologies of, 48–51, *49*
Synthetic drugs, 232
Syringes, *13,* 15

T

Tachyarrhythmias, 51
    ICD for, 126
Tachycardia, 2, 22
    adrenal crisis and, 182
    allergies and, 154, 155
    anginal episode and, 100, 103
    diabetic ketoacidosis (DKA) and, 172
    pacemaker malfunction, 126
    seizures and, 79
    shock and, 61
    substance abuse and, 230, 232
    ventricular, 104, 126
Tachypnea, 2, 23
    aspirations, foreign body, 114
    diabetic ketoacidosis (DKA) and, 171–172
    heart failure and, 115
Tamponade, 61
Tea bags, 208, *208*
Teeth
    fractured, 76
    loss of, 87
    socket, 207–208
Temperature, 21
    body, 26
    measuring and recording, 2, 26, *26*
TENS. *See* Transcutaneous electrical nerve stimulators (TENS)
Tetanus, 74
Tetany, 67
Thermometer, 15
Thiazides, 31
Thiopental sodium, 233
Thready pulse, 23, 59, 59*t*
Thrombogenic episodes, 209
Thrombolytic therapy, 91
Thrombosis disorders, 209
Thrombotic cerebrovascular accident, 87, 87*t,* 89, 89*t,* 210
Thrombus, 67, 87, 100, 104
Thyroid emergencies, 189–192
Thyroid gland, 187, *187*
Thyroiditis, 188

Thyroid storm
    overview, 191
    signs and symptoms of, 191–192, 192*t*
    treatment of, 192
Thyrotoxicosis, 188
Thyroxine, 188, *188*
TIA. *See* Transient ischemic attack (TIA)
Tinnitus, 35
Tissue death, 12
Tobacco use, 98
Toothbrushes, battery-operated, 127, *128*
Topical anesthetics, 152
Toxemia, 191
Toxicology screening, 75
Toxins, 58, 153
Toxoplasmosis, 74
Tranquilizer, 189, 191
Transcutaneous electrical nerve stimulators (TENS), 127, *127*
Transient ischemic attack (TIA), 87
Transient loss of consciousness (TLoC). *See* Syncope
Trauma, 61, 74, 207, 210
Triazolam, 234
Tricyclic antidepressants, 157
Triglycerides, 97, 99
Tuberculosis, 180
Tumors, 67, 74
Type 1 diabetes, 166, 167
    See also Diabetes mellitus (DM)
Type 2 diabetes, 166, 167
    See also Diabetes mellitus (DM)

U

Ultrasonic cleaning baths, 127, *127*
Ultrasonic scaler, 127, 225
Unstable angina (UA), 100–101
Uremia, 73, 74
Urinalysis, 75
U.S. Department of Health, 31

V

Valsalva maneuver, 49
Variant angina, 101
Vasoconstrictors
    cocaine as, 231, 232
    dysrhythmia and, 128
    hemophilia and, 208